# Antidiabetic Plants in India and Herbal Based Antidiabetic Research

T. Pullaiah
*Department of Botany*
*Sri Krishnadevaraya Univerisity*
*Anantapur - 515 003, Andhra Pradesh*

&

K. Chandrasekhar Naidu
*Department of Botany*
*Andhra University*
*Visakhapatnam - 530 003, Andhra Pradesh*

2022

Regency Publications
*A Division of*
Astral International Pvt. Ltd.
New Delhi – 110 002

*First Published, 2012*
*Reprinted, 2022*

ISBN: 978-81-87498-67-4 (Hardbound)

*Publisher's note:*

*Every possible effort has been made to ensure that the information contained in this book is accurate at the time of going to press, and the publisher and author cannot accept responsibility for any errors or omissions, however caused. No responsibility for loss or damage occasioned to any person acting, or refraining from action, as a result of the material in this publication can be accepted by the editor, the publisher or the author. The Publisher is not associated with any product or vendor mentioned in the book. The contents of this work are intended to further general scientific research, understanding and discussion only. Readers should consult with a specialist where appropriate.*

*Every effort has been made to trace the owners of copyright material used in this book, if any. The author and the publisher will be grateful for any omission brought to their notice for acknowledgement in the future editions of the book.*



*Published by* : **Regency Publications**
*A Division of*
**Astral International Pvt. Ltd.**
– ISO 9001:2015 Certified Company –
4736/23, Ansari Road, Darya Ganj
New Delhi-110 002
Ph. 011-43549197, 23278134
E-mail: info@astralint.com
Website: www.astralint.com

# PREFACE

This book is a compilation work and embodies a fairly comprehensive information of the fundamental aspects of diabetes, herbal based antidiabetic research and antidiabetic plants in India. This book will promote research aspirations in botanists and particularly beginners in the area of medical botany. It also provides information to the pharmacy students and researchers in identifying antidiabetic agents from natural resource and in standardizing herbal formulations/crude drugs. It provides information briefly about the important work done in antidiabetic research and a detailed account on the work done during 1995 to 2002 encompassing more than 200 references.

This book also provides brief information about diabetes, especially pertaining to NIDDM; different antidiabetic agents and management of NIDDM. Information about animal models used in the screening of plant extracts, experimental protocols in antidiabetic research is also given in detail.

This book also offers information about the antidiabetic plants available in India, brief description about the plant, it's distribution in India, flowering fruiting season, vernacular names, methods of propagation with a brief account of the herbal use in treating diabetes.

January 2003

T. Pullaiah
K. Chandrasekhar Naidu

# CONTENTS

# CONTENTS

CHAPTER 1

# INTRODUCTION

Diabetes is a chronic disorder of carbohydrate, fat and protein metabolism. It is characterized by dangerously high level of serum glucose known as hyperglycemia or elevated blood glucose. There are two major types of diabetic diseases, designated as Type-I and Type-II.

Type-I: Insulin dependent Diabetes Mellitus (IDDM) or Juvenile—onset diabetes accounts for about 10% of diabetes. The main symptoms include high blood sugar, excessive thirst, frequent urination, increased appetite, fatigue, weight loss, poor wound healing, blurred vision etc. The only treatment of this type available is insulin injections. The risk of hypoglycemia is greatly increased. About 1.8 million people in the United States are affected by Type-I diabetes with an estimated 18 million persons affected world wide.

Type-II: Non-insulin dependent diabetes (NIDDM) in 90% of all diabetics. The classic symptoms being polyphagia (frequent hunger), polyuria (frequent urination), polydipsia (frequent thirst); other symptoms might include weight loss, poor wound healing, dry mouth, itchy skin, blurred vision, fatigue, impotence, recurrent infection etc. The major chronic complications of Type-II diabetes mellitus include accelerated macrovascular disease, retinopathy, renal disease neuropathy etc. Type-II diabetes affects 15 million people in the United States and approximately 150 million diabetics around the world. Diabetes is said to be the seventh leading cause of death in the United States. There are four classes of oral glucose-lowering agents other than insulin and in use to treat Type-II diabetes. They are sulfonylureas, biguanides, glucosidase inhibitors and thiazolidinediones. Each of these treatments has its drawbacks, ranging from the developing of resistance and adverse effects to lack of responsiveness in large segments of the patient population. Moreover none of these glucose-lowering agents adequately controls the hyperlipidemia that frequently met with this disease.

A change in diet, lifestyle and exercise will help greatly in management of diabetes at the initial stages with lesser impact at later stages. Several minerals have been found to benefit diabetics either due to deficiencies or because of the beneficial effect on glucose metabolism.

Plant—based products have been popular all over the world for centuries. In diabetics, some herbal alternatives are proven to provide symptomatic relief and assist in the prevention of the secondary complications of the disease. Some herbs have also been proven to help in the regeneration of beta cells and in overcoming insulin resistance. In addition to maintain normal blood sugar level, some herbs are also reported to possess antioxidant and cholesterol lowering action.

So, herbal medication is the most commonly used alternative therapy for diabetes treatment. Alternatives are needed because of inability of current therapies to contribute normoglycemia and prevention of diabetic complications. The enormous costs of modern treatment and dependency of 85–95% of rural population in developing countries on traditional medicine for their primary health care necessitates the alternative strategies for the prevention and treatment of diabetes. Moreover herbs are known for their safety, efficacy, cultural acceptability and lesser side effects besides maintaining normoglycemia in diabetics. However, their safety and efficacy need to be further evaluated by experimental and clinical studies. Preparation of standardized medicinal herbs is urgently needed for future studies and therapies. To date, over 600 traditional plant treatments for diabetes have been reported but only a small number of these have received scientific and clinical evaluation to assess their efficacy. However, the hypoglycemic effect of some herbal extracts have been confirmed in human and animal models of Type-II diabetics and conventional drugs have also been derived from the active molecules of these medicinal plants. For example, metformin, a less toxic biguanide and potent oral glucose-lowering agent, was developed from the plant *Galega officinalis* and used to treat diabetes.

In recent years researches have been extended to examine antidiabetic activity and to identify alternate treatment strategies that pose less of a risk for diabetics. Yet there is a clear, urgent need for the intensified search to identify the antidiabetic agents from plant sources to combat seriousness of the problem.

India is very rich in herbal and medicinal plant wealth with suitable geoclimatic conditions. It has well documented and well practical knowledge for traditional herbal medicine.

Discovery of drug requires a systematic and well designed approach on the correct plant to reach the expected goals with in the expected time. The two techniques involved in the bioassay assessment programme are *in vivo* and *in vitro* studies. For the study of hypoglycemic and antihyperglycemic activity through *in vivo*, it is necessary to employ animals and diabetic humans. Rodents or rabbits treated with Alloxan/Streptozotocin are the suitable models for *in vivo* antidiabetic study.

The need of basic information about the availability of antidiabetic plants in India for Research workers for their scientific pursuits are keenly felt. In this book Animal models, experimental protocols, methods of estimation of different parameters, previous work done on the subject particularly during 1995 and 2001, important bio-active constituents isolated, availability of antidiabetic plants, their distribution, flowering seasons, their local and trade names, parts used, description along with illustrations for some of the plants etc. are given for about 596 antidiabetic plants available in India. It is hoped that it can serve as a useful tool for the selection and collection of potential plants for discovery of desirable/expected antidiabetic agents and drug development for the treatment of diabetics.

CHAPTER 2

# DIABETES—NEED AND SCOPE FOR HERBAL BASED ANTIDIABETIC RESEARCH

## DIABETES OVERVIEW

Diabetes is a chronic disorder of metabolism of carbohydrates, protein and fat due to absolute or relative deficiency of insulin secretion and with varying degrees of insulin resistance. It is often accompanied after a period of time by specific micro and macro vascular, neuropathic and nephropathic complications. Diabetes is characterized by hyperglycemia (elevated blood glucose). The blood glucose levels of a healthy man are 80 mg/dl on fasting and up to 160mg/dl in the postprandial state. According to national diabetes data group (NDDG 1979), NIDDM is diagnosed when a patient has random blood sugar > 200mg/dl on two occasions and has a fasting plasma glucose > 140mg/dl or a sustained elevation of plasma glucose concentration ≥ 200mg/dl after an oral glucose load of 75gms. at two hours and one other between 0 time and 2 hours ≥ 200mg/dl.

Most of the food we eat is broken down into simple sugar called glucose. This glucose is the main source of fuel to get energy for the body. After digestion the glucose reaches our blood stream where it is available for body cells to utilize for energy. But insulin is needed for the glucose to get into the cells. Insulin is a hormone secreted by the pancreas. It is the duty of the pancreas to secrete the adequate amount of insulin, to transport glucose from blood into different cells of the body. If the said pancreas does not produce enough insulin or the produced insulin does not work properly, the glucose can not get into the body cells. So glucose stays in the blood. This makes blood sugar level become high causing diabetes. Thus, the body loses its main source of fuel for energy even though the blood contains huge amounts of glucose. This high-level blood glucose levels for longer periods cause many complications to the different systems of the body.

The world health organization (WHO, 1985) classified diabetes into six types.

1. Insulin Dependent Diabetes Mellitus (IDDM)
2. Non-Insulin Dependent Diabetes Mellitus (NIDDM)
   a) Obese; b) Non-obese
3. Malnutrition related diabetes mellitus (MRDM)
4. Diabetes associated with other conditions and symptoms
   a) Pancreatic disease
   b) Diseases of hormonal etiology
   c) Drug induced or chemical induced diabetes
   d) Abnormalities of insulin or its receptors
   e) Certain genetic syndromes
   f) Miscellaneous
5. Gestational Diabetes Mellitus (GDM)
6. Impaired glucose tolerance (IGT)
   a) Obese; b) Non-obese; c) Associated with certain syndromes.

The high incidence of NIDDM in India appears to be relatively recent development (due to change in the type of food intake and modernization in their life style). This necessitates to develop the potential herbal remedy to improve the well-being of persons with diabetes. Hence the discussion is limited to the NIDDM only.

## NON-INSULIN DEPENDENT DIABETES MELLITUS: (NIDDM OR TYPE-II OR MATURITY-ONSET DIABETES)

It occurs predominantly in older people over age 40 years. Type-II diabetes is most common accounting for even 90% of all cases of diabetes. Development of Type-II diabetes seems to be multifactorial such as Genetic, Obesity, high caloric intake, environmental chemical factors etc. About 80% of people with Type-II diabetes are with overweight (obese).

In NIDDM, the pancreas usually produces insulin, but for some reason, the body can not use the insulin effectively. NIDDM represents a variety of diabetic states. Insulin secretion is usually sufficient to oppose the ketogenic action of glucagon but not to prevent hyperglycemia. Three factors are involved in the development of obesity and insulin resistance resulting NIDDM. They are:

a) Free fatty acids (produced by breakdown of fat)
b) Leptin (a protein produced by fat cells)
c) Tumor necrosis factor or TNF (a component of immune system).

NIDDM is characterized by insulin resistance (diminished tissue sensitivity to insulin) and impaired beta-cell function (delayed or inadequate insulin release).

**Symptoms of NIDDM**

a) Frequent urination (Polyuria)
b) Unusual thirst (Polydipsia)
c) Frequent hunger (Polyphasia)
d) Weight loss
e) Unhealed wounds
f) Feeling tired
g) Frequent fungal infection
h) Foot lesions
i) Balanitis etc.

**Short Term Complications**

a) Hyperglycemia (High blood sugar)
b) Hypoglycemia (Low blood sugar)
c) Imbalance of excess sugar in the blood and inadequate quantity of water, potassium and sodium.

**Long Term Complications**

a) Hypertension (High blood pressure)
b) Dislipidemia (High levels of cholesterol and Triglycerides in the blood)
c) Vascular complications (Micro, macro vascular, coronary artery disease and atherosclerosis)
d) Cardiomyopathy (Functional disturbances of the myocardium due to cardic dilatation)
e) Neuropathy (Nerve)
f) Nephropathy (Kidney)
g) Retinopathy (Vision)
h) Foot disease etc.

**NIDDM Management**

Correction of hyperglycemia and the maintenance of normal blood glucose concentration are the most important aspects in management. If blood sugar levels maintains closely to the normoglycemia one can avoid risk of complication for diabetes. NIDDM therapy involves modification of life style, diet, exercise and use of oral hypoglycemic agents. In one third of the patients it can be controlled through diet, exercise and weight loss. The rest of the patients need oral medication that stimulate the pancreas to secrete more insulin or to increase the body's cell sensitivity to the insulin.

***1. Important Oral Anti-diabetic Drugs***

Oral hypoglycemic agents are used in patients with NIDDM, unresponsive to dietary control or in those in whom dietary control was initially successful but has now failed. They are:

a) *Sulphonylurea*
First generation—Tollbutamide, Chlorpropamide.
Second generation—Glibenclamide, Glipizide, Gliclazide.

b) *Biguanides:* Metformin, Phenformin

c) *Inhibitors of alpha-glucosidase:* Acarbose

d) *Insulin*

Type-II diabetes patients are not dependent upon exogenous insulin for survival. Insulin may be required at times for control of transient, stress-induced hyperglycemia or hyperglycemia that persists in spite of other therapy.

Other antibiabetic drugs are included in Table 1.

**Table 1.Classification of Drugs Currently Available for Management of Diabetes Mellitus**

| Classification | Drugs available |
|---|---|
| (A) Insulin and insulin-analogues | |
| Ultra short acting analogue | Lispro insulin |
| Short acting | Regular insulin |
| Intermediate acting | NPH/zinc insulin |
| Premixed (regular and NPH) | 30/70, 50/50, 25/75 |
| (B) Insulin releasers (action on beta cells) | |
| (a) Shorter duration of action | Repaglinide, Glipizide, Tollbutamide |
| (b) Intermidiate duration of action | Gliclazide—early insulin peak<br>Glibenclamide—delayed insulin peak |
| (c) Longer duration of action | Glimepiride—poor secretagogue |
| (C) Insulin sensitisers (enhance insulin action on target tissue) | |
| Biguanide | Metformin, Phenformin |
| Glitazones | Pioglitazone, Rosiglitazone |
| Sulfonyl urea | Glimepiride |
| (D) Suppressor of hepatic glucose production | |
| Biguanide• | Metformin |
| Glitazone | Pioglitazone |
| (E) Interfere with carbohydrate absorption from gut | |
| α—glucosidase inhibitor | Acarbose |
| Fenugreek and other fibre in diet | |
| (F) Lower hepatic insulin in-resistance | Phenobarbitone, Metformin |
| (G) Lipid lowering drugs | |
| Fabric acid derivatives | |
| Docosahexanoic acid and Eicosapentanoic acid | Benzafibrate, phenofibrate |
| (Help to lower insulin resistance in the presence of dislipidemia) | |

### 2. Diet in Diabetes

Change in diet is the important factor in the management of diabetes. Eating right helps to keep blood sugar, blood lipids and blood pressure under control, which help from complications. Elimination of all simple carbohydrates and inclusion of a high fiber diet is desirable. The calorie contents of the food is important in planning diet. High calorie food consumption leads gaining obesity, glucose intolerance, dyslipidemia, coronary artery diseases, atherosclerosis etc. So an ideal diabetic diet includes calorie content, fiber content, glycemic index and physical form of food. The high carbohydrate, high fiber diet is highly recommended.

### 3. Exercise and Weight Reduction in NIDDM

Physical activity is an important factor in controlling blood sugar levels. Exercise can prevent the onset of NIDDM and it regulates the blood glucose for those already suffering from diabetes. Exercise promotes the entry of glucose into the cells thereby lowers blood sugar levels. Exercise also prevents the cardiovascular disease, reduces cholesterol levels and weight.

### 4. Mineral Supplements

There are also nutritional supplements that can be useful in treating diabetes. Several mineral supplements have been found beneficial to people with diabetes, either because of potential deficiencies or because of the beneficial effect on glucose metabolism. Among the most important vitamins and minerals for supplementation are Vitamin-$B_3$, $B_{12}$, Vitamin-C, Vitamin-E, Chromium, Magnesium, Manganese, Phosphorus, Potassium, Selenium, Vanadium, Zinc, Bioflavonoids, essential fatty acids and Co-enzyme $Q_{10}$.

### 5. Herbal Remedies

Although different methods of treatment currently available for Diabetes mellitus it is difficult to maintain normoglycemia, prevention of diabetic complications and different pathological aspects except in the method of pancreatic transplantation. But, it is very expensive and difficult to get the required donor. So, there is a clear need for alternate sources of drugs and strategies for diabetes therapy and it is found that, the best strategy will be the study of traditional antidiabetic plants for prevention, and therapy of diabetes. Because, many botanical products have found to possess beneficiary effects in controlling diabetes by stimulating insulin secretion and actions improving insulin binding, inhibition of glucose absorption etc. Several botanical supplements have been studied and used as potential therapeutic agents in the management of diabetes and its related complications. To date, over 600 traditional plant treatments for diabetes have been reported in India but only a small number of these have received scientific and medical evaluation to assess their efficacy. The antidiabetic effect of some herbal extracts has been confirmed in human and animal models of Type-II diabetes. The following are the most studied in this connection and commonly used medicinal herbs for treatment of diabetes.

*Gymnema sylvestre*, *Trigonella foenum-graecum*, *Pterocarpus marsupium*, *Aloe vera*, *Momordica charantia*, *Azadiractha indica*, *Panax* sps., *Syzigium cumini*, *Allium* sps., *Phyllanthus emblica*, *Coccinia cordifolia* etc. (Gupta,1994).

Inclusion of pectin-rich fruits and vegetables can be regarded as one of the primary prevention strategies of hyperlipidemia. Eleven pectins were screened among which pectins from *Carica papaya*, *Coccinia indica*, *Lycopersicon esculentum* and *Cucumis* sps. showed highly significant hypolipidemic activity in albino rats, while others were less significant or insignificant in their action (Kumar et al., 1993, 1997).

### *6. Need and Scope of Alternative Remedy*

Due to the modernization of life-style, NIDDM is becoming a major health problem in developing countries. Even in the developed countries the rate of mortality due to diabetes is more alarming. It is the seventh leading cause of death in the United States. In India every fourth man is a diabetic or has the chance of becoming a diabetes patient. Indians with big bellies central obesity make them more prone to diabetes. Life expectancy is drastically reduced by NIDDM in developing countries where its prevalence is increasing due to modernization in their life style and inadequate treatment. With increasing incidence of Diabetes mellitus in rural population throughout the world there is a clear need for the development of alternate strategies for Diabetes therapy as the current therapies are proving to be inadequate to combat all the metabolic aberrations of the disease. The high cost and poor availability of current therapies for many of the rural population in India necessitates the need for the development of indigenous, inexpensive botanical sources for antidiabetic and antihyperlipidemic crude or purified drugs.

Herbal medicines are being used by about 80% of the world population particularly in the developing countries for primary health care. The natural products shall be considered as the best in primary health care because of better cultural acceptability, safety, efficacy, potent, inexpensive and lesser side effects. Several herbal medicines and supplements have been studied as potential therapeutic agents in the management of diabetes and its related complications. Hundreds of plants have been studied for their potential blood glucose lowering properties. In recent years many developed countries have shown growing interest in alternative or complementary system of medicine for management of diabetes. Several plant species have been used in traditional medicine to treat symptoms of diabetes since several hundred years.

None of the presently available sulfonylureas completely normalize insulin secretion and action (Back Bielsen et al., 1988). A scientific investigation of traditional herbal remedies for diabetes may provide valuable leads for the development of alternate drugs and therapeutic strategies. The bioactive extracts and compounds need to be standardized on the basis of active principle along with fingerprints. This can be achieved by judicious and rationally designed interdisciplinary research programmes. Cost efficient, potent and less or no side effect of drugs of plant origin have been achieved through compound formulations either in their natural or semi processed form. But it definitely requires proper standardization, efficacy and dose regimen for therapeutic use. The herbal remedies can act as good adjuvant drug to reduce the requirement of insulin or sulphonyl urea derivatives.

The plant kingdom is a wide field to look for an effective oral hypoglycemic agents as more than 1300 plant species have been used ethnopharmacologically or experimentally to treat symptoms of diabetes mellitus throughout the world. India is one of the 12 mega biodiversity centers having over 45,000 plant species comprising 15,000–18,000 flowering plants, 23,000 fungi, 2,500 algae, 1,600 lichens, 18,000 bryophytes and others are microorganisms (Kamboj, 2000). Many of these plants are having therapeutic properties and used in traditional medicine. India is the largest grower of *Plantago ovata, Cassia senna, Ricinus communis, Aloe barbadensis, Allium sativum, A. cepa, Piper longum, Withania somnifera, Gossypium herbaceum* etc. The export of crude extracts/drugs in bulk amounts of *Commiphora mukul, Azadirachta indica, Rauvolfia serpentina, Catharanthus roseus, Adhatoda vasica, Zingiber officinale, Juglans regia, Tinospora cordifolia, Holarrhena pubescens, Emblica officinalis, Terminalia chebula, T. bellirica* etc are richly available in India and are being used in several herbal formulations (Bhakuni, 1997). Interestingly all these happened to be potential antidiabetic plants.

India is well suited for development of drugs from medicinal plants, because India has a rich traditional knowledge and heritage of herbal medicines both for use in preventive and curative subjects. During recent years many organizations have intensified their search for new antidiabetic drugs from herbs. Since the diabetes is listed in the thrust areas for investigation to secure effective remedy, several institutions like CDRI, IICT, RRL, Jammu are engaged in research largely in addition to the several universities in the exploration of herbal drugs for their use in diabetes treatment. However, search for antidiabetic agents needs to be intensified because of the vast population suffer severely from this disease.

## THE MAIN OBJECTIVES OF THIS BOOK ARE

1. To promote research aspirations in botanists and beginners in the area of medical botany. Botanist played a very important role in the chemotaxonomic studies. So it becomes necessary to isolate and estimate the concentration of chemotaxonomic marker of each plant. The role of botanists in recent times is further extended to screen the various extracts and fractions of the plants for various medicinal activities. He is also a competent person to carry out these studies since he possesses a sound biological knowledge and obtained experience even in animal handling.
2. To identify and isolate biologically active leads from natural resources for the treatment of NIDDM.
3. Through standardized herbal medicines using active compounds, to make India to export sizable crude herbal drugs as herbal medicines are in great demand in the developed world for primary health care because of their efficacy, safety and lesser side effects for NIDDM.

### REFERENCES

Back-Bielsen, H.O. Hother-Nielsen and O. Pedersew. 1988. Mechanism of action of sulphonylureas with special reference to the extra-pancreatic effect: An Overview. *Diabetic Med.* **5**: 613–620.

Bhakuni, D.S. 1997. Some aspects of aromatic and Medicinal plants, *J. Indian Chem. Soc.*, **74**: 349–356.

Gupta, S.S. 1994. Prospectus and perspective of natural plant products in medicine. *Indian J. Pharmacol.* **26**: 1–12.

Kamboj, V.P. 2000. Herbal medicine. *Curr. Sci.* **78**: 35–39.

Kumar. G.P., S. Sudheesh, B. Ushakumari, A.K. Valsa, S. Vijayakumar, C. Sandya and N.R. Vijayalakshmi.1997. A comparative study on the hypolipidimic activity of eleven different pectins. *J. Food. Sci. Technol.* **34**: 103–107.

Kumar. G.P., S. Sudheesh and N.R. Vijayalakshmi. 1993. Hypoglycemic effect of *Coccinia indica*: mechanism of action. *Planta Med.* **59**: 330–332.

National diabetes data group. 1979. Classification and diagnosis of DM and other categories of glucose intolerance. *Diabetes.* **28**: 1039–1057.

Seshiah, V. 1997. A handbook on Diabetes mellitus. All Indian publishers & distributors, Chennai

WHO. 1985. Technical report India on Diabetes mellitus. **727**: 1–113.

CHAPTER 3

# ANIMAL MODELS USED IN THE SCREENING OF PLANT EXTRACTS/ COMPOUNDS FOR ANTIDIABETIC ACTIVITY

To study the hypoglycemic and antihyperglycemic activities one need to employ animals with normoglycemia and/or induced hyperglycemia. The two important aspects involved in this bioassay study are selection of animal model and management of animal stock.

## ANIMAL MODEL

The use of animal model to mimic human disease has become very popular. In animal models experiments can be performed that are not possible in humans. In biological screens it enables us to know the active molecules or gene products that suppress the disease. In pre-clinical drug discovery research trials with complementary/supplementary approaches, if necessary with animal models, would be useful. It is cheaper, reduce the time involvement and money spent on understanding the molecular basis of human disease. Generally, the drug that suits the animals naturally suits human system since there is closeness in many physiological and pathological conditions (if not all) in both the systems. Although Hamsters, Rabbits, Dogs, Guinea pigs, Monkeys etc. are used as experimental animals, the Mice/Rat (Rodent) and Rabbit models are widely used in antidiabetic bioassay assessment and pre-clinical drug identification trials to understand better the gene product function and to identify potential drug targets. Technology is available for introduction of new DNA sequences into the germ line to get transgenic mouse and rats. Moreover, breeding cycle in mouse and rats is short, easy to breed, manipulate and can be genetically engineered.

Roles of specific genes can be known easily in identified genetic models. Since the area of interest here is antidiabetic study, the discussion is limited to the use of mouse, rats and rabbits only.

## Advantages of Animal Models for Anti-diabetic Study

To study the hypoglycemic and antihyperglycemic activities animals are employed with normoglycemia and or induced diabetic state. Animal models with physiological and pathological changes of each diabetic subtype are helpful to understand characters of disease better and to identify effective drug. Experimentation that is not possible in humans would be conducted with different NIDDM animal models. This gives information to us in the identification of new factors involved in the regulation of food intake and of genes that might contribute to these conditions. The synteny between rodent and human genes allows transfer of information to facilitate identification of homologous genes. Several distinct autosomal and polygenic rodent genetic models are available. Different chemicals and environmental factors, which impact on the development of diabetes, can be worked out.

Animal models related diabetic study would be broadly classified into two types.

### *a) IDDM Animal Models*

Chemically induced Type-I diabetes is the commonly used animal model. NOD mouse and the BB diabetic rats are the genetic models.

### *b) NIDDM Animal Models*

These are of three types. (a) Genetic NIDDM; (b) Chemically induced NIDDM; and (c) Surgical NIDDM models.

a) Genetic NIDDM models are produced by spontaneous mutations, selective breeding or genetic engineering. These models exhibit characters of glycemia, insulinemia and obesity.
b) Chemically induced NIDDM models can be obtained by alloxan, streptozotocin (STZ) or certain chemical treatments. So that type-II diabetes model can be achieved with expected pathology.
c) Surgical NIDDM can be obtained by removal of pancreatic mass to a lesser or greater extent.

## Source and Management of Animals

Use of good quality animals is essential for obtaining good and reproducible results in the testing of drugs. Setting up of animal facility for production of good quality animals is a costly affair. So it is advised to procure the experimental animals from Breeding Centres, commercial breeders or Laboratory animals centres. The best source of this kind is National Center for Laboratory Animal Sciences, National Institute of Nutrition, Hyderabad. Although there are several private commercial breeders and animal sellers, it is advised to procure animals from Government institutes in order to get the animals of expected standards. To meet the growing demand for quality Laboratory animals, Indian Council of Medical Research, Government of India, established National Center for Laboratory Animal Sciences. Different species and strains of genetically defined animals are bred in this facility by adopting the most advanced techniques. This National facility supplies the required number and desirable strain of animals to the users. Animals purchased from this facility are free from all parasites and pathogenic microbial organisms.

The basic requirements which need to be maintained are mentioned in the Table. 2.

**Table 2. Housing and Environmental Requirements for Animals in Laboratories as per INSA Guidelines**

| Physical Conditions | Mouse | Rat | Rabbit |
|---|---|---|---|
| Average Adult weight | 25–30 g | 200–300 g | 2.0–2.5 kg |
| Type of housing | Cage | Cage | Cage |
| Floor area per animal (Sq. cm) | 65–100 | 150–100 | 3700–4600 |
| Cage height minimum (cm) | 13 | 18 | 36 |
| Room Temperature (O°C) | 22–24 | 22–24 | 20–22 |
| Relative Humidity (%) | 45–55 | 50–55 | 40–50 |
| Suitable bedding material in the cages | Paddy husk or saw dust | Paddy husk or saw dust | — |
| Nesting material | Paper cutting | Paper cutting | Cotton/paper |
| Ventilation air changes per hour | 10–12 | 10–12 | 10–12 |
| Light intensity (LUX) Florescent tube light | 300–400 | 300–400 | 300-400 |
| Photocycle (Light:Dark) | 12:12 | 12:12 | 12:12 |
| Noise level (avoid high frequency sounds) | 65 decibel | 65 decibel | 65decibel |
| Filtration | | | |
| Microfilters can remove bacteria & fungal spores | 0.1–0.3 μm | 0.1–0.3 μm | 0.1–0.3μm |

## NUTRITIONAL REQUIREMENTS

Species vary in their nutritional requirements. Although the needs of rats and mouse are close, each species has its own feeding regimen. The dietary requirements are not the same at every period of the animal's life. All animals need certain basic substances in their diet, but in different proportions. The basic requirements are protein, fat, carbohydrate, vitamins, salts and minerals. Animal should be provided clean feed. Water should be free of all pathogenic organisms. Table 3 shows the diet composition for Rodents and Rabbits recommended by the National Institute of Nutrition, Hyderabad.

**Table 3. Diet Composition for Rodents and Rabbits**

| Type of animal | Rodents | Rabbits |
|---|---|---|
| a) Wheat flour | 22.3 % | 61.3 % |
| b) Roasted Bengal gram flour | 60.0 % | 28.2 % |
| c) Skim milk powder | 5.0 % | 0.0 % |
| d) Casein | 4.0 % | 1.0 % |
| e) Refined oil | 4.0 % | 5.0 % |
| f) Salt mixture with starch | 4.0 % | 4.0 % |
| g) Vitamin and choline mixture with starch | 0.5 % | 0.5 % |
| h) Vitamin C | — | 50.0 mg/100 mg |

### *Scale of Diet*

| | |
|---|---|
| Rat | : 5–20 gms/day |
| Mouse | : 5 gms/day |
| Rabbit | : 50–100gms/day (depending up on the breed) |
| Extra diet for rabbits | : Bengal gram 20gms and Lucerne grass 100 gms. |

The maximum period of storage of diet before consumption should not exceed more than one month, because most of the ingredients that go to make up a diet are liable to undergo deterioration on storage.

## HYGIENE

Maintenance of hygienic conditions with regard to the animal house and cages is very important aspect. Cleaning and sterilization of cages, diet, water containers and disinfection of animal house needs to be undertaken periodically.

## ETHICAL PROTOCOLS

All animal procedures are in compliance with Breeding of and Experiments on Animals (control and supervision) Rules, 1998 by subsection (1) of section 17 of the prevention of cruelty to Animals Act, 1960 (59 1960) under the notification of the Government of India, Ministry of Environment and

Forests No. S.O. 789 (E) dt. 8-9-1998 and in the Gazette of India. In exercise of the powers conferred by sub section (1) (1A) and (2) of section (17) of the prevention of the cruelty to animal act, 1960 (59 of 1960), the committee for control and supervision of experiments on animals amended some of the rules on 18.12.2000, vide number S.O. 168(E). Some of the important aspects of this rule are:

a) No establishment shall perform any experiment on animals unless it is registered. For getting registration one has to apply to the member Secretary, Committee for the purpose of control and supervision of experiments on animals, Ministry of social justice and empowerment, Govt. of India, Room No. 209, D'Wing, Sastry Bhavan, New Delhi-110001.
b) Every establishment shall appoint an Institutional Animal Ethics Committee with the specified composition.
c) Every registered establishment before acquiring animals or conducting any experiment on animals, shall apply for permission of the committee or the Institutional animals ethics committee, furnishing particulars about name of the species to be used, number, experimental protocols etc. and shall obtain the permission before conducting experiment.
d) Experiments shall be performed with due care and humanity. Experiments shall also be performed in every case by or under the supervision of a person duly qualified in that behalf.
e) Every establishment /Institutional animal ethics committee shall maintain a record of the animals under its control and custody in the specified format.

In addition to these, one has to follow the rules strictly specified in Breeding of and experiments on Animals (control and supervision) Rules, 1998.

## REFERENCES

Blake, J.A. et al. 2000. The mouse Geome Database (MGD); expanding genetic and genomic resources for the laboratory mouse. Nucleic Acids Res. **28**: 108–111.

Chagnon, Y.C. and C. Bouchard, 1996. Genetics of obesity: *Advances from rodent studies, Trends Genet.* **12**: 441.

Hrabe de Angelis, M. and R. Balling, 1998. Large scale ENU screens in the mouse; genetics meets genomics, *Mutat. Res.* **400**: 25–32.

In the Gazette of India, Extraordinary Part-II section-3 subsection (ii). Ministry of social justice & Empowerment notification–breeding of and experiments on animals (control and supervision) Rule, 1998. S.O. No: **1074** and S.O. No: **168**(E).

Ktorza, A. et al. 1997. Are animal models of diabetes relevant to study of the genetics of non-insulin dependent diabetes in humans? *Diabetes Metab.* **2**: 38.

CHAPTER 4

# BIOASSAY ASSESSMENT AND EXPERIMENTAL PROTOCOL

A thorough Phytochemical and Pharmacological study of traditional anti-diabetic plants is essential for the development of new botanical anti-hyperglycemic agents. There would be number of obstacles in this search for antidiabetic agents but one has to work with sustainable interest to reach the expected goals. It requires longer time to complete all the pharmacological, toxicological and clinical tests. The foremost step in this is identification of most potential antidiabetic plants. This is mainly based on the literature evidence and online search. The other factors to be taken into account while choosing a plant are: (a) wide traditional use (b) significant antihyperglycemic activity (c) availability of plant source (d) easy identity of plant (e) no or less toxicity etc.

The extract is prepared from the plant thus selected and then be subjected to bioassay tests for hypoglycemic activity and toxicity. Through this method one can identify more natural, antidiabetic and therapeutically potential extracts or crude drugs. From the extracts, compounds can be isolated through chromatographic methods. Finally, activity of individual compounds needs to be tested. Those compounds which show most significant activity would then be subjected to toxicological studies. Final steps in the process of antidiabetic drug development from plant sources will be the evaluation of identified drugs for safety and efficacy through clinical trials. Then they would be formulated as a suitable dosage form. The overall research design is given in a circuit form as in Fig. 1. Protocol used in identification and isolation of antidiabetic compounds from plant sources is also given in stepwise form.

For assessment of biological activity of plant extracts/compounds diabetic animal models are required with desired pathology resembling human diabetes. To achieve such desired animal models in a short span of time, use of chemicals is the alternative to induce diabetes in experimental animals. Alloxan, Streptozotocin (STZ), 2, 4-dinitrophenol and diazoxide are the important chemical agents that are used in induction of Diabetes. Hormones such as epinephrine, corticotropin, glucogon, anterior pituitary extract somatotropin etc. are used for induction of diabetes. Genetically induced diabetic animals have also been used in the screening of plant constituents, but it is difficult to get such animals with desired characters.

**Stepwise protocol in isolation and identification of antibiabetic compounds from plant sources:**

1. Identification of plants with antidiabetic activity basing on literature survey and on-line search.
2. Plants thus chosen will be collected and subjected to shade drying and powdering
3. Extraction with various solvents of increasing polarity (from hexane to alcohol) using Soxhlet apparatus.

   or

   Extraction with alcohol and then fractionating the alcoholic extract (in aqueous phase) with various organic solvents like petroleum ether, ether, ethylacetate and n-butanol.
4. Performing simple chemical tests on the extracts prepared to establish groups of compounds like alkaloids, steroids, terpenoids, flavonoids, glycosides, anthrquinones etc.
5. Screening of extracts for antidiabetic activities using animal model like rats, mice or rabbits. If the extracts possess significant activities then they will be further investigated as per the following.
6. Study of the Thin Layer Chromatography (TLC), Paper Chromatography (PC) Profile of the extract to know the complexity and number of components present (finger printing of extract).
7. Subjecting the extracts to column chromatography over absorbents like silica gel or alumina as a method for separating the pure crystalline/oily compounds by gradient elution method (Hexane, 5,10,15,25,35,50 and 75 % Ethylacetate in Hexane, pure ethylacetate, 1,5,10 and 15 % Methanol in Ethylacetate) followed be TLC, PC, filtration, crystallization etc.
8. Screening the pure compounds and in some cases fractions to the same type of activities as done under point 5 above to establish the type of compound/fraction responsible for the claimed activity.
9. Identification of crystalline/oily pure compounds by spectroscopic techniques including UV, IR, NMR, MS, m.p. and Co-TLC. Finally confirmed by chemical tests, if necessary.
10. Toxicity studies on animals and finally clinical trials as per the protocol laid down to assess the feasibility of using these compounds as drugs.
11. Preparation of semisynthetic derivative of the leads discovered to have antidiabetic drugs for better pharmaceutical and therapeutic acceptability.

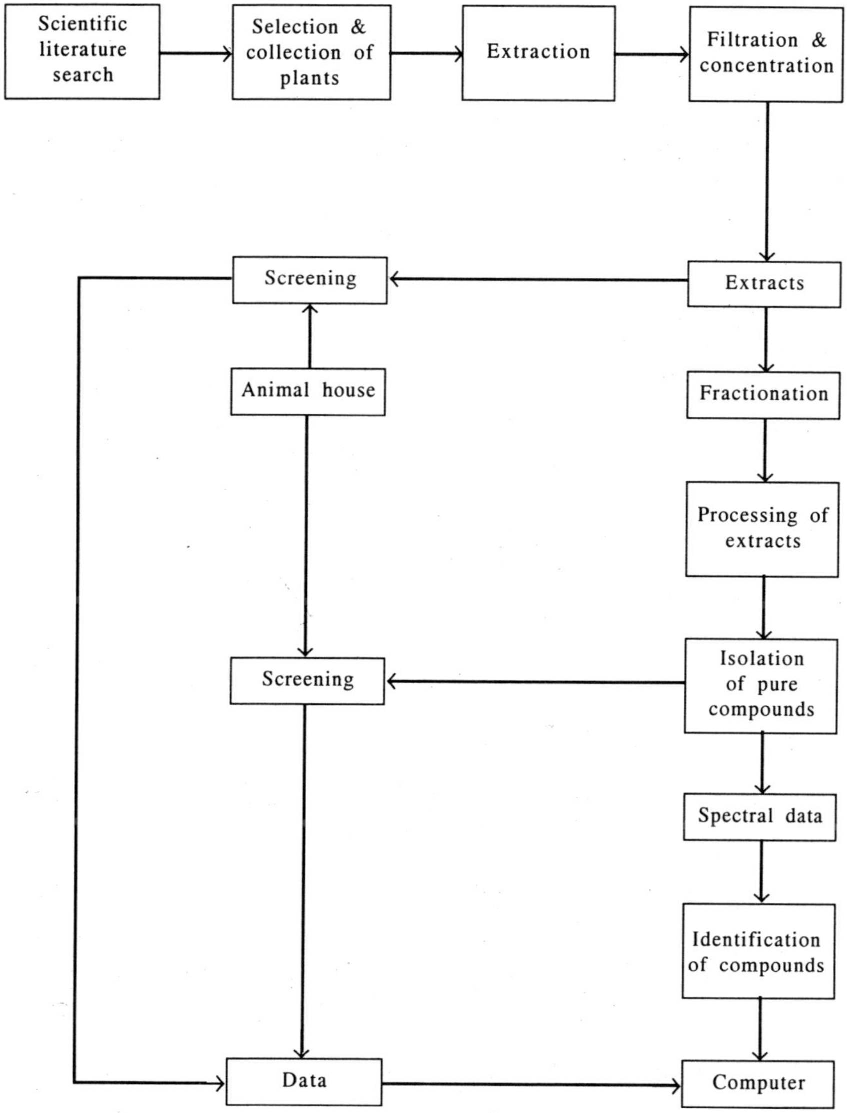


Figure 1: Diabetic Research Design

Alloxan, a cyclic urea, was the first agent reported to produce diabetes in animal models. But the mortality rate is high with alloxan, due to severe hyperglycemia and ketoacidosis at early stages. Later STZ has come into light and proved as the best agent to produce diabetes, because it has greater selectivity of β-cells and lower rate of mortality. Moreover STZ animals do not develop Ketonuria or rise Free fatty acids (FFA) in plasma and show normal level of myocardial glycogen. STZ causes permanent damage to the β-cells and establishes irreversible diabetes. So it is advised to choose STZ to induce diabetes.

STZ [2 deoxy-2-(3 methyl-3-nitrosourea) 1-D-glucopyramose] was discovered in 1963 from fungus *Streptomyces achromogenens*. Structurally it consists of a glucose molecule with highly reactive nitrosourea side chain that initiates cytotoxic action. The glucose moiety causes specific binding to membrane receptor to cause β-cell damage. Three major phenomena are responsible for β-cell damage. (a) process of methylation, (b) free radical generation and (c) formation of nitric oxide.

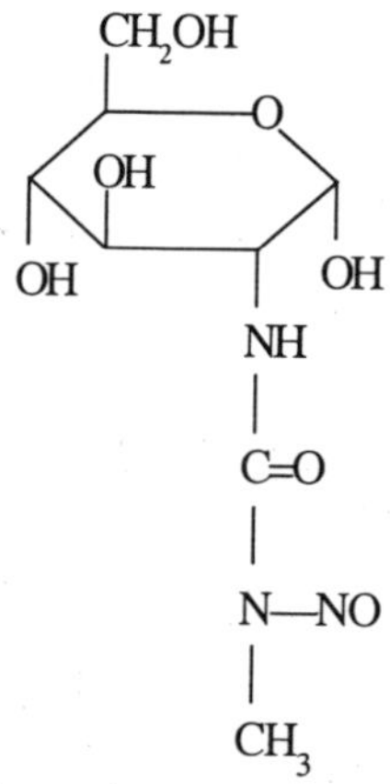


Streptozotocin

Although dose range suggests from 30–100 mg/kg/bw by different investigators in different strains, a single intravenous dose of 40–45 mg/kg/bw is enough to induce diabetes in Sprague Dawley male rats. However, there is variability in the severity of diabetes produced by several investigators in different groups of rats when route of administration and dose of STZ are constant. So it is better if one has to workout the suitable dose of STZ to the experimental animal if necessary to produce desired pathology. Since this chapter is providing only preliminary procedure for bioassay assessment in antidiabetic study, discussion is confined only to the rat model.

The following parameters, shown in Table 4, need to be studied to know the activity of an extract/compound. Other parameters with narrower interests in connection with antidiabetic research for the targeted drug discovery are not discussed here.

**Table 4. Diagnostic Values**

| | | |
|---|---|---|
| a. Blood glucose levels | | 70–126mg/dl (normal) on fasting<br>140–200 mg/dl (borderline)<br>< 200 mg/dl (normal)<br>> 200 mg/dl (high)<br>2 hours post prandial |
| b. Triglycerides on fasting | 200 mg/dl | 2.26 mmol/L (normal) |
| | 200–400 mg/dl | 2.26–4.52 mmol/L (borderline) |
| | 400–1000 mg/dl | 4.52–11.29 mmol/L (high) |
| c. Cholesterol (total) | < 200 mg/dl | < 5.2 mmol/L (normal) |
| | 200–239 mg/dl | 5.2–6.2 mmol/L (borderline) |
| | > 240 mg/dl | > 6.2 mmol/L (high) |
| d. Glycosylated heamoglobin | Hb A1 (%) | Up to 8.5 (normal)<br>8.5–10.5 (borderline)<br>> 11.0 (high) |
| | Hb $A1_c$ (%) | Up to 6.0 (normal)<br>6.0–8.5 (borderline)<br>> 9.0 (high) |

Selection of animals, induction of diabetes, recruitment of animals into the study, dose regimen, data collection and data analysis are the major events in the bioassay assessment programme.

## SELECTION OF ANIMALS

Select only healthy male Sprague-Dawley or albino rats measuring 180–200 gms. Approximately a minimum number of 35 rats needs to be taken for a batch (keeping in view the mortality and severity of diabetes) the animals must be fed with high fat diet for two weeks for induction of NIDDM. Then confirm the insulin resistance by measuring serum insulin and Triglycerides levels.

### Induction of Diabetes using STZ

#### *Preparation of STZ*

The animals must be kept for fasting 16 hours before STZ administration. In order to induce diabetes, animals must be weighed to determine the amount of STZ to be given. STZ is not stable in solution form. So, solution be made fresh whenever it is required. But it is stable for 15 minutes at pH 4.5. STZ must be prepared at a dose level of 40–45 mg/kg/bw in citrate buffer 0.1 M with the pH adjusted to 4.5. The STZ thus prepared must be administered based on the route selected immediately (within 5 minutes) as the half-life of STZ is 35 minutes.

### *Route of Administration of STZ*

After high fat diet and overnight fasting (preferably 16 hours), the rats are anesthetized with a combination of 65 mg/kg/bw ketamine and 7 mg/kg/bw xylazine intramuscularly. Insulin resistant rats are made into diabetic rats by injecting freshly prepared Streptozotocin 40 mg/kg/bw in citrate buffer 0.1 M with pH 4.5 into the tail vein with temporary indwelling insulin syringe slowly. The route of administration can be intravenous, intra peritoneal or sub-cutaneous. If the intravenous route is selected to facilitate easy administration, apply xylene to the tail or expose the tail to electric lamp for brief period at the place of injection for dialation of vein. Intravenous delivery of STZ is ideal when compared to the other two methods. Care must be taken while administering the STZ to the rats. The diet and water is then kept accessible to the rats after the STZ administration.

Hyperglycemia develops with in 24–48 hours and remains at 3–4 times higher than normal levels of blood glucose. But stable glucose value will be achieved after 4 days of induction of diabetes. There would be a reduction of 50% and 95% plasma and pancreatic insulin levels respectively. β-cell necrosis followed by β-cell degeneration occur within 3 days after administration of STZ in adult rats establishing irreversible diabetes.

## Recruitment of the Animals into the Study

After 4 days of STZ administration, blood glucose levels must be tested to determine the diabetic condition. Basing on their blood glucose levels ranging from 300–500 mg/dl, animals need to be recruited for the study. As far as possible the rats which have uniform diabetic glucose levels are selected. The diabetic animals are divided into 4 groups of 7 animals each. First, second, third and fourth group of animals to be meant for vehicle, low dose, high dose and metformin treatments respectively. The weights of animals are recorded on the first day. The diet is removed at 7 AM on the day of the study and blood glucose, Triglycerides, Cholesterol and insulin levels may be estimated before first treatment of the extract/compound for control values through one of the convenient colorimetric methods. (Methods of estimation are given at the end of this chapter). Instead of the colorimetric method glucose strip method can also be used. Although using strip is easy and quick method to estimate different parameters, but cost involved is very high. If it is decided to use strip method to estimate, glucose, triglycerides, cholesterol one should use this method throughout the experiment and also in any future repeats.

**Dose Regimen is as follows**

In case of rats, it is always better if the administered volume restricted to 1 ml.

- Vehicle: (Vehicle/twice a day) n = 7
- Low dose: (x mg/kg/bw/twice a day) n = 7
- High dose: (5x mg/kg/bw/twice a day) n = 7
- Metformin compound to be tested (250 mg/kg/bw/twice a day) n = 7.

Treatment shall be given twice a day. First treatment will be at 10 AM immediately after the 0' hour estimations and second treatment will be between 4 and 5 PM.

**Data Collection**

Duration of the study is for two weeks if it is an extract and the data is to be collected at 7 different points. One-week study is enough if one wishes to work with pure compound and it requires collection of data at 4 different points only. At the end of the study ethonize the rats.

***Data Collection Schedule is as follows***

*1st day*

- 0' hour estimation of blood glucose, serum insulin, TG and cholesterol for all the four groups of rats is to be done before first treatment.
- First treatment will be soon after completion of the 0' hour estimations preferably at 10.00 AM.
- Again estimate the required parameters 4 hours after the first treatment. Second and sixth hour estimations are also to be done if necessary.
- Second treatment will be in the evening.

So these estimations are required on every alternate day. Body weights also need to be measured on these days. In the rest of the days treatment needs to be given to the rats as per the schedule (twice a day).

**Experimental Design for Acute Study**

In this study, blood samples are to be collected just before the treatment and at the time periods of 1, 2, 3, 4, 6, 8, 10, 12, 14, 16, 20 & 24 hours after treatment for estimation of blood glucose only. As this design remains frequent collection of blood samples, usually rabbits are used since it is difficult to collect the blood samples frequently from small animals like rats and mouse.

**Data Analysis**

Express the data in mean ± S.E. Analyze data by student 't' test.

## METHODS OF ESTIMATION OF DIFFERENT PARAMETERS

### (A) Blood Glucose Estimation

There are several methods for estimation of blood glucose. *viz.* Nelson—Somogyi method and GOD/POD method, Strip method etc,.

#### *(i) Nelson-Somogyi Method*

In this method blood was deproteinised by a mixture of Barium hydroxide and Zinc sulphate, which gives a filtrate containing practically no reducing substances other than glucose. The filtrate obtained was heated in boiling water bath with alkaline copper reagent. The alkaline copper was reduced to Cuprous copper by glucose in the blood. Disodium hydrogen arsenate was added to the cooled reaction mixture. The Cuprous copper was oxidized to cupric state by Disodium hydrogen arsenate and the reduced Disodium hydrogen arsenate gives a green to blue color and this was measured at 520 nm. in visible spectrophotometer (Hawk's, 1976).

*Procedure for preparation of reagents*

Barium hydroxide solution:

Dissolve 90gms. of $Ba(OH)_2.8H_2O$ in distilled water and dilute to 2000 ml in a graduated cylinder. Filter if cloudy and store in well-stoppered container.

Zinc Sulphate solution:

Dissolve 100gms. of $ZnSO_4.7H_2O$ in distilled water, dilute to 2000 ml in a graduated cylinder and mix.

It is important that these two solutions exactly neutralize each other.

Alkaline copper reagent:

Solution-A: Dissolve 50 gms. of anhydrous sodium carbonate, 50gms. of Rochelle salt, 40 gms. of Sodium bicarbonate and 400 gms of anhydrous Sodium sulphate in about 1600 ml of distilled water and dilute to 2 Liters. Mix and filter if not clear, sediment forms in a few days, filter again.

Solution-B: Dissolve 150 gms. of $CuSO_4.5H_2O$ in distilled water and dilute to 1 Liter. Add 0.5 ml of concentrated Sulphuric acid and mix.

On the day of experiment, take 4 ml of solution B in a 100 ml graduated cylinder dilute to 100 ml with solution A and mix.

*Arsenomolybdate color reagent*

Dissolve 100gms. of Ammonium molybdate in 1800ml of distilled water. Add 84 ml of concentrated Sulphuric acid with stirring. Dissolve 12gms. of Disodium ortho-Arsenate ($Na_2H_2SO_4$. $7H_2O$) in 100 ml distilled water and add this with stirring to the acidified Molybdate solution. Keep the mixture in an incubator at 37° C for 1 to 2 days.

*Standard glucose solutions*

Dissolve 1.0 gm of anhydrous glucose in about 10 to 15 ml of 0.2 % Benzoic acid solution, then transfer it to 100 ml volumetric flask, dilute to the mark with Benzoic acid solution. This solution contains 10 mg of Glucose per 1 ml. From this prepare the dilutions which gives 20, 40, 80, 100, 120 mg/ml respectively. Then these concentrations are transferred to Folin-Wu tubes. Prepare the blank with 2 ml of distilled water. Then add 1 ml of alkaline copper sulphate reagent to each of the Folin-Wu tubes and cover the top of each tube with a marble. These tubes are heated in a boiling water bath for 20 minutes. They are cooled under tap water for one minute. To each tube add 1 ml of Arsenomolybdate color reagent and mix gently without shaking. Then measure the optical density color development at 520 nm, against the blank.

*Estimation of glucose in the blood sample*

*Deprotinization:*

Place 1 ml of blood sample in a 50 ml of flask. Add 9.5 ml of Barium hydroxide solution, with constant mixing, add 9.5 ml of Zinc sulphate solution and mix by rotation. Shake vigorously and filter on a filter paper, collect the filtrate.

*Measurement of glucose concentration*

Measure 0.5 ml of the Barium-Zinc filtrate into a Folin-Wu tube. Add 1 ml of alkaline Copper sulphate reagent and cover the top of the each tube with a marble. Then heat the tube in a boiling water bath for 20 minutes and then cool it under tap water for one minute. Then add 1 ml of Arsenomolybdate color reagent and mix gently without shaking.

Then measure the optical density of color development at 520 nm against blank. The concentration of the glucose in the blood can be known from the standard graph constructed using different known concentrations of glucose (Nelson and Somogyi, 1944).

### *ii) GOD/POD Method (Glucose Kit Method)*

This is one stepped, simple and rapid method. In this method, glucose is oxidized by the glucose oxidase which gives D-gluconic acid and hydrogen peroxide. Hydrogen peroxide in the presence of the peroxidase oxidizes phenol, which combines with 4 amino-antipyrine to produce a red colored quinoneimine dye. The intensity of the color produced is proportional to glucose concentration in the sample and this can be measured at 505 nm in visible spectrophotometer (Philip D Mayne, 1994; Trinder, 1969).

$$\text{D-glucose} + H_2O + O_2 \xrightarrow{GOD} \text{D-gluconic acid} + H_2O_2$$

$$H_2O_2 + \text{4-Aminoantipyrine} + \text{Phenol} \xrightarrow{POD} \text{Quinoneimine dye} + H_2O$$

Collect the blood (3 drops) from the tip of the rat tail directly into the microcentrifuge tubes by tail sliceing with surgical blade. Serum/Plasma should be separated from the blood cells at the earliest preferably within 30 minutes by centrifugation. Less than 10 mg/ml Sodium fluoride is preferred as anticoagulant due to its anti-glycolytic activity. Excess usage of Sodium fluoride is not advisable since it inhibits the color development. Serum glucose concentration is generally stable for about 8 hours at room temperature. Then serum glucose levels can be estimated by calorimetric method at a wavelength of 505 nm. Sample and reagent volumes needs to be 10 ml and 1 ml respectively. Pipette into clean and dry test tubes labeled as blank (B), standard (S) and test (T).

| **Parameters** | **B** | **S** | **T** |
|---|---|---|---|
| Reagent | 1.0 ml | 1.0 ml | 1.0 ml |
| Distilled water | 0.01ml | — | — |
| Standard | — | 0.01 ml | — |
| Sample | — | — | 0.01 ml |

Mix well and keep for 20 minutes at room temperature. Then measure the absorbance of test (T), standard (S) against blank (B) on a spectrophotometer at 505 nm.

Calculations:

$$\text{Glucose concentration in mg \%} = \frac{\text{Absorbance of test}}{\text{Absorbance of standard}} \times 100$$

### *(iii) Strip Method*

Quantitative determination of blood glucose in the range of 60–600 mg/dl can be done by using test strips meant for blood glucose estimation with the Accutrend (Roche group) reflection photometer or using any other brands of glucometer.

## (B) Estimation of Triglycerides

### *(i) Enzymatic Spectrophotometric Method*

Triglycerides in the serum or plasma can be measured by enzymatic spectrophotometric method (glycerol phosphate oxidase / peroxidase).

*Procedure*

Pipette into labelled test tubes after getting the reagent to room temperature.

| Parameters | Blank | Standard | Sample |
|---|---|---|---|
| Triglyceride standard | — | 10.0 ml | — |
| Sample | — | — | 10.0 ml |
| Reagent | 1.0 ml | 1.0 ml | 1.0 ml |

Mix thoroughly and incubate the tubes for 15 minutes at room temperature. Measure the absorbance (A) of the standard and sample at 500 nm against the blank. The color is stable for about 2 hours.

Calculations:

$$\frac{\text{(A) Sample}}{\text{(A) Standard}} \times 2100 = \text{triglycerides mg/dl.}$$

### *(ii) Peroxidase—Coupled Method*

Triglycerides are measured using Triglyceride GB reagent on Roche COBAS FARA centrifugal analyzer. In this method, free glycerol is eliminated in an initial blank reaction that differs from the final reaction by the omission of lipase and 4-aminophenazone. The initial reaction is followed by enzymatic hydrolysis of triglycerides with lipase and determination of the liberated glycerol by an enzymatic, colorimetric reaction of peroxide and 4–aminophenazone to form color that is directly proportional to the amount of triglycerides present in the sample (Mc Gowan et al., 1983).

### *(iii) Strip Method*

Quantitative determination of triglycerides in the range of 70–600 mg/dl (0.8–6.86 mmol/L) can be made by using test strips meant for triglycerides estimation with the reflection photometer Accutrend GCT (Roche group) or using any other reflection photometer.

## (C) Estimation of Free Fatty Acids

### *(i) Half Micro Test*

Free fatty acids in serum or plasma can be measured by enzymatic colorimetric assay. The principle involved in this method is, free fatty acids are in the presence of the enzyme acyl-CoA synthetase (Acyl CS), converted by adenosine-5-triphosphate (ATP) and coenzyme A (CoA) into acyl coenzyme A (Acyl CoA), resulting in adenosine-5-monophosphate (AMP) and pyrophosphate being produced. Acyl CoA reacts with oxygen in the presence of Acyl CoA oxidase to form 2,3-enoyl-Co enzyme A (enoyl CoA). The resulting hydrogen peroxide converts 2, 4, 6-tribromo-3-hydroxy-benzoic acid and 4-aminoantipyrine to a red dye in the presence of peroxidase. The dye is measured in the visible range at 546 nm (Shimizu et al., 1980; Harris, 1974).

*Procedure*

| Pipette into cuvettes | Blank | Sample |
|---|---|---|
| Reaction mixture | 1.00 ml | 1.00 ml |
| Sample | — | 0.05 ml |
| Redistilled water | 0.05 ml | — |
| *Mix and bring to 25°C and keep for about 10 minutes.* | | |
| Add n-ethyl-maleinimide-solution (ii) | 0.05 ml | 0.05 ml |
| *Mix and read absorbance of the solutions ($A_1$).* | | |
| Reaction mixture B (iii) | 0.05 ml | 0.05 ml |
| *Mix and wait until the end of the reaction at 25°C (15 minutes) and read absorbance of the solution ($A_2$)* | | |

*Calculation*

Calculate the absorbance differences ($A_2$-$A_1$) for both blank and sample. Substract the absorbance difference of the blank ($DA_b$) from the absorbance difference of the sample ($\Delta A_s$). This gives $\Delta A$.

$$\text{Concentration, } C = \frac{V}{\epsilon \times d \times v} \times \Delta A$$

where V = Final volume (ml); v = Sample volume (ml); d = Light path (cm); $\epsilon$ = Absorption coefficient of the dye stuff at 546 nm:19.3 $[1 \times c^{-1}]^3$.

Concentration, $C = \frac{1.15}{19.3 \times 1 \times 0.05} \times \Delta A$ (nmol free fatty acids/1 serum, plasma)

### *(ii) Enzymatic Method*

To quantify fatty acids using acyl-coA synthetase in biological fluid in coupling the formation of activated fatty acid with free enzymatic reactions, which lead to a fluorimetric detection of NADH consumption (Jebens et al., 1992). This method is very simple and inexpensive and well suited for automation. The presence of up to 10 nmoles fatty acids in the sample tube is accurately determined.

## D) Insulin Estimation

### *Radioimmunoassays*

The sensitivity of radioimmunoassay is greater than that of other assays. The following could be determined by radio immunoassay.

(a) Total Immunoreactive Insulin (IRI)
(b) Non-Extracted Immunoreactive Plasma Insulin (NEIRI)
(c) Free Plasma Insulin (Free IRI)
(d) Acute Insulin Sensitivity (KITT)

Insulin was performed by the coated tube RIA method. In this solid phase RIA, insulin specific antibody is immobilized on the wall of a polypropylene tube. Radiolabelled antigen and antigen from the sample compete for a limited number of antibody binding sites. The amount of labeled antigen bound to antibody is inversely proportional to the amount of insulin in the sample (Yalow and Berson, 1964).

## E) Estimation of Cholesterol

### *Cholesterol Kit (DRL) Method*

After collection of blood sample, it is to be allowed to clot with stirrer. The serum is separated from the collected blood by centrifugation. Then the serum cholesterol is estimated using cholesterol kit through spectrophotometer at 560nm.

$$\text{Total cholesterol in mg \%} = \frac{\text{Absorbance of test}}{\text{Absorbance of standard}} \times 200$$

### *(ii) Strip Method*

Quantitative determination of cholesterol in the range of 150–300 mg/dl (3.88–7.75 mmol/L) can be done by using test strips with the help of Acutrend GC/GCT (Roche group) reflectance photometer or using any other reflectance photometer.

## REFERENCES


Dulin, W.E. and B.M. Wyse. 1969. Studies on the ability of compounds to block the diabetogenic activity of STZ. *Diabetes*, **18**: 459.

Ganda, O.P., A.A. Rossini, and A.A. Like. 1976. Studies on STZ diabetes. *Diabetes*, **25**: 595.

Harris, R.J. 1974. *Pediatr*. **84**: 578–584.

Hawk's, 1976. Physiological Chemistry, Bernard L. Oser, Blood analysis. 14th edition Tata McGraw-hill Publishing Co. New Delhi. pp.1054–1056.

Jebens, E. et al. 1992. *Scand. J. Clin. Lab. Invest.* **52**:717.

Mc Gowan, M.W., J.D. Artiss, D.R. Strandbergh and B. Zork. 1983. A peroxidase—coupled method for the colorimetric determination of serum triglycerides. *Clin. Chem*. **29**: 538–542.

Philip D. Mayne. 1994. 'Carbohydrate Metabolism'. In: Clinical chemistry in Diagnosis and Treatment. *ELBS*. 195–217.

Shimizu, S., Y. Tani, H. Yamada, M. Tabata and T. Murachi. 1980. Enzymatic determination of serum—free fatty acids a colorimetric method. *Anal. Biochem*. **107**: 193–198.

Nelson, N. and M. Somogyi, 1944. A photometric Adoption of the Somogyi method for the determination of glucose. *J. Biol. Chem*. **153**: 375–380.

Trinder, P. 1969. Determination of glucose in blood using glucose oxidase with an alternative oxygen receptor. *Ann. Clin. Biochem*. **6**: 24.

Yalow, R.S. and S.A. Berson. 1964. Immunoassay of plasma insulin. *Meth. Biochem. Anal*. **12**: 69.

CHAPTER 5

# RESEARCH WORK DONE ON THE FEW IMPORTANT ANTIDIABETIC PLANTS

Before the advent of insulin injection and other pharmaceutical preparations, healers relied heavily upon herbs to treat diabetes. Isolation of active principles of diverse chemical groups from plant sources such as morphine, strychnine, quinine, emetine, muscarine etc. necessitated studies of their action by animal experimentations. This was started by the French school with Francis Magendie and Claude Bernard, who studied most of the isolation principles and this was the starting point of modern pharmacology. Later, German, English and American workers and their joint endeavours in the field of Pharmacology, have brought this branch of science to its present stage. Plant products investigated for anti-diabetic effect have been exhaustively reviewed (Aiman, 1970; Hauda and Chawla, 1989; Ivorr et al. 1989; Gupta, 1994; Marles and Farnsworth, 1995). Hence discussión is limited to the work done from 1995 to 2001 except a few instances. It is observed that some of the plant extracts restrict the rise of blood sugar caused by the pituitary hormones responsible for inhibiting peripheral utilization of glucose and causing glycogenolysis in maturity onset diabetes. Some plants have been reported to promote regeneration of Beta cells of Langerhans in pancreas, lowers haemoglobin in A1c, cholesterol and triglyceride levels. Hundreds of plant species have been studied for their potential blood glucose lowering, hypocholesterolemic, hypotensive, antioxidant etc. properties and isolated number of active constituents. The important constituents among them are given below (Wang and Ng, 1999; Marles and Farnsworth, 1995).

**Hypoglycemic Products**

Polysachharide peptides
Alkaloids
Glycopeptides
Triterpenoids
Peptides
Aminobutyric acid derivatives
Steroids
Flavonoids
Lipids
Phenolics
Coumarins
Iridoids
Alkyldisulfides
Guanidine
Xanthones

**Hypotensive Compounds**

Flavonoids
Diterpenes
Alkaloids
Glycosides
Polysaccharides
Proteins

**Hypocholesterolemic Compounds**

Beta-Carotene
Lycopene
Cycloartenol
Beta-sitosterol
Sitostanol
Saponins
Soyabean protein
Indoles
Dietary fiber
Propionate
Mevinolin (beta-hydroxy-beta-methylglutaryl coenzyme A reductase inhibitor)
Polysaccharides

**Antithrombotic Compounds**

Heparins
Flavonoids
Tocotrienols
Statins
Garlic compounds

**Antiatherosclerotic Compounds**

Statins
Garlic compounds etc.

Although number of herbs are reported to possess some degree of antidiabetic activity, a significant amount of research as well as traditional usage is confined only to a few useful plants, some of which have been given here.

## *Gymnema sylvestre* (Retz) R.Br. ex Schult. **(Gurmar, Gymnema): Asclepiadaceae**

This herb is original 'Sugar destroyer'. *Gymnema* stimulates the pancreatic beta cells to produce more insulin in Type-II diabetes and enhances the ability of insulin to decrease blood glucose, increase glucose uptake and utilization by peripheral tissue (Bhaskaran, et al. 1990; Shanmugasundaram et al., 1990a,b; Shanmugasundaram et al., 1983). *Gymnema* may also decrease cholesterol and glucose absorption from the gastro intestinal tract (Shimuzu et al., 1997; Preuss et al., 1998), *Gymnema* reduces the activities of glycogen phosphorylase, gluconeogenic enzymes and sorbitol dehydrogenase (Tim Kaczmar, 1998).

The bioactive constituents of *Gymnema* are gymnemic acid (triterpenoid saponins mixture), gymnosides a (1) and b, gymnemic acid V (7), stigmosterol, Quercitol (sterols), betaine, trimethylamine, choline (amino acid derivaties) (Murakami et al., 1996; Kapoor, 1990).

In clinical trials *Gymnema* decreased fasting and postprandial blood glucose levels 19–35% and 21% respectively in addition to haemoglobin A1C by 29–35% (Shanmugasundaram et al., 1990b; Bhaskaran, 1990; Khare et al. 1983). In another clinical study 22 diabetic patients were able to discontinue the use of their oral hypoglycemic drugs and maintain their blood glucose levels with the extract alone when gymnema is used (400mg/ day) for a period of 18–20 months. The remaining patients were able to maintain with reduced conventional drugs (Bhaskaran, et al. 1990).

## *Trigonella foenum-graecum* L. **(Fenugreek): Fabaceae**

Several studies with fenugreek seeds have shown the hypoglycemic properties in both animal and human diabetic subjects. This is due to its high content of soluble fibre. In most of the studies fenugreek was very effective at lowering LDL cholesterol and triglyceride levels (Zia et al., 2001; Gomez Mary et al., 1998; Abdel-Barry et al., 1997; Ali et al., 1995; Khosla et al., 1995; Sharma et al., 1990; Sharma, 1986).

The bioactive compounds that are isolated from the seeds are fenugreekine (Steroidal sapogenin–peptide ester), disosgenin (saponins), trigonelline, gentianine, carpine (alkaloids), 4-hydroxyisoleucine (amino acid), galactomannan, scopoletin (coumarins), niacin (nicotinic acid), phytic acid and a-tocopherol and vitamin-E (Sauvaire et al. 1998; Haefel et al. 1997; Marles and Farnsworth, 1995; Ali et al.,1995).

Clinical studies of fenugreek has confirmed that it lowers the fasting (30%) and postprandial blood glucose levels (20–35%), haemoglobin A1c (12%), cholesterol and triglyceride levels (Chandra and Aruna, 1997; Sharma et al., 1996, 1990; Puri et al., 1994 and Madar et al., 1988).

***Momordica charantia*** **L. (Bitter gourd): Cucurbitaceae**

Bitter gourd has been extensively used in folk medicine as a remedy for diabetes. Blood sugar lowering action of the fresh juice or extract of the unripe fruit has been clearly established in both experimental and clinical studies (Khan, 1998; Ali et al., 1993; Srivastava et al., 1988, 1993; Karunanayake et al., 1990). *M. charantia* may stimulate insulin release and decrease hepatic glucose output. It also enhances the glucose utilization in the liver, utilization of insulin by peripheral tissue and decreases glucose absorption from intestine (Ahmad et al., 1999; Baldwa, et al., 1977; Sarkar et al. 1996; Srivastava, 1993; Akhtar, 1982; Welihinda et al. 1982, 1986; Khannan and Jain, 1981). An insulin like protein polypeptide-P, isolated from *M. charantia* fruit showed hypoglycemic effect and decrease of haemoglobin A1c when injected in diabetic subjects (Baldwa et al., 1977, Ng et al., 1986). Oral administration of a n-butanol fraction extract (30mg/kg) decreased the blood glucose level by 34% at 3rd hour after administration and increased glucose utilization (Sarkar et al, 1996; Higashino et al., 1992). In another study serum gamma-glutamyl transferase and alkaline phosphatase concentrations were elevated following oral administration of both the fruit and the seed extract (Tennekoon et al., 1994).

The bioactive constituents that are isolated from the fruit and seeds include charantin (steroid glucoside) and polypeptide 'P' (insulinomimetic peptide). Charantin is more potent than the drug tolbutamide (Marles and Farnsworth, 1995).

***Pterocarpus marsupium*** **Roxb. (Vijayasar): Fabaceae**

Extract of the bark and the heartwood decreased fasting (~ 30mg/dl), postprandial blood glucose (~ 45mg/dl) and haemoglobin A1c (0.4%). The bioactive constituents are believed to be epicatechin (flavonoid), marsupium (benzofuranone), pterosupin (dihydrochalcone) and liquiritigenin (stilbene) (Marles and Farnsworth, 1995).

Marsupin and pterostilbene of heartwood of *P.marsupium* significantly lowered the blood glucose level of hyperglycemic rats and the effect was comparable to that of metformin (Manickam et al., 1997).

***Allium cepa*** **L. and *Allium sativum* L. (Onion and Garlic): Liliaceae**

Clinical studies showed that onion and garlic have significant blood sugar, cardiovascular and lipid lowering effects (Shukla et al., 2000; Agarwal, 1996; Marles and Farnsworth, 1995; Sharma et al., 1977). The sulfur-containing compounds of garlic enhances the circulating insulin efficiency (Fetrow and Avila, 1999). S-allyl cysteine sulphoxide (SACS) present in garlic decreases fasting blood glucose and lowers serum cholesterol levels in diabetic rats similar to glibenclamide and insulin action (Sheela et al., 1995; Sheela and Augusti, 1992). Allyl and related sulfoxides are inhibiting thiol group enzymes (Augusti, 1996). Onion and garlic prevents atherosclerosis and isoprenaline induced myocardial necrosis (Saxena et al., 1980; Kumar et al., 1979). Garlic has cardiovascular protective activity and antidiabetic effect (Dasture and Kulkarni, 1999).

The bioactive constituents are allyl propyl disulphide (APDS), diallyl disulphide oxide (allicin), S-allyl cysteine sulphoxide (SACS), S-allyl mercaptocysteine and certain flavonoids (Marles and Farnworth, 1995).

### *Panax quinquefolius* (Ginseng) Araliaceae

*Panax* root has been studied in Type-2 diabetes subjects. Ginseng supplements significantly improved blood glucose level, haemoglobin A1c (Vuskan et al., 2000; Sotaniemi et al., 1995). Ginseng may increase glucose absorption, glucose transport and promotes the insulin secretion (Yuan et al., 1998; Ohinishi et al., 1996; Hasagawa et al. 1994).

The active constituents of ginseng root are ginsenosides (Marles and Farnsworth, 1995). The dose used in clinical trials in subjects with diabetes is 200mg/kg/day and 3000mg/kg/day (Volger et al., 1999).

### *Aloe vera* (L.) **Burm.** f. **(Aloe) Liliaceae**

The dried sap of the aloe plant is one of the several traditional remedies used for diabetes. The pulp of Aloe gel has been used orally to treat Type-II diabetes and hyperlipidemia. The active constituents are believed to be glucomannan (Polysaccharides) and vitamins, saponins, B-sitosterol and amino acids. Aloe gel decreased fasting blood glucose, haemoglobin A1c and triglyceride levels (Ernst, 1997; Bunyapraphatsara et al., 1996; Yongchiayudha et al., 1996).

*A. vera* leaf pulp extract showed hypoglycemic activity on IDDM and NIDDM rats, the effectiveness being enhanced for Type–II diabetes in comparison with glibenclamide (Okyar et al., 2001; Volger and Ernst, 1999).

### *Lagerstroemia speciosa* (Banaba) Lythraceae

Extract of leaves showed a significant decrease in total hepatic lipid (65%) contents. This is due to a reduction in the accumulation of triglycerides (Suzuki et al., 1999). In another study extract of leaves lowered the serum insulin and total cholesterol levels in mice (Kakuda et.al., 1996; Miyajiet et.al., 1999; Yogendra Mishra et.al., 1990). The hypoglycemia effect of colosic acid was found in both the *in vitro* and *in vivo* assays (Murakami et al., 1993). The inhibitory effect of banaba on postprandial hypoglycemic is due to the inhibition of α-amylase and α-glycosidases in rats (Suzuki et al., 2001).

Table 4

| Plant name and Family | Extract | Active constituents responsible for the activity | Activities | Authors and Years |
|---|---|---|---|---|
| 1 | 2 | 3 | 4 | 5 |
| *Abroma angusta* Sterculiaceae | Aqueous extract | — | 4 gms/kg of aqueous extract for 16 weeks resulted in significant fall in fasting blood glucose, total and LDL cholesterol and T.G. levels in diabetic rats | Ali Hussain and Mala Rao, 2001 |
| *Abutilon indicum* (L.) Sweet Malvaceae | Leaf extract | — | Alcohol and water extracts of *A. indicum* leaves 400 mg/kg showed significant hypoglycemic effect in normal rats 4 hours after administration (23.1% and 26.95% respectively) | Seetharam et al., 2002 |
| *Acanthopanax senticosus* Araliaceae | — | Saponin | Showed hypoglycemic activity | Sui et al., 1994 |
| *Aegle marmelos* (L.) Correa ex Roxb. Rutaceae | Leaf extract | — | Showed Potential hypo-glycemic activity and regeneration of damaged pancreas | Das, 1996; Sachdewa et al., 2001 |
| *Aesculus hippocastanum* L. Hippocastanaceae | — | Escins, la, lb, 11a and 11b | Hypoglycemic activity in the oral glucose tolerance test in rats | Yoshikawa et al., 1996 |
| *Anacardium occidentale* L. Anacerdiaceae | Aqueous leaf extract | — | A dose of 400 mg/kg/bw reduced blood sugar levels in both normal and alloxan induced rabbits | Esimone et al., 2001 |
| *Anemarrhena asphodeloides* Liliaceae | — | 1.Pseudoprototins saponin A III from rhizome<br>2. Mangiferrin | Significant hypoglycemic activity in STZ induced diabetic mice. MF and MG lowered the blood glucose level of KK-AY-mice and improved hyper insulemenia after oral administration | Nakashina et al., 1993; Ichikri et al., 1998 |

| | | | | |
|---|---|---|---|---|
| | | (MF) and its glucosides (mangiferrin-7-0-?-D-glucoside) (M.G.) | | |
| *Aronica melanocarpa* Elliot | — | Anthocyanin | Prevented generation of free oxygen radicals, decrease of peroxidation of lipids, unsaturated fatty acids | Jankowhi et al., 1999 |
| *Bauhinia megalandra* Fabaceae | Aqueous extract of leaves | — | Reduced glucose levels in diabetic patients. This is due to inhibition of glucose-6-phosphatase. | Gonalez-Mujica et al., 1998 |
| *Bauhinia forticata* L. Fabaceae | Decoction | — | STZ diabetic rats treated with decoction showed a significant reduction in serum and urinary glucose and urinary urea. | Pepato et al., 2002 |
| *Barleria prionitis* L. Acanthaceae | Alcoholic and aqueous extract | — | Alcoholic and aqueous extracts of leaf and root caused significant fall in blood glucose level in diabetic rats. | Geetham and Wahi, 2001 |
| *Beta vulgaris* L. Chenopodiaceae | — | Beta vulgo-rosides II, III and IV | Exhibited hypoglycemic activity in an oral glucose tolerance test in rats | Yoshikawa et al., 1996 |
| *Biophytum sensitivum* DC. Oxalidaceae | Leaf extract | — | Leaf extract showed fall in plasma glucose by 36.9% and improvement in the oral glucose tolerance test | Puri and Baral, 1998 |
| *Caesalpinia bonducella* Fleming Caesalpiniaceae | Aqueous and 50% ethanolic extracts | — | Both extracts produced significant anti-hyperglycemic, anti-hypercholesterolemic and anti-hypertriglyceridemic effects in STZ diabetic rats | Sharma et al., 1997 |
| *Cannabis sativa* L. Cannabinaceae | Ethanolic extract of the fruit | | Fruits posses a more significant anti-hyperglycemic activity than Gliclazide | Aslam et al., 2000 |
| *Capparis decidua* Capparidaceae | Fruit powder | — | Lowers alloxan induced lipid peroxidation (LPO) and alters superoxide dismutase (SOD) and catalase (CAT) enzymes activity to reduce oxidative stress | Yadav et al., 1997a |

| 1 | 2 | 3 | 4 | 5 |
|---|---|---|---|---|
| *Cassia fistula* L. Fabaceae | Ethanolic extract of the roots | — | The 95% ethanolic extract of the roots lowered the blood sugar level up to 30% after 2 hours in fasted albino rats | Vaishanava, 1993 |
| *Catharanthus roseus* (L.) Don Apocynaceae | Fresh leaf paste and extract | | Significant fall in blood sugar in STZ induced diabetic rats | Goyal et al. 1999, Chattopadhyay, 1999a |
| *Cimicifuga duhurica* Ranunculaceae | | Isoferulic acid from rhizome | Antihyper glycemic action in spontaneous diabetic rats has been reported | Liu et al., 1999 |
| *Cissus sicyoides* L. Vitaceae | Leaf extract | — | Potential hypoglycemic activity in hereditary, STZ induced Diabetic and normal rats. | Mori et al., 2001 |
| *Citrullus colocynthis* (L.) Schrad. Cucurbitaceae | Fruit extract | — | Insulino tropic effect | Nonila et al., 2000 |
| *Cleome droserifolia* Capparaceae | Plant extract | — | Plant has hypoglycemic effect suppression to hepatic glucose output and hypocholesterolemic effect | Nicola et al., 1996 |
| *Coccinia indica* Wight & Arn. Cucurbitaceae | Leaf preparation | | Protective influence against hyperlipedemia and hypoglycemia in NIDDM patients | Kamble et al., 1996 Kumar et al., 1997 Kalpana and Srinivas, 1997 |
| *Commiphora myrra.* Burseraceae | Ethanolic extract of resin | — | The active fraction of petroleum ether extract showed effects on blood glucose and body weights | Ubillas et al., 1999 |
| *Coriandrum sativum* L. Apiaceae | Aqueous extract of coriander | — | Increased 2-deoxy glucose transport, glucose oxidation and incorporation of glucose into glycogen. Coriander has anti-hyperglycemic insulin— releasing and insulin—like activity | Gray and Fatt, 1999 |
| *Cryptolepsis sanguinolenta* Asclepidaceae | — (Indoloquinolone alkaloid) | Cryptolepine | Oral treatment has antihyperglycemic effect declines in plasma insulin concentration and increases glucose uptake by 3T3-L1 cells | Luo et al., 1998a |

| | | | | |
|---|---|---|---|---|
| *Cuminum nigrum* Apiaceae | — | Flavonoid fraction of seeds | Flavonoids have been reported to possess insulin triggering and/or insulin-like properties | Ahmad et al., 2000 |
| *Curcuma longa* L. Zingiberaceae | Herbal medicine | — | Positive results were observed in the management of diabetes mellitus with ayurvedic herbal medicine | Rajagopalan and Sasidharan, 2000 |
| *Cyamopsis tetragonaloba* (L.) Taub. Fabaceae | Petroleum ether extract | — | 20 days treatment significantly decreased blood glucose and blood urea levels and increased the serum proteins and obumin levels | Bhandari and Sharma, 1999 |
| *Eclipta alba* (L.) Hassk. Euphorbiaceae | Herbal formulation | — | Decrease in STZ—hyperglycemia | Bhattacharya et al., 1997 |
| *Enicostemma littorale* Gentianaceae | Aqueous extract | — | Treatment with aqueous extract decreased in glucose, cholesterol and triglyceride levels and increases in insulin sensitivity and provides nephroprotection in diabetic rats | Murali et al., 2002 |
| *Eucalyptus globulus* Labill. Myrtaceae | Aqueous extract of eucalyptus | — | Represents an effective anti hyperglycemic dietary adjunct for the treatment of diabetes. | Gray and Flatt, 1998 |
| *Ficus benghalensis* L. Moraceae | — | Leucodeliphinidin derivative & some new compounds | Its action is closely similar to that of an ED of Glebineclamide. Active hypoglycemic constituents were isolated and some of them stimulated blood insulin levels in NIDDM patients | Geetha et al., 1994; Shukla et al., 2000; Mukherjee et al., 1998 Kumar et al., 1994; and Augusti et al., 1994 |
| *Olea europaea* L. Oleaceae | — | Iridoid Ole | Shows hypoglycemic effects in normal and alloxan, diabetic rats | Trovato et al., 1994 |
| *Globulairia alypum* Globulariaceae | Leaves | — | The hypoglycemic activity of this plant has been suggested to be mediated through enhancement of peripheral metabolism of glucose and increase insulin release | Skin et al., 1999 |
| *Hibiscus rosa-sinensis* L. Malvaceae | Leaf extract | — | 250 mg/kg/bw showed significant (37%) glucose lowering effect in glucose induced hyperglycemic rats | Sachdewa, et al. 2001 |

| 1 | 2 | 3 | 4 | 5 |
|---|---|---|---|---|
| *Hintonia latifolia* (copalchi) | — | Coutareagenin (neoflavonoid) | Reduction of diabetic evaluated blood sugar levels. | Korec et al., 2000 a, 2000 b |
| *Inula racemosa* Hook. Asteraceae | Alcoholic extract of the root | — | Lowers blood glucose and enhances liver glycogen; hypoglycemic response may be at peripheral level by potentiating the insulin sensitivity | Yamini Tripati and Padmaja Chaturvedi, 1995 |
| *Larrea tridentata* | — | Nordihydro guaiaretic acid (Masoprocal) Lip-oxygenase inhibitor | Lower plasma glucose concentration in Type – 2 diabetes mouse models | Luo et al., 1998 b |
| *Mangifera indica* L. Ancardiaceae | Extract | — | Exhibited ??Amylase inhibitory activity | Prashanth et al., 2001 |
| *Medicago sativa* Fabaceae | Luerne in the diet (62.5 g/kg) and drinking water (2.5 g/kg.) | — | Reduced the hyperglycemia, insulin releasing and insulin like activity | Gray and Flatt, 1977 |
| *Momordica cymbalaria* Hook. Cucurbitaceae | Fruit powder | — | Significant reduction in fasting blood glucose serum cholesterol and triglycerides in the treated diabetic rats | Kameswara Rao et al., 1999 |
| *Morus nigra* *Morus alba*. Moraceae | Leaf and bark extracts | — | A single oral dose 500 mg/kg reduced blood glucose in alloxan reduced diabetic mice | Hosseinzadeh et al., 2000 |
| *Musa sapientum* L. Musaceae | Chloroform extract of flower | — | Significant reduction in blood glucose and glycosylated Hb. Decrase in thioburbuturic acid reactive substances and the increase in reduced glutathione, glutathione peroxidase and inhibited the antioxident | Pari and Umamaheswari, 2000 |
| *Myrcia multiflora* DC Myricaceae | — | Flavanone glucosides, myrciacitrins – I acetophenone glucosides, myrciaphenone— B | Found to show potent inhibitory activities on aldose reductase and alphaglucosidase in diabetic mice. | Yoshikawa et al., 1997 a, b, c. |

| | | | | |
|---|---|---|---|---|
| *Nelumbo nucifera* Gaertn. Nelumbonaceae | Ethanolic extract of rhiyome | — | Reduced the blood sugar level of normal, glucose fed hyperglycemic and induced diabetic rats | Mukherjee et al., 1997 |
| *Ocimum sanctum* L. Lamiaceae | Alcoholic leaf extract | — | Lowering of blood sugar level in normal, glucose fed hyperglycemic and induced diabetic rats | Chattopadhyay 1993, 1999; Bhattacharya et al., 1997 |
| *Ophiopogon japonicus* Liliaceae | — | Polysaccharides | The isolated polysaccharides from this plant significantly lowered blood sugar by 54% at 11 h after administration | Zang et al., 1993 |
| *Opuntia megacantha* Cactaceae | Leaf extract | — | Reduced blood glucose elevation in plasma urea and creatinine concentrations and the reduction of plasma Na+ concentration. | Bwititi et al. 2000 a, 2000 b, Musabayane, 2000 |
| *Pandanus odorus* Ridl. Pandanaceae | — | 4 – hydroxy–benzoic acid from roots | Hypoglycemic effect in normal rats | Peungvicha et al., 1998 |
| *Parmentiera edulis* Bignoniaceae | — | Lactucin-8-0-methyl acrylate of fruit | The compound lowers blood sugar levels after administration to alloxan-diabetic mice. | Perez et al., 2000 |
| *Pascalium decompositum* | Methanolic and aqueous extract of roots | — | Precipitate (WMP) obtained through maceration of water extract with methanol showed significant hypoglycemic activity in mild diabetic rats | Alarcon Aguilar and Jimenez Estrade, 2000 |
| *Polygala senegal* L. var. *latifolia* Polygalaceae | n-butanol extract of rhlizome | E and Z – senegasaponins a and b Senegins II–IV (1 & 2) | Showed a significant decrease in the glucose level of diabetic mice (KK.AY). Hypoglycemic effect was identified as a triterpenoid glycoside senegin-II. Compounds senegins II–IV, 1 and 2 significantly lowered the glucose levels. | Kako et al., 1996; Yoshikawa et al., 1995. Kako et al., 1997 |
| *Polygonatum officinalis* Liliaceae | Rhizome methanolic extract | — | Enhanced insulin sensitivity and hypoglycemic activity | Miura and Kato, 1995 |
| *Polyscias fruticosa* Araliaceae | Ethnolic and n-butanol leaf extracts | — | 250 mg/kg/bw and 500 mg/kg/bw extracts showed effective antihyper glycemic activity in STZ induced diabetic rats | Divakar and Bensita, 1998 |

| 1 | 2 | 3 | 4 | 5 |
|---|---|---|---|---|
| *Pongamia pinnata* (L.) Pierre Fabaceae | Powder of flowers | — | In NIDDM patients, treatment with the powder produced a dose-dependent decrease in the blood glucose levels. | Akhtar and Akhtar, 1999 |
| *Portulaca pilosa* Portrulacaceae | Whole plant | — | It has anti-diabetic properties | Das, 1999 |
| *Psidium guajava* L. Myrtaceae | — | Glycon from Fruit | Glycon isolated from the fruit markedly reduced blood sugar level on I.P. injection to normal and alloxan produced hypoglylemic rabbits. | El-Badrawy et al., 1999 |
| *Pterocarpus santalinus* L. Fabaceae | Bark extract | — | Ethanolic fraction at the dose of 0.25 g/kg body weight showed maximum anti-hyperglycemic activity | Rao et al., 2001 |
| *Punica granatum* L. Punicaceae | Extract | — | Exhibited ?? Amylase inhibitory activity | Prashanth et al., 2001 |
| *Pycranthus angolensis* Myristicaceae | — | Pycrathuguinone A and B | The compounds A and B are the representatives of a novel terpenoid type quinone skeleton and both compounds possess significant anti-hyperglycemic activity | Fort et al., 2000 |
| *Rubus imperialis* Rosaceae | Methanolic extract of leaves, roots and stems and ethyl acetate fraction from roots | — | Hypoglycemic activity | Kanegusuku et al., 2002 a, b |
| *Salacia oblonga* Wall. Celastraceae | Methanolic extract of the root | Diterpene, Triterpene and Kotalagenin 16-acetate. | Inhibitary activity on the increase in serum glucose level in rats | Matsuda et al. 1999 a, 1999 b, 2000. |
| *Salacia reticulata* L. Celastraceae | — | Kotalanol (alpha – glucosidase inhibitor) | Kotalanol has more potent inhibitory activity against sucrose than salacinol and acarbose | Yoshikawa et al., 1998 |

| | | | | |
|---|---|---|---|---|
| *Sida cordifolia* L. Malvaceae | Methanolic extract | — | Hypoglycemic activity | Kanth and Diwan, 1999 |
| *Sida cordifolia* L. Malvaceae | Methanotic extract of root | — | Methanolic extract of root was found to possess significant hypoglycemic activity | Ravikanth and Diwan, 1999 |
| *Smilax glabra* Roxb. Liliaceae | Methanolic extract of Rhizome | — | Significantly lowered the blood glucose of KK-AY mice due to raised insulin sensitivity | Fukunaga et al., 1997 |
| *Suaeda fruticosa* Chenopodiaceae | Aqueous extract | — | The aqueous extract at a dose of 192 mg/kg/bw produced a significant decrease in blood glucose and plasma cholesterol in diabetic rats | Benwahhoud et al., 2001 |
| *Swertia japonica* Gentianaceae | — | Bellidifolin | Bellidifolin showed a potent and dose dependent hypoglycemic activity in STZ induced diabetic rats | Basnet et al., 1995 a,b |
| *Teramnus labialis* (Roxb.) Benth. Fabaceae | — | Fraxidincoum-arin | Showed antihyper glycemic activity | Fort et al., 2000 |
| *Tinospora cordifolia* (Willd.) Miers ex Hook. f. Menispermaceae | Aqueous root extract | — | Significant reduction in blood glucose and brain liquids. Increase in body weight, total haemoglobin and hepatic hexokinase. Lowers hepatic glucose-6-phosphatase and serum acid phosphatase, alkaline phosphatase and lactate dehydrogenase in diabetic rats. | Stanely et al. 2000 |
| *Tinospora crispa* Menispermaceae | Extract | — | Significant anti-hyperglycemia, which is due to stimulation of insulin release via modulation of beta-cell $Ca^{2+}$ concentration. | Noor and Ashcroff, 1998 |
| *Xanthium strumarium* L. Asteraceae | — | Caffeic acid | Increase of glucose utilization by caffeic acid seems to be responsible for the lowering of plasma glucose. | Hsu et al., 2000 |
| *Zizypus jujuba* Lamk. Rhamnaceae | Leaf decoction | — | Plasma glucose levels decreased significantly in hyperglycemic rats | Erenmemisoglu, 1995 |

***Tinospora cordifolia* (Willd.) Miers ex Hook.f. (Gulonga) Menispermaceae**

Oral administration of an aqueous *T.cordifolia* root and leaf extracts 5.0 gm/kg to alloxan diabetic rats caused a significant reduction in blood glucose and brain lipids. The extract caused an increase in body weight, total haemoglobin and hepatic hexokinase. It lowers cholesterol, phospholipids, free fatty acids, hepatic glucose-6-phosphatase and serum acid phosphatase, alkaline phosphatase and lactate dehydrogenase in diabetic rats (Stanely et al., 2000; Prince and Menon, 1999; Stanley et al., 1999; Battacharya et al., 1997). Leaves of *T.cordifolia* have an insulin-like action and can significantly reduce the blood glucose in diabetic rabbits (Wadood et al., 1992).

***Syzygium cumini* (L.) Skeels. Myrtaceae**

Oral administration of 2.5 and 5.0 g/kg body weight of the aqueous extract of the seed for 6 weeks resulted in a significant reduction in blood glucose and an increase in total haemoglobin. It also prevented decrease in body weight and decreased free radical formation. The decrease in thiobarbituric acid reactive substances and increase in reduced glutathione, superoxide dismutase and catalase clearly shows the antioxidant property of the seed extract (Prince et al., 1998).

***Azadirachta indica* A. Juss. (Neem) Meliaceae**

*A.indica* leaf extract blocks significantly the inhibitory effect of serotonin on insulin secretion mediated by glucose and extract was found to have the most potent blood sugar lowering activity (Chattopadhyay, 1999 a, b). Leaf extract blocked the action of epinephrine which is responsible for reduction in pheripheral utilization of glucose and glucogenolytic effect (Chattopadhyay, 1996).

Information about the other plants is given in the Table 5. This review is limited to the years 1995 and 2001 because earlier information can be found in the review of Marles and Farnsworth (1995).

## REFERENCES

Abdel—Barry, J.A., I.A. Abdel-Hussain and M.H. Al-Hakiem. 1997. Hypoglycemic and antihyperglycemic effects of *Trigonella foenum-graecum* leaf in normal and alloxan induced diabetic rats. *J. Ethnopharmacol.* **58**: 149–155.

Agarwal, K.C. 1996. Therapeutic actions of garlic constituents. *Med. Res. Rev.* **16**: 111–124.

Ahmad, M., M.S. Akhtar, T. Malik and A.H. Gilani. 2000. Hypoglycemic action of the flavonoid fraction of *Cuminum nigrum* seeds. *Phytotherapy Research* **14**: 103–106.

Ahmad, N., M.R. Hussain and K.S. Bennoor. 1999. Effect of *Momordica charantia* extracts on fasting and postprandial serum glucose levels in NIDDM patients. *Bangladesh Med. Res. Counc. Bull.* **25**: 11–13.

Aiman, R. 1970. Recent research in indigenous antidiabetic medicinal plants: An overall assessement. *Indian J. Physiol. and Pharmcol.* **14**: 65–76.

Akhtar, M.S. 1982. Trial of *Momordica charantia* Linn. powder in patients with maturity—onset diabetes. *JPMA*, **32**: 106–107.

Aktar, M.S. and P. Aktar. 1999. Hypoglycemic effect of dried (Sukhchain) *Pongamia pinnata* flowers in normal volunteers and NIDDM Patients. *Hamdard Medicus.* **42**: 33–36.

Alarcon—Aguilar, F.J., M. Jimenz-Estrada, R. Reyes—Chilpa and R. Roman-Romor. 2000. Hypoglycemic effect of extracts and fraction from *Pascalium decompositium* in health and Alloxan-diabetic rats. *J. Ethnophancol.* **72**: 21–27.

Ali Hussain, H.E.M. and J.K. Mala rao. 2001. Preliminary studies on the hypoglycemic effect of *Abroma angusta* in Alloxan diabetic rats. *Indian J. Clinical Biochem.* **16**: 77–80.

Ali L. et al. 1993. Studies on hypoglycemic effects of fruit pulp, seed and whole plant of M*omordica charantia* on normal and diabetic model rats. *Plant Med.* **59**: 408–411.

Ali, L., A. Azad Khan, Z. Hassan, M. Mosihuzzaman, N. Nahar T. Nasreen, M. Nur-e-Alam and B. Rokeya. 1995. Characterization of the hypoglycemic efforts of *Trigonella foenum-graecum* seed. *Planta Med.* **61**: 358–360.

Augusti, K.T. et al., 1994. Effect of leucopelargonium derivative from *F. bengalensis* Linn. *Indian J. Med. Res.* **99**: 82–86.

Augusti, K.T. 1996. Therapeutic Values of onion (*Allium cepa* L.) and garlic (*Allium sativum* L.). *J. Ethnopharmacol.* **53**: 5–9.

Aslam, M., E.Y. Sezik and E. Yesilada. 2000. Anti-hyperglycemic effect of *Cannabis sativa* L. fruits. *J. Faculty of Pharmacy of Gazi University.* **17**: 89–93.

Baldwa, V.S., C.M. Bhandari, A. Pangaria and R.K. Goyal 1977. Clinical trial in Patients with Diabetes Mellitus of an insulin like compound obtained from a plant source. *Upsala J. Med. Sci.* **82**: 39–41.

Basnet, P., S. Kadota, M. Shimiju, Y. Takata, M. Kobayashi and T. Namba. 1995a. Bellidifolin stimulates glucose uptake in rat-1 fibroblasts and Ameliorates Hyperglycemia in STZ—induced Diabetic rats. *Planta Med.* **61**: 402–405.

Basnet, P., S. Kadota, M. Shimizer and T. Namba. 1995b. Bellidifolin: a potent hypoglycemic agent in STZ induced diabetic rats from *Swertia japonica. Phytochemistry* **39**: 997–999.

Benwahhoud, M., H. Jouad, M. Eddouks and B. Lyoussi. 2001. Hypoglycemic effect of *Suaeda fruticosa* in STZ induced diabetic rats. *J. Ethnopharmacol.* **76**: 35–38.

Bhandari, U. and J.N. Sharma. 1999. Effect of Petroleum ether extract of guar gum in STZ—induced hyperglycemic rats. *Pharmaceutical Biol.* **37**: 248–250.

Bhaskaran, K., B. Kizar Ahmath, K.R. Shanmugasundaram and E.R. Shanmugasundaram. 1990. Antidiabetic effect of a leaf extract from *Gymnema sylvestre* in non-insulin-dependent diabetes mellitus. *J. Ethnopharmacol* **30**: 295–305.

Bhattacharya, S.K., K.S. Satyan and A. Chakrabarthi. 1997. Effect of Trasina, an Ayurvedic herbal formation on pancreatic islet superoxide dismutase activity in hyperglycemic rats. *Indian J. Exp. Biol.* **35**: 297–299.

Bunyapraphatsara, N., S.V. Yongchiayaudha, and O. Chokechaijaroenporn 1996; Antidiabetic activity of *Aloe vera* L. Juice, 11. Clinical trial diabetes mellitus patients in combination with glibenclamide. *Phytomed.* **3**: 245–248.

Bwititi, P., C.T. Musabayane and C.F. Nhachi 2000 a. Effects of *Opuntia megacantha* on blood glucose and kidney function in STZ diabetic rats. *J. Ethnopharmacol.* **69**: 207–215.

Bwititi, P., C.T. Musabayane and C.F. Nhachi. 2000 b. Effects of *Opuntia megacantha* on blood glucose and kidney function in STZ diabetic rats. *J. Ethnopharmacol*; **69**: 247–252.

Chandra, V. and K. Aruna. 1997. Glycemic and Cholesterolaemic effect of sprouted fenugreek on diabetic subjects. *Ind. J. Nutr. Diet.* **34**: 246–251.

Chattopadhyay, R.R. 1993. Hypoglycemic effect of *Ocimum sanctum* leaf extract in normal and STZ diabetic rats. *Indian J. Exp. Biol.* **31**: 891–893.

Chattopadhyay, R.R. 1996. Possible mechanism of antihyperglycemic effect of *Azadirachta indica* leaf extract part IV. *Indian J. Exp. Biol.* **34**: 341–345

Chattopadhyay, R.R. 1999 a. A comparative evaluation of some blood sugar lowering agents of plant origin. *J. Ethnopharmacol.* **67**: 367–372.

Chattopadhyay, R.R. 1999 b. Possible mechanism of *Azadirachta indica* leaf extract: Part V. *J. Ethnopharmacol.* **67**; 373–376.

Das, A.V., P.S. Padayatti and C.S. Paulose. 1996. Effect of leaf extract of *Aegle marmelos* (L.) Correa ex Roxb. on histological and ultrastructural changes in tissues of STZ induced diabetic rats. *Indian J. Exp. Biol.* **34**: 341–345.

Das, S. 1999. Medical importance of *Portulaca pilosa* and its conservation. South East Asian Seminar on Herbs and Herbal Medicines Patna, P. **112**: 16–19. January.

Dasture, A.V. and P.H. Kulkarni. 1999. Therapeutic excellence of garlic (*Allium sativum*). *Deerghayu International.* **57**: 28–32.

Divakar, M.C. and M.B. Bensita. 1998. Screening of various leaf extracts of *Polyscias fruiticosa* Harms for their antidiabetic activity. *Indian J. Nat. Prod.* **14**: 24–28.

El-Badrawy, E.E.Y. 1999. Hypoglycemic effect of the glycan isolated from Guava fruit (*Psidium guajava*). *VDLUFA—Schriftenr* **52**: 203–206.

Erenmemisoglu, Aydin, Kelestimur, Fahirettin, A. Koker, Hulusi, Ustun, Huseyin Tekol, Yalcin, Ustadal and Muzaffer. 1995. Hypoglycemic effect of *Zizyphus jujuba* leaves. *J. Pharm. Pharmacol.* **47**: 72–74.

Ernst, E. 1977. Plants with hypoglacemic activity in humans. *Phytomed.* **4**: 73–78.

Erimone, C.O., J.M. Okonta and C.O. Ezugwu, 2001. Blood sugar lowering effect of *Anacardium occidentale* leaf extract in experimental rabbit model. *J. Natural Remedies*, **1**: 60–63.

Fetrow, C.W. and J.R, Avila, 1999. Professional's Handbook of complementary and Alternate medicine. Springhouse, PA: Springhouse Corporation.

Fort, D.M., K. Rao, S.D. Jolad, J. Luo, T.J. Carlson and S.R. King. 2000. Anti-hyperglycemic activity of *Teramnus labialis* (Fabaceae). *Phytomedicine* **6**: 465–467.

Fort, D.M., P. Ubillas Rosa, R. Mendez, J.L. Chen, T.T.H.C. Ianiro, C.B. Hasbun, C. Reimar, J. Luo, J.R. Michael, M. Iwu, T.J. Carlson, S.R. King, D.E. Bierer and R. Cooper. 2000 Novel Anti-hyperglycemic terpenoid quinines from *Pycranthus angulensis*. *J. Org. Chem.* **65**: 6534–6539.

Fukunaga, T., T. Miura, K. Furuta and A. Kato. 1997. Hypoglycemic effect of the rhizomes of *Smilax glabra* in normal and diabetic mice. *Biol Pharm Bull.* **20**: 44–46.

Geetha B.S., B.C. Mathew and K.T. Augusti. 1994. Hypoglycemic effect of leucodelphinidin derivative isolated from *Ficus bengalensis* L. *Indian J. Physio. Pharmacol.* **38**: 220–222.

Geetham, M. and A.K. Wahi. 2001. Antidiabetic activity of *Barleria prionitis* Linn. *J. Natural Remedies.* **1**: 64–66.

Ghannam, N., M. Kingston, I.A. Al-meshaal, M. Tariq, N.S. Parman and N. Woodhouse. 1986. The antidiabetic activity of aloes: Preliminary clinical and experimental observations. *Hormon Res.* **24**: 288–294.

Gomez, M.P.J. Bhaskar and Geetha. 1998. Antidiabetic effects of Fenugreek seed extract on anabas testudinens with special reference to carbohydrate metabolism. *J. Ecotoxicol. Environ Monit.* **8**: 103–106.

Gonalez–Mujica, F., N. Motta and Becerra. 1998. Inhibition of hepatic neoglucogenesis and glucose-6-phasphatase by aqueous extract of *Bauhinia megalandra* leaves. *Phytotherapy Research.* **12**: 291–293.

Goyal, D.K. and S.K. Tiwari. 1999. Study on *Vinca rosea* Linn. in Madhumeha. *J. Res. Ayurveda and Sidda*. **20**: 93–100.

Gray, A.M. and P.R. Fatt. 1997. Pancreatic and extra-Pancreatic effects of the traditional anti-diabetic plant, *Medicago sativa* (lucerne). *J. Nutr.* **127**: 1923–1928.

Gray, A.M. and P.R. Fatt. 1998. Antihyperglycemic action of *Eucalyptus globulus* are associated with pancreatic and extra-pancreatic effects in mice. *Journal Nutr.* **128**: 2319–2322.

Gray, A.M. and P.R. Fatt, 1999; Insulin—releasing and insulin-like activity of the traditional anti-diabetic plant *Coriandrum sativum*. *J. Ethnopharmacol.* **67**: 103–109.

Gupta, S.S. 1994. Prospects and perspectives of natural plant products in medicine. *Indian J. Pharmacol.* 26:1–12.

Haefele C. et al. 1997. Characterization of a dioxygenase from *Trigonella foenum-graecum* involved in 4-hydroxyisoleucine biosyntheses. *Phytochem.* **44**: 563–566.

Hauda, S., A.S. Chawla and Maninder. 1989. Hypoglycemic plants: A review. *Fitoterapia*. **60**: 195.

Hasagawa, H., S. Matsumiya, C. Murakami, T. Kurokawa, R. Kaasi, S. Ishibashi and K. Yamazaki. 1994. Interactions of ginseng extract, ginseng separated fractions, and some triterpenoid saponins with glucose trasporters in sheep erythrocytes. *Planta Med.*, **60**: 153–157.

Higashino, H., A. Suzuki and K. Pootakham. 1992. Hypoglycemic effects of *Momordica chanantia* and *Phyllanthus niruri* extracts in STZ induced rats. *Nippon yakurigaku zasshi*, **100**: 415–421.

Hosseinzadeh, H. and A. Sadheghi. 1999. Antihyperglycemic effects of *Morus nigra* and *Morus alba* in mice. *Pharm. Pharmacol.* **9**: 63–65.

Hsu, F.L., Y.C. Chen and J.T. Cheng. 2000. Caffeic acid as active principle from the fruit X*anthium strumarium* to lower plasma glucose levels in diabetic rats. *Planta Medica*. **66**: 228–230.

Ichiki, Hroydki, Miura, Toshihiro, Kubo, Masayoshi, Ishihara, Eriko, Komatsu, Yashuhiro, Tanigawa, Keiichiro, Okada and Minoru. 1998. *Bio. Pharm. Bull.* **21**: 1389–1390.

Ivorra, M.D., M. Paya and A. Villar. 1989. A review of natural products and plants as potential antidiabetic drugs. *J. Ethanopharmacol.* **27**: 243

Jankoski, A., J. Niedworok and B. Jankoshi. 1999. The influence of *Aronica melanocarpa* Elliot of experimental diabetes in the rats. *Herba polonica*, **45**: 345–353.

Kako, M., T. Miura, Y. Nishiyama, M. Ichimaru, M. Moriyasu and A. Kato. 1997. Hypoglycemic activity of some triterponeoid glucoside. *J. Nat Prod.* **60**: 604–605.

Kako, M., T. Miura, Y. Nishiyama, M. Ichimaru, M. Moriyasu and A. Kato. 1996. Hypoglycemic effect of the rhizomes of *Polygala senegal* in normal and diabetic mice and its main component, the triterpenoid glycoside senegin-II. *Planta Med.* **62**: 440–443.

Kakuda, T., I. Sakane, T. Takihara, Y. Ozaki, H. Takeuchi and M. Kuroyanagi. 1996. Hypoglycemic effect of extracts from *L. speciosa* leaves in diabetic KK-AY mice. *Biosci Biote Bioche*. **60**: 204–208.

Kalpana,P. and K. Srinivas. 1997. Plant foods in the management of diabetes mellitus. Vegetables as potential hypoglycemic agents. *Nahrug*. **41**: 68–74.

Kamble, S.M., G.S. Jyotishi, P.L. Kamalakar and S.M. Vaidya. 1996. Efficacy of *Coccinia indica* W & A in diabetes mellitus. *J. Res. Ayurveda and sidda*. **17**: 77–84.

Kameswara Rao, B., M.M. Kesavulu, R. Giri and C. Appa Rao. 1999. Antidiabetic and hypolipidemic effect of *Momordica cymbalaria* Hook. Fruit powder in alloxan-diabetic rats. *J. Ethnopharmacol* **67**: 103–109.

Kanegusuku, M., J.C. Benassi, R.C. Pedrosa, R.A. Yunes. V.C. Filho, A.A. Maia, M.M. De-Souza, F. Delle Monache and R. Niero. 2002. Cyto-toxic, hypoglycemic activity and phytochemical analysis of *Rubus imperialis* (Rosaceae) *Z. Naturforsch,* **57**: 272–276.

Kanth, V.R., and P.V. Diwan. 19... Analgesic, anti inflammatory and hypoglycemic activities of *Sida cordifolia. Am. J. Clin Nutr.* **69**: 647–655.

Kapoor, L.D. 1990. Handbook of Ayurvedic Medicinal plants. CRC press Inc.

Karunanayake, E.H. et al. 1990. Effect of *Momordica charantia* fruit juice on streptozotocin—induced diabetes in rats. *J. Ethnopharmacol* **30**: 199–204.

Khan, R.A. 1998. A Study of Karela *Momordica charantia* on blood glucose. *Hamdard medicus* **42**: 56–61.

Khanna, P. and S.C. Jain. 1981; Hypoglycemic activity of polypeptide-P from a plant source. *J. Nat. Prod.* **44**: 648–655.

Khare, A.K., R.N. Tondon and J.P. Tewari 1983. Hypoglycemic activity of an indigenons drug *Gymnema sylvestre* in normal and diabetic persons. *Ind. J. Physiol. Pharmac,* 257–258.

Khosla P, et al. 1995. Effect of *Trigonella foenum-graecum* (fenugreek) on blood glucose in normal and diabetic rats. *Indian J Physiol Pharmacol.* **39**: 173–174.

Korec, R., K. Heiny Sensch and T. Zoukas. 2000. Effects of the neoflavanoid countareagenin, one of the antidiabetic active substances of *Hintonia latiflora,* on STZ—induced diabetes mellitus in rats. *J. Nutr.* **130**: 164–170.

Kumar. A, B. Bhasin, V.K. Kulshrestha, S.R. Arora, and D.N. Prasad. 1979. Comparative study of anti-atherosclerotic activity of *Allium cepa* and *Allium sativam* and *Commiphora mukul* in rats and rabbits. *Indian J. Pharmacol* **11**: 61.

Kumar, G., P.S. Sudheesh, B. Ushakumari, A.K. Valsa and S. Vijayalakshmi, 1997. A comparative study on the hypolipidemic activity of eleven different pectins. *J. Food Sci Technol.* **34**: 103–107.

Kumar, R.V. et al. 1994. Insulin sparing action of a leucocyanidin derivative isolated from *Ficus bengalensis* Linn. *Indian J. Biochem. Biophys.* **31**: 73–76.

Liu, I.M., T.C. Chi, F.L. Hsu, C.F. Chen and J.T. Cheng. 1999. Isoferulic acid as a active principle from the Rhizome of *Cimicifuga dahurica* to lower plasma glucose in diabetic rats. *Planta Medica.* **65**: 712–714.

Luo, J., et al. 1998 a. *Cryptolepis sanguinolenta*: an ethnobotanical approach to drug discovery and the isolation of a potentially useful new-antihyperglycemic agent. *Diabet Med.* **15**: 367–374.

Luo, J., et al. 1998 b. Masoprocal (nordihydro guaiaretic acid): a new antihyperglycemic agent isolated from the creosote bush (*Larrea tridentata*). *J. Dairy Sci.* **81**: 1608–1618.

Madar, Z., R. Abel, S. Samish and J. Arad. 1988. Glucose lowering effect of Fenugreek in non-insulin dependent diabetics. *Eur J Clin Nutr.* **42**: 51–54.

Manickam, M., M. Ramanathan, M.A. Jahromi, J.P. Chansouria and A.B. Ray. 1997. Antihyperglycemic activity of phenolics from *Pterocarpus marsupium. Pharmazic.* **52**: 645–646.

Marles, R.J. and N.R. Farnsworth. 1995. Antidiabatic Plants and their active constituents. *Phytomedicine* **2**: 137–189.

Matsuda, H., T. Murakami, K. Yashiro, J. Yamahara and M. Hoshikawa, 2000. Antidiabetic principles of natural medicines IV. Aldose reductase and alpha-glucosidase inhibitors, from the roots of *Salacina oblonga* Wall. (Celastraceac): Structure of a new friendelane-type triterpene, Kotalagenin 16-acetate. *Eur J. Clin Nutr.* **54**: 380–385.

Miura, T., and A. Kato. 1995. The difference in hypoglycemic action between *Polygonati sibricum* rhizome and *P. officinalis* rhizome. *Biol. Pharm. Bull.* **18**: 1605–1606.

Miyaji, N., M. Kazama, H. Ina, K. Yamada and T. Yamakawa. 1999; Influence of Banabakuwa extracted powder on plasma glucose level in rats. *J. Traditional Medi.* **16**: 208–211.

Mori et al. 2001. Effect of *Insulina* leaf extract on development of diabetes. Comparison between Normal, STZ—induced diabetic rats and Heriditory diabetic mice. Nipponsiyo, showkuryo. *Gakkaishu*, **64**: 197–203.

Mukhrjee P.K., K. Saha, M. Pal and B.P. Saha, 1997. Effect of *Nelumbo nucifera* rhizome extract on blood sugar level in rats. *Planta Med.* **63**: 558–560.

Murakami, C., K. Myoga, R. Kasai, K. Ohtani, T. Kurokawa, S. Ishibashi, F. Dayrit, W.G. Padolina and K. Yamasaki. 1993. *Chem.. Pharma. Bull.* **41**: 2129–2131.

Murakami, N., T. Murakami, M. Kadoya, H. Matsuda, J. Yamahara and M. Yoshikawa. 1996. New hypoglycemic constituents in gymnemic acid from *Gymnema sylvestre. Biol Pharm Bull.* **19**: 364–366.

Murali, B., U.M. Upadhaya and R.K. Goyal. 2002. Effect of chronic treatment with *Enicostemma littorale* in NIDDM rats. *J. Ethnopharmacol.* **81**: 199–204.

Musabayane, C.T. 2000. Effect of *Opuntia megacantha* on blood glucose and kidney function in STZ diabetic rats. *J. Ethnopharmacol.* **69**: 247–252.

Ng, T.B., C.M.Wong, W.W.Li and H.W.Yeung. 1986. Insulin-like molecules in *Momordica charantia* seeds. *J. Ethnopharmacol*, **15**: 107–117.

Nicola W.G., K.M. Ibrahim, T.H. Mikhail, R.B. Girgis and M.E. Khadr. 1996. Role of the hypoglycemic plant extract *Cleome droserifolia* in improving glucose and lipid metabolism and its relation to insulin resistance in fatty liver. *Biol Pharm Bull.* **20**: 44–46.

Nonila, R., R. Gross and H. Rchid. 2000. Insulino tropic effect of *Citrullus colocynthis* fruit extracts. *Planta Medica* **66**: 418–423.

Noor, H. and S.J.K. Aschroff. 1998. Pharmaceutical characterisation of the antihyperglycemic properties of *Tinospora crispa* extract. *J. Ethnopharmacol.* **62**: 7–13.

Ohinishi, Y., S. Takagi, T. Miura, M. Usami, M. Kako and E. Ishara. 1996. Effect of ginsing radix on GLUT2 protein content in mouse liver in normal and epinephrine-induced hyperglycemic mice. *Biol. Pharm. Bull.*, **19**: 1238–1240.

Okyar, A., A. Can, N. Akev and G. Baktir. 2001. Effect of *Aloe vera* leaves on blood glucose level in Type-I & Type-II diabetic rat models. *Phytotherapy Research.* **15**: 157–161.

Pari, L. and J. Umamaheswari, 2000. Antihyperglycemic activity of *Musa sapientum* flowers: effect on lipid perioxidation on Alloxan diabetic rats. *Phytotherapy Research*, **14**: 136–138.

Pepato, M.T., E.H. Keller, A.M. Baviera, I.C. Kettelhut, R.C. Vendramini and I.L. Brunethi. 2002. Antidiabetic activity of *Bauhinia forticata* decoction in STZ diabetic rats. *J. Ethnopharmacol.* **81**: 191–197.

Perez. R.M., C. Perez, M.A. Zavala, S. Perez, H. Hernandez and F. Lagunes. 2000. Hypoglycemic effect of Lactucin-8-0-methylacrylate of *Parmentiera edulis* fruit. *J. Ethnopharmacol.* **71**: 391–394.

Pery, R.M., C. Perz and M.A. Zavala. 2000. Hypoglycemic effect of lactucin-8-0-methyl acrylate of *Parmentiara edulis* fruit. *J. Ethnopharmacol.* **71**: 391–394.

Peungvicha, P., R. Temsiririskkul, J.K. Prasain, Y. Tezuka, S. Kodota, S.S. Thirawarapan and H. Watanabe. 1998. 4-hydroxybenzoic acid: a hypoglycemic constituent of aqueous extract of *Pandanus odorus* root. *J. Ethnopharmacol.* **62**: 79–84.

Prashanth, D., R. Padmaja and D.S. Samjulla. 2001. Effect of certain plant extracts on α-amylase activity. *Fitoterapia* **72**: 179–181.

Preuss, H.G., S.T. Jarrell, R. Scheckenbach, S. Lieberman and R.A. Anderson, 1998. Comparative effects of chromium, vanadium and *Gymnema sylvestre* on sugar induced blood pressure elevation in SHR: *J. Am Coll Nuts.* **17**: 116–123.

Prince, P.S., V.P. Menon and L. Pari. 1998. Hypoglycemic activity of *Syzigium cumini* seeds: effect on lipid peroxidation in alloxan diabetic rats. *J. Ethnopharmocal* **61**: 1–7.

Prince, P.S. and V.P. Menon 1999. Antioxidant activity of *Tinospora cordifolia* roots in experimental diabetes. *J. Ethnopharmacol.* **65**: 277–281.

Puri, D and N. Baral. 1998. Hypoglycemic effect of *Biophytum sensitivum* in the alloxan diabetic rabbits. *Indian J. Physiol. Pharma.* **42**: 401–406.

Puri, D., K.M. Prabhu and P.S. Murthy, 1994. Hypocholesterolemic effect of the hypoglycemic principle of fenugreek seeds. *Indian J. Clin. Biochem.* **9**: 13–16.

Rao, B.K., R. Giri, M.M. Kesavulu and C. Appa Rao. 2001. Effect of oral administration of bark extracts of *Pterocarpus santalinus* L on blood glucose level in experimental animals. *J. Ethropharmacol.* **74**: 69–74.

Ravikanth, V. and P.V. Diwan. 1999. Analgesic anti inflammatory and hypoglycemic activity of *Sida cordifolia. Phytotherapy Research.* **13**: 75–77.

Sachdewa, A., D. Raina, A.K. Srivatsava and L.D. Khemani. 2001. Effect of *Aegle marmelos* and *Hibiscus rosa-sinensis* leaf extract on glucose tolerance in glucose induced Hyperglycemic rats. *J. Env. Biol.* **22**: 53–57.

Sauvaire, Y. et al. 1998. 4-hydroxyisoleucine: a novel amino acid potentiator of insulin secretion. *J. Nat Prod.* **61**: 397–400.

Sarkar, S., M. Pranava and R. Marita. 1996. Demonstration of the hypoglycemic action of *Momordica charantia* in a validated animal model of diabetes. *Pharmacol Res.* **33**: 1–4.

Saxena, K.K., B. Gupta, V.K. Kulshrestha, R.K. Shrivastava and D.N. Prasad, 1980. Effect of garlic pretreatment on isoprenaline induced myocardial necrosis in albino rats. *Indian J. Physoil and Pharmacol* **24**: 233.

Seetharam, Y.N., G. Chalageri, S.R. Setty and Bheemachar. 2002. Hypoglycemic activity of *Abutilon indicum* leaf extracts in rats. *Fitoterapia* **73**: 156–159.

Shanmugasundaram E.R., C. Paneerselvam, P. Samudram, and K.R. Shanmugasundaram, 1983. Enzyme changes and glucose utilization in diabetic rabbits: the effect of *Gymnema sylvestre* R. Br. *J. Ethnopharmacol.* **7**: 205–234.

Shanmugasundaram E.R., K.L. Gopinath, K.R. Shanmugasundaram, and V.M. Rajendran 1990a. Possible regeneration of the islets of Langerhans in streptozotocin—diabetic rats given *Gymmema sylvestre* leaf extracts. *J. Ethnopharma.* **30**: 265–279.

Shanmugasundaram, E.R., G. Rajeswari, K. Baskaran, B.R. Rajesh, K.R. Shanmugasundaram and B. Kizar Ahmath. 1990b. Use of *Gymnema sylvestre* leaf extract in the control of blood glucose in insulin dependent diabetes mellitus *J. Elthnopharma.* **30**: 281–294.

Sharma K.K., et al. 1977. Antihyperglycemic effect on onion: effect on fasting blood sugar and induced hyperglycemia in man. *Ind. J. Med Res.* **35**: 422–429.

Sharma R.D.. 1986. Effect of fenugreek seeds and leaves an blood glucose and serum insulin responses in human subjects. *Nutr Res* **6**: 1353–1364.

Sharma, R.D., A. Sarkar, D.K. Hazra, B. Mishra, J.B. Singh, S.K. Sharma, B.B. Maheswari and D.M. Maheswari. 1996. Use of fenugreek seed powder in the management of non-insulin dependent diabetes mellitus. *Nutr. Res.* **16**: 1131–1339.

Sharma, R.D., T.C. Raghuram and N.S. Rao. 1990. Effect of fenugreek seeds on blood glucose and serum lipids in type-I diabetes. *Eur J. Clin. Nutr.* **44**: 301–306.

Sharma, S.R., S.K. Dwivedi and D. Swarup. 1997. Hypoglycemic, antihyperglycemic and hypolipidemic activities of *Caesalpinia bonducella* seeds in rats. *Diabetes Care*, **20**: 1774–1780.

Sheela C.G., and K.T. Augusti, 1992. Antidiabetic effects of S–allyl cysteine sulphoxide isolated form *Allium sativum* Linn. *Ind. J. Exper. Biol.* **30**: 523–526.

Sheela, C.G., K. Kumud and K.T. Angusti. 1995. Anti-diabetic effects of onion and garlic sulfoxide amino acids in rats. *Planta Med.* **61**: 356–357.

Shimuzu K., A. Lino, J. Nakajima, K. Tanaka, S. Nakajyo, N. Urakawa, M. Atschi, T. Wada, and C. Yamashita. 1997. Suppression of glucose absorption by some fractions extracted from *Gymnema sylvestre* leaves. *J. Vet. Med. Sci.*; **59**: 245–251.

Shukla, R., S.B. Sharma, D. Puri and P.S. Murthy. 2000. Indegenous drug for diabetes mellitus. *J.K. Science*. **2**: 128–131.

Skin, F., A. Kuaya, J.T. Jaouhari, H.B. Lazrek, M. Jana and H.E. Amri. 1999. Hypoglycemic activity of *Globularia alypum* leaves in rats. *Fitoterpia* **70**: 382–389.

Sotaniemi, E.A., E. Haapakoski and A. Rautio. 1995. Ginseng therapy in NIDDM patients. *Diabetes Care*. **18**: 1373–1375.

Srivastava, Y. et al. 1988. Effect of *Momordica charantia* Linn. Pomous aqueous extract on cataractogenesis in murine alloxan diabetics. *Pharmacy Res. Comm.* **20**: 201–209.

Srivastava, Y., H. Venkata Krishna-Batt, Y. Verma and K. Venkaiah. 1993. Antidiabetic and adaptogenic properties of *Momordica charantia* extract: an experimental and clinical evaluation. *Phytotherapy Res.* **7**: 285–289.

Srividya, N. and S. Periwal. 1995. Diuretic, hypotensive and hypoglycemic effect of *Phyllanthus amarus*. *Indian J. Exp. Biol.* **33**: 861–864.

Stanely. M., P. Prince, V.P. Menon and G. Gunasekharan 1999. Hypolipidemic action of *Tinospora cordifolia* roots in alloxan diabetic rats. *J. Ethnopharmacol.* **64**: 53–57.

Stanely, M., P. Prince and V.P. Menon 2000. Hypoglycemic and other related actions of *Tinospora cordifolia* roots in alloaxan-induced diabetic rats. *J. Ethnopharmacol,* **70**: 9–15.

Sui. D.Y., Z.Z. Lu, S.H. Li and Y. Cai. 1994. Hypoglycemic effect of saponin isolated from leaves of *Acanthopanax senticosus*. *Chung Kuo Chung Tsa Chih.* **19**: 638–685.

Suzuki, Y., K. Yuko, K. Hayashi, M. Kaguhiko, Iwao, T. Kakuda and Takumi. 2001. Effect and mode of action of banaba (*L. speciosa*) leaf extract on postprandial blood glucose in rats. *Gakkaishi.* **54**: 131–137.

Suzuki, Y., T. Unno, M. Ushitani, K. Hayashi and T. Kakuda. 1999. Antiobesity activity of extracts from *Lagerstroemia speciosa* L. leaves on female KK—Ay mice. *J Nutr Sci Vita.* **45**: 791–795.

Tennekoon, K.H., S. Jeevathayaparan, P. Angunawala, E.H. Karunanayake and K.S. Jayasinghe. 1994. Effect of *Momordica charantia* on key hepatic enzymes. *Br. J. Nutr.* **72**: 731–743.

Tim Kaczmar. 1998. Herbal support for diabetes management. *Clinical nutrition insights* **6**: 1–4.

Trovato, A., A.M. Forestieri, L. Lank, R. Burbera, M.T. Monforte and E.M. Galiti. 1994. Hypoglycemic activity of different extracts of *Olea europaea* L in rats. *Planta Med. Phytother.* **26**: 300–308.

Ubillas, R.P., Mendez, D. Christopher, S.D. Joland, L.J. King, R. Steven, T.J. Carlson and D.M. Fort. 2000. Antihyperglycemic Furanosesquiterpens from *Commiphora myrrha* **92**: 75–93.

Vaishnava, M.M., A.K. Tripati and K.R. Gupta. 1993. Constituents of *Cassia fistula* roots. *Fitoterapia.* **64**: 93.

Vogler, B.K. and E. Ernst. 1999. *Aloe vera*: A systematic review of its clinical effectiveness. *Br. J. Gen. Proc.* **49**: 823–828.

Vogler, B.K., M.H. Pittler and E. Ernst. 1999. The efficacy of ginseng. A systematic review of randomised clinical trials. *Eur J Clin Pharmacol.* **55**: 567–575.

Vuskan, V., J.L. Sievenpiper, V.Y.Y. Koo, T. Francis, U. Belijan-Zdrakovic, Z. Xu and E. Vidgen. 2000. American ginseng (*Panax quinquefolius* L) reduces postprandial glycemia in non-diabetic subjects with type 2 diabetes mellitus. *Arch Int Med.* **160**: 1009–1013.

Wadood, N., A. Wadood and S.A. Shah, 1992. Effect of *Tinospora cordifolia* on blood glucose and total lipid levels of normal and alloxan-diabetic rabbits. *Planta Med.* **58**: 131–136.

Wang, H.X., and T.B. Ng. 1999. Natural products with hypoglycemic, hypotensive, hypocholesterolemic, antiatherosclerotic and antithrombotic activities. *Life Sci.* **65**: 2663–2677.

Welihinda, J., et al. 1982. The insulin—releasing activity of the tropical plant *Momordica charantia. Acta Biol. Med. Germ.* **41**: 1229–1240.

Welihinda, J., E.H. Karunanayake, M.H.R. Sheriff and K.S.A. Jayasinghe. 1986. Effect of *Momordica charantia* on the glucose tolerance in maturity onset diabetes. *J. Ethanopharmacol.* **17**: 277–282.

Yadav, P., S. Sankar and D. Bhatnagar, 1997a. Action of *Capparis decidua* against alloxan—induced oxidative stress and diabetes in rat tissue. *Pharmacol Res.* **36**: 221–228.

Yadav, P., S. Sankar and D. Bhatnagar. 1997b. Lipid peroxidation and antioxidant enzymes in erythrocytes and tissues in aged diabetic rats. *Indian J Exp. Biol.* **35**: 295–296.

Yamini, B. Tripathi and Padmaja Chaturvedi. 1995. Assessment of endocrine response of *Inula racemosa* in relation to glucose homeostasis in rats. *Indian J. Exp. Biol.* **33**: 686–689.

Yogendra Mishra, M.S.Y. Khan, R. Zafar and S.S. Agarwal. 1990. Pharmacological and phytochemical studies on *Lagerstroemia speciosa* L. *Indian J. Pharma. Sci.* **52**: 58.

Yongchiayudha. S., V. Rungpitarangsi, N. Bunyapraphatsara and O. Chokechaijaroenporn, 1996. Antidiabetic activity of *Aloe vera* L. Juice I, clinical trial in new cases of diabetes mellitus. *Phytomed.* **3**: 241–243.

Yoshikawa, M., T. Murakami, E. Harada, N. Murakami, J. Yamahara and H. Matsuda. 1996. Bioactive saponins and glycosides VII, on the hypoglycemic Principles from the root cortex of *Aralia elata* Seem: Structure related hypoglycemic activity of oleanolic acid oligoglycoside. *Planta Med.* **62**: 440–443.

Yoshikawa, M., T. Murakami, M. Kadoya, H. Matsuda, O. Muraoka, J. Yamahara and N. Murakami. 1996. Medicinal foodstuff. III. Sugarbeet. (1): Hypoglycemic oleanolic acid oligoglycosides, betavulgarosides I, II, III and IV from the root *Beta vulgaris* L. chenopodiaceae. *Br. J. Nutr.* **76**: 63–73.

Yoshikawa, M., T. Murakami, T. Veno, M. Kadoya, H. Matsuda, J. Yamahara and N. Murakami. 1996. Bioactive saponins and glycosides I. Senegae radix (1): E-senegasaponins a and b and z—senega saponins a and b, their inhibitory effect on alcohol absorption and hypoglycemic activity. *J. Ethnopharmacol.* **50**: 13–17.

Yoshikawa, M., T. Murakami, K. Yashiro and H Matsuda Kotalanol. 1998. A potent alpha—glucosidase inhibitor with thiosugar sulfonium sulfate structure from antidiabetic ayurvedic medicine *Salacia reticulata. Indian J. Physiol Pharmacol.* **42**: 401–406.

Yoshikawa, M., H. Shimada, N. Nishida, Y.L, I. Toguchida, J. Yamahara and H. Matsuda. 1998. Antidiabetic principles of natural medicines II. Aldose reductase and alpha—glucosidase inhibitors from Brazilian natural medicine, the leaves of *Myrica multiflora* DC. Structures of myricacitrins I and II and myricaphenones A and B. *Biosci Biotechnol Biochem.* **62**: 28–33.

Yuan, C.S., J.A. Wu, T. Lowell and M. Gu. 1998. Gut and brain effects of American ginseng root on brainstem neuronal activities in rats. *Am. J. Chin. Med.* **26**: 47–55.

Zia, T., S.N. Hasnain and S.K. Hasan. 2001. Evaluation of the oral hypoglycemic effect of *Trigonella foenum-graecum* L. (methi) in normal mice. *J. Ethnopharmacol.* **75**: 191–195.

CHAPTER 6

# ANTIDIABETIC PLANTS IN INDIA

## ABBREVIATIONS USED IN THE TEXT

Ass: Assamese
Ben: Bengali
Guj: Gujarathi
Hin: Hindi
Kan: Kannada
Mal: Malayalam
Mar: Marathi
Ori: Oriya
Pun: Punjabi
Tam: Tamil
Tel: Telugu

* * *

**Abelmoschus esculentus** (L.) Moench

Syn: *Hibiscus esculentus* L.

Family: Malvaceae

Annual erect herb, up to 2m tall, covered with hairs. Leaves alternate, cordate, palmately lobed, coarsely toothed, scabrous. Flowers yellow with a crimson centre. Fruit capsule, 6–8-ribbed, seeds many.

Cultivated throughout India.

Sanskrit: Bhenda

Local names: *Ben*: Dhoras; *Guj*: Binda, *Hin*: Bhindi, Bhindi-Tori, *Kan*: Bendekayi; *Mal*: Venta; *Mar*: Bhendi; *Tam*: Ventai; *Tel*: Bendakaya.

Trade name: Lady's finger.

Propagation: by seeds

Uses: Fresh seedless tender fruits 2, are given twice daily as a specific medicine to cure diabetes.

**Abelmoschus manihot** (L.) Medikus

Syn: *Hibiscus manihot* L.
*Hibiscus pungens* Roxb.

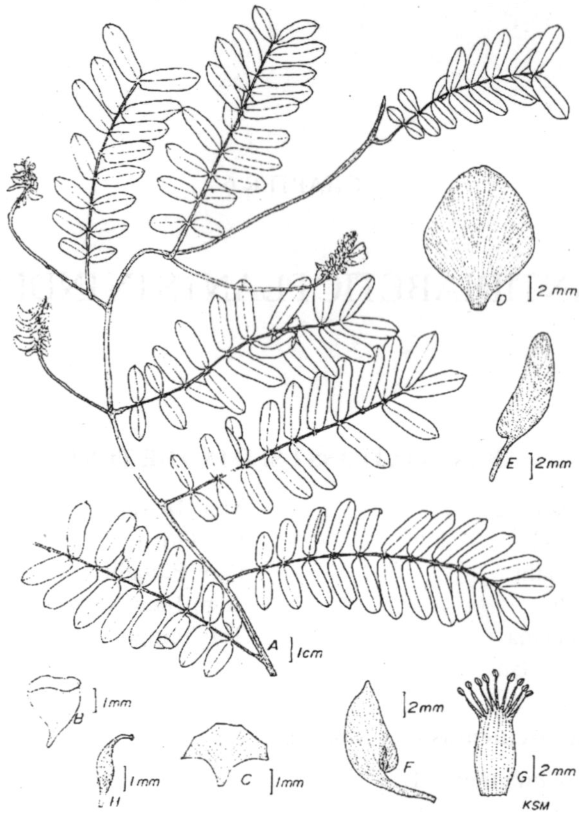


Fig. 1: *Abrus precatorius* L.
A. Twig; B. Calyx; C. Calyx split open; D. Standard petal; E. Wing petal; F. Keel petal; G. Staminal column; H. Pistil.

Family: Malvaceae.

Perennial, simple or sparingly branched, strigose and weakly prickly undershrubs, up to 3m tall. Leaves broadly ovate. Flowers yellow with a deep purple or chocolate base within, in terminal racemes. Fruit capsule, ovoid-oblong.

Rare in Andhra Pradesh, Assam, West Bengal, Nagaland, Manipur, Tripura and Orissa.

Fl.& Fr.: Aug–Jan.

Local names: *Ass*: Usipag; *Guj*: Kantalo bhindo; *Mar*: Jangali bhendi, ranbhendo.

Propagation: by seeds.

Uses: The mucilage has hypoglycemic activity. The viscous substance Abelmosan A, B and C are isolated from the roots. These substances are useful as antidiabetic and for prevention of liver failure.

**Abrus precatorius** L.

Syn: *Glycine abrus* L.

Family: Fabaceae (Papilionaceae)

An annual woody twiner. Leaves even pinnate, leaflets 7–12 pairs, oblong. Flowers rose to pink in axillary racemes, Fruit pod, oblong, pubescent, 5–10-seeded, seeds subglobose; blood red with a black lateral blotch around the hilum. Varieties with different coloured seeds-i.e., pure white seeds, pure red seeds and all black seeds also occur.

Common all over India on hedges and bushes.

Sanskrit: Gunja.

Local names: *Ben*: Chun-hali, Kundi; *Guj*: Chanothi; *Kan*: Ganji, Gulganju, Guluganji, Madhuka; *Mal*: Kunni, Kunnikuru; *Mar*: Chanoti, Gunchi, Gunja; *Tam*: Gundumani; Kuntumani; *Ori*: Gunja, Runj; *Tel*: Gurivinda, Gurivinja, Guruginja.

English: Wild Liquorice

Trade name: Indian Liquorice, Rosary Pea.

Propagation: Through seeds.

Uses: Used for treatment of Diabetes (Marles and Farnsworth, 1995). Aqueous extract of leaves lowers the glucose level.

**Abutilon indicum** (L.) Sweet

Syn: *Sida indica* L.

Family: Malvaceae

Perennial, woody, densely tomentose undershrub, up to 1m tall. Leaves broadly ovate-orbicular, deeply cordate, pubescent. Flowers orange yellow, axillary, solitary. Fruit schizocarp, depressed-globose, tomentose. Seeds black, tubercled.

Common in hedges and wastelands all over India.

Sanskrit: Atibala.

Local names: *Ben*: Jhampi, Petari; *Guj*: Dabali, Khapat; *Hin*: Jhampi, Kanghi, Khangani; *Kan*: Srimudrigida; *Mal*: Jhonkaped, Uram; *Mar*: Chakrabhenda, Kangori, Mudra, *Ori*: Nakochono; *Tam*: Perum tutti, Ponnai thutti, Thuttli; *Tel*: Thuthurubenda, Papidlakaya, Kammalaku.

Trade name: Country mallow.

Propagation: Through seeds.

Uses: The plant possess antidiabetic properties (Setha Ram et al., 2002).

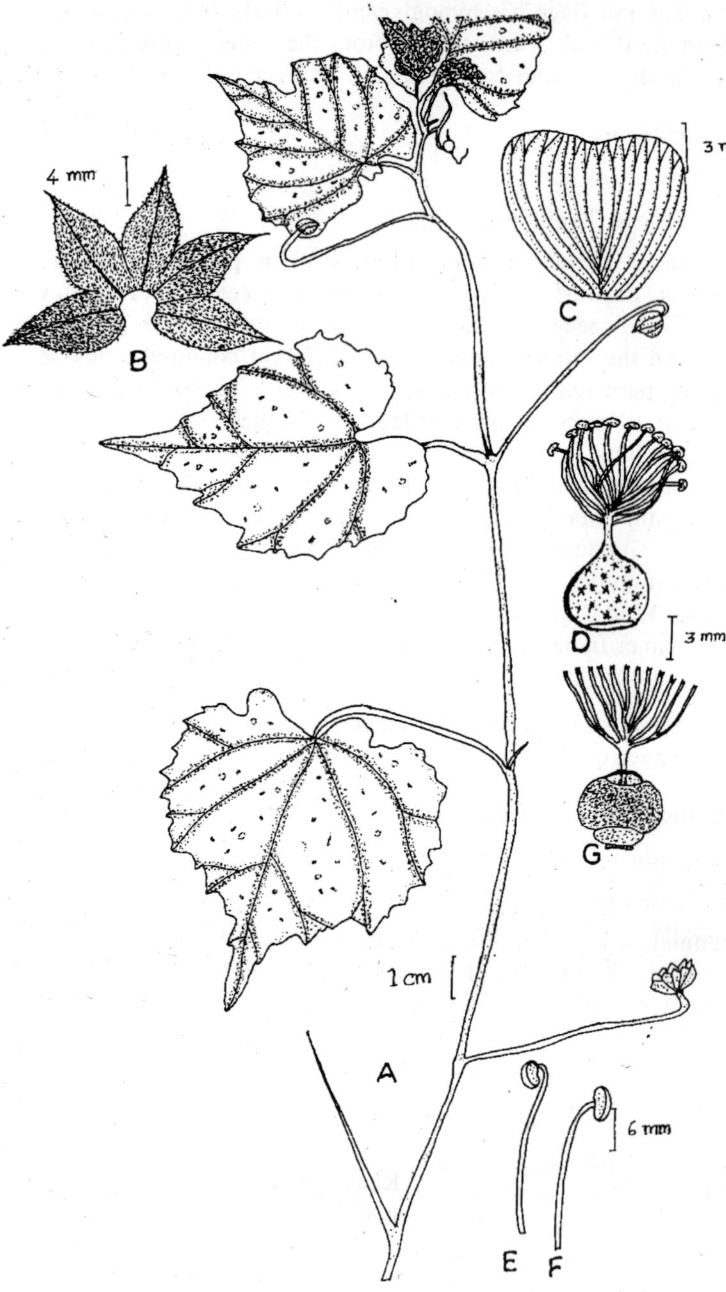


Fig. 2: *Abutilon indicum* (L.) Sw.
A. Twig; B. Calyx split open; C. Petal; D. Staminal column; E & F. Stamens; G. Pistil.

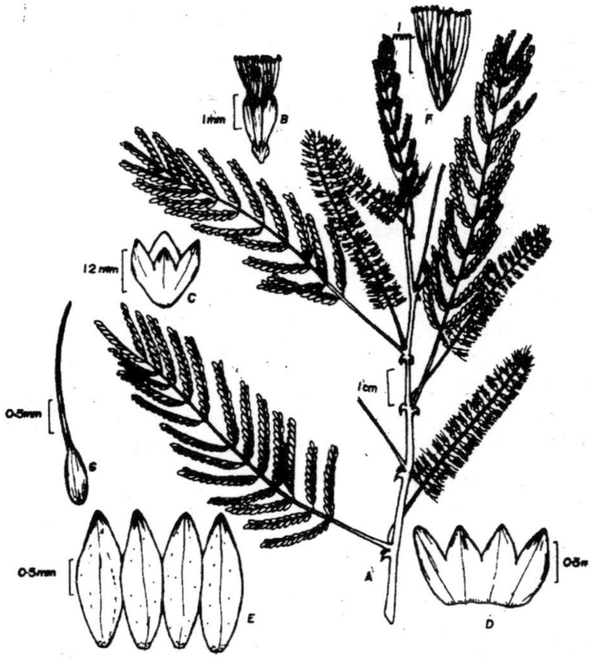


Fig. 3: *Acacia catechu* (L.f.) Willd.
A. Twig; B. Flower; C. Calyx entire; D. Calyx split open; E. Corolla split open; F. Staminal column; G. Pistil.

**Acacia catechu** (L.f.) Willd.

Syn: *Mimosa catechu* L.f.

Family: Leguminosae (Fabaceae).

Shrub like armed trees, 4–5m tall, young branchlets dark brown to purple, 2 curved stipular spines. Leaves 2-pinnate, pinnae 10–15 pairs, leaflets 20–40 pairs, elliptic-oblong. Flowers light greenish-yellow in axillary spikes. Pod flat, thin, straight, glabrous, dark-brown, shining, seeds 4–10, greyish brown, shining.

Occasional in dry deciduous forests in South India, Assam, Bihar, Delhi, Orissa, Rajasthan and West Bengal.

Sanskrit: Khadira.

Local names: *Ass*: Khoria; *Ben*: Khayar; *Guj*: Kherio-baval; *Hin*: Khair, Khaira; *Mal*: Karinnali; *Mar*: Kankachu; *Ori*: Khoiru; *Pun*: Khair; *Tam*: Othalei, Kasukkati, Karunkali; *Tel*: Nalla sandra, Kachu.

Trade name: Cutch tree, Black Catechu, Pegu Catechu.

Fl. & Fr.: August–November

Uses: Bark and heart wood used in the treatment of Diabetes.

**Acacia ferruginea** DC.

Family: Mimosaceae

Deciduous tree, up to 10m tall, armed with prickles. Leaves pinnate, pinnae 6–8, leaflets 15–25 pairs, oblong. Flowers creamy-white in axillary spikes. Fruit pod, seeds 3–6.

Fl. & Fr.: February–June.

Peninsular India, Delhi, Rajasthan, West Begal.

Uses: Stem bark useful in the treatment of diabetes.

**Acacia melanoxylon** R. Br.

Family: Mimosaceae

Large evergreen tree. Leaves bipinnate, the rachis modified into a phyllode. Flowers in globose heads in axillary racemes. Fruit pod, linear.

Introduced and naturalized.

Trade name: Australian black wood.

Uses: Seeds used to treat diabetes.

**Acacia modesta** Wall.

Family: Mimosaceae

Moderate sized, thorny tree, up to 9m tall. Leaves bipinnate, pinnae 4–6 pairs. Flower heads greenish. Fruit pod, 6–8-seeded.

Sub-Himalayan tract and outer Himalayas.

Uses: Seeds showed hypoglycemic activity in normal rats.

**Acacia nilotica** (L.) Willd. ex Del.

Syn: *Acacia arabica* auct non (Lam.) Willd.
*Mimosa arabica* Lam.

Family: Leguminosae (Fabaceae).

Armed tree, up to 15m tall, bark dark brown or black, longitudinally fissured or deeply cracked. Leaves bipinnate, pinnae 4 pairs, leaflets 15–20 pairs, oblong. Flowers golden yellow in axillary globose heads. Fruit pod, moniliform, whitish tomentose, constricted between seeds, seeds 8–12, dark brown, compressed, shining.

Common all over India, in waste lands, hedges and tank bunds.

Fl.: June–September, Fr.: ripen in April–May.

Sanskrit: Barburah.

Local names: *Ben*: Babul; *Guj*: Babaria, Baval; *Hin*: Babul, Kikar; *Kan*: Gobbli Jaali; *Mal*: Kari velam; *Mar*: Babhul; *Ori*: Bambuda; *Tam*: Karu velam, Kariram; *Tel*: Nallatumma.

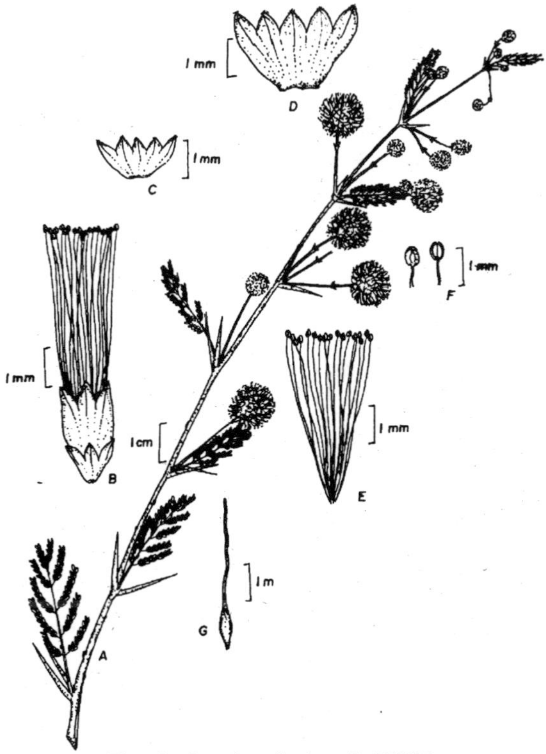


Fig. 4: *Acacia nilotica* (L.)Willd.
A. Twig; B. Flower; C. Calyx split open; D. Corolla split open;
E. Staminal column; F. Anthers; G. Pistil.

Trade name: Babul, Indian Gum Arabic.
Propagation: By seeds.

Uses: Bark is used for treatmnet of diabetes (Marles and Farnsworth, 1995).

**Acacia polyacantha** Willd.

Syn: *Acacia suma* (Roxb.) Buch.-Ham. ex Voigt.
*Mimosa suma* Roxb.

Family: Mimosaceae

Tree, up to 15m tall, armed with stipular spines. Leaves alternate, pinnate, pinnae 15–25 pairs, leaflets 50–60 pairs, elliptic. Fruit pod, seeds 5–8, black.

Fl. & Fr.: March–October.

Uses: Seeds used in the treatment of diabetes.

**Acacia senegal** (Willd.)

Syn: *Acacia verek* Guill. & Perr.

Family: Mimosaceae

Small, deciduous thorny tree, up to 6m tall. Leaves bipinnae with stipular spines, pinnae 6–10. Flowers yellowish, fragrant in axillary spikes. Fruit pod.

Throughout India.

Sanskrit: Svetakhadira.

Local names: *Guj:* Corodio vabul.

Uses: Stem bark used to treat diabetes.

**Acalypha wilkesiana** Muell.-Arg.

Family: Euphorbiaceae

Monoecious shrub, up to 4m tall. Leaves elliptic or ovate, mottled. Flowers reddish in spikes.

Grown in gardens for ornament.

Trade name: Copper leaf, Fire-dragon, Jacob's coat, Beefsteak plant.

Uses: Aerial parts useful in the treatment of diabetes.

**Achillea millefolium** L.

Family: Asteraceae

Perennial herb, to 1m tall. Leaves alternate, oblong, aromatic. Flowers white in dense terminal heads. Fruit achene, compressed.

Common in temperate and alpine areas in Himalayas like Chamba, Kangra, Mandi, Kullu, Shimla, Lahul-spiti and Kinnaur between 2000 and 3800m.

Trade name: Milfoil, Common Yarrow.

Uses: Plant used for curing diabetes (Marles and Farnsworth, 1995)

**Achyranthes aspera** L.

Family: Amaranthaceae

Annual erect herb, up to 1m tall. Leaves orbicular-obovate. Flowers greenish-white in terminal spikes. Fruit utricle, ovoid.

Common weed of wastelands and hedges throughout India.

Fl. & Fr.: All round the year.

Sanskrit: Apamarga.

Local names: *Ass & Ben*: Apang; *Guj*: Aghedo, Aghedi; *Hin*: Chir-chira, Apag, Chichra, Chir-chitta, Latjira; *Kan*: Utrnigida, Uttrane; *Mal*: Katalati,

Puthkunda; *Mar*: Aghadha, Aghara; *Ori*: Apamaranga; *Tam*: Nayuruvi; *Tel*: Uthareni.

Trade name: Prickly-chaff Flower.

Propagation: by seeds.

Uses: Plant is used for curing diabetes

**Aconitum moschatum** (Bruehl) Stapf

Family: Ranunculaceae

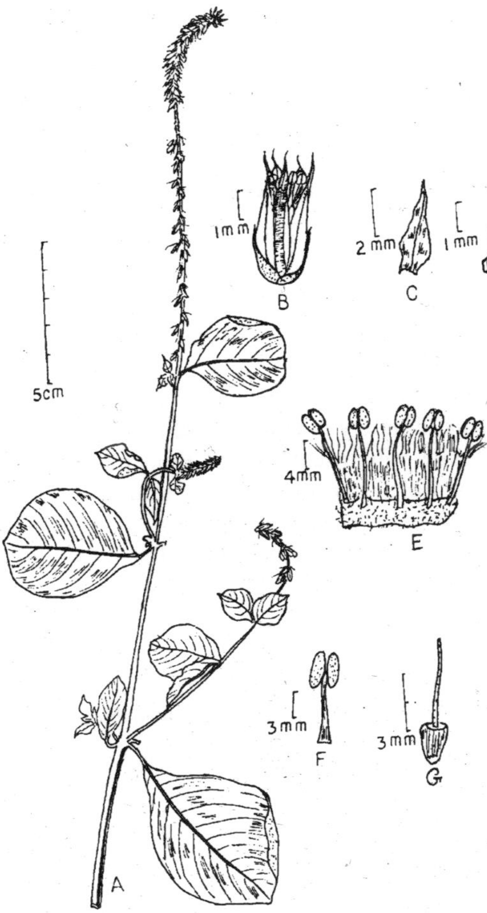


Fig. 5: *Achyranthes aspera* L.
A. Twig; B. Flower; C. Bract; D. Bracteole; E. Staminal tube opened; F. Stamen; G. Pistil.

Perennial herbs, up to 70cm tall, roots cylindric. Leaves few, arising from collar, lamina orbicular-cordate or subreniform, palmately 5-partite. Flowers in racemes, variegated, purple outside, yellowish green at lower part. Fruit follicles.

Endemic to Jammu & Kashmir.

Fl. & Fr.: August–September.

Uses: Plant useful in treating diabetes.

**Aconitum violaceum** Jacq. ex Stapf

Syn: *Aconitum multifidum* Royle

Family: Ranunculaceae

Biennial herb up to 35cm tall, roots paired, tuberous. Leaves very few, 1 or 2 on the hypogeous stem and 1 or 2 higher up on the stem, lamina orbicular, cordate or reniform, deeply 5-partite. Flowers blue or violet in a short raceme or a corymb. Fruit of follicles.

Rare in Alpine zones of Jammu & Kashmir.

Uses: Plant useful in treatment of diabetes.

**Acorus calamus** L.

Family: Araceae

Semi aquatic herb with a creeping and branched aromatic rhizome. Leaves bright green, arranged alternately in two vertical rows on the rhizome. Flowers light brown in sessile cylindrical spadix. Fruit oblong berry.

It is found wild or cultivated through out India.

Sanskrit: Vacha, Ugragandha, Bhuta nashini.

Local names: *Ben*: Bach; *Guj*: Vekhand; *Hin*: Bach, Ghorbach; *Kan*: Baje, Vasa; *Mal*: Vayambu, Vashampa; *Mar*: Vekhand; *Tam*: Vasambu, Cirakkoli; *Tel*: Vasa.

Trade name: The sweet Flag.

Propagation: by division

Native of south Asia and Central and Western North America.

Uses: Rhizome useful for curing diabetes (Marles and Farnsworth, 1995).
*Note*: Item banned for export.

**Actiniopteris radiata** (Swartz.) Link

Syn: *Actiniopteris australis* (L.f.) Link

Family: Actiniopteridaceae

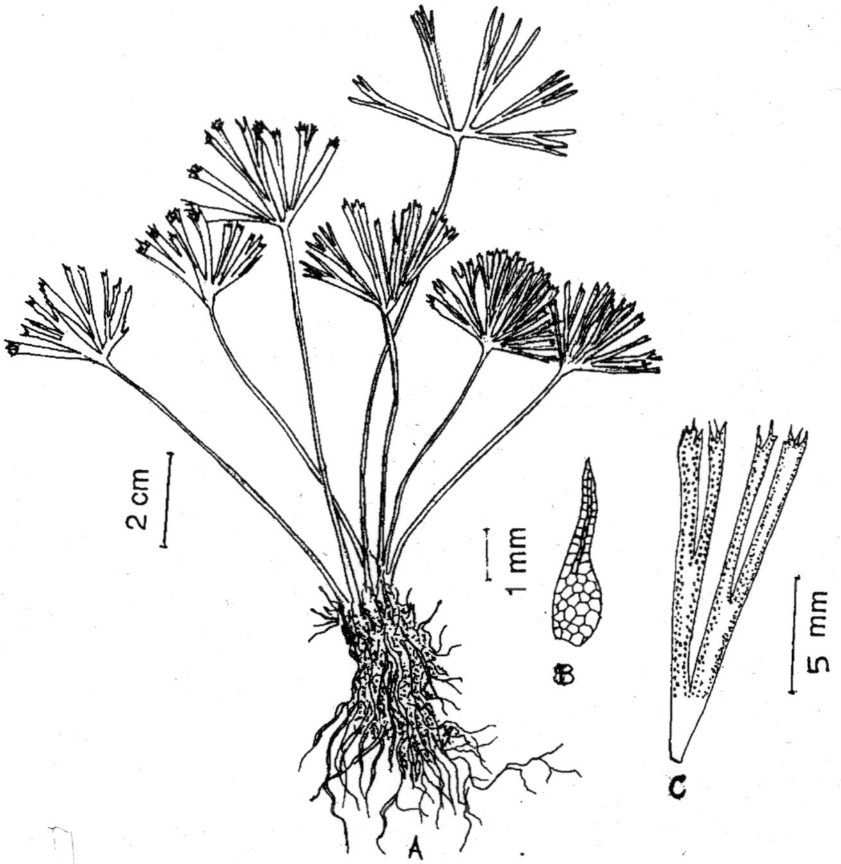


Fig. 6: *Actiniopteris radiata* (Sw.) Link
A. Habit; B. Rhizome scale; C. Few segments of lamina enlarged showing sori.

Terrestrial fern. Rhizome very short. Lamina fan-shaped, all arising from the rhizome, pinnae clustered, deeply dissected, lobes linear, glabrous. Sori arranged in two rows on the lower side of the pinnae lobes.

Throughout India below the elevation of 1200m, in moist crevices of rocks.

Local names: *Hin*: Mayurasikhi, Morpamkhi; *Kan*, *Mal* & *Tel*: Mayurasikha; *Tam*: Mayilatumshikhai.

Trade name: Peacock's tail.

Propagation: by spores

Uses: Whole plant useful for curing diabetes (Marles and Farnsworth, 1995).

**Actinodaphne angustifolia** Nees

Syn: *Actinodaphne hookeri* Meissnn.

Family: Lauraceae

Moderate-sized tree, up to 6m tall. Leaves variable in shape. Flowers unisexual, male flowers clustered or shortly racemose, female flowers umbellate or in sub-racemose clusters. Fruit berry, globose, red when ripe.

Found in the evergreen forests of Eastern and Western Ghats, Sikkim and North-East India.

Local names: *Kan*: Galwara, Hoggodgimara; *Mal*: Malavirinji; *Mar*: Gulchal, Pichli; *Ori*: Jarchampa, Judambo; *Tam*: Thali.

Uses: Leaves used to treat diabetes.

**Actinodaphne madraspatana** Bedd. ex Hook.f.

Family: Lauraceae.

Medium sized tree, branchlets pubescent. Leaves elliptic-lanceolate, coriaceous, shining above. Flowers dioecious, yellowish from the naked branches, male flowers in clusters, female flowers umbellate. Fruit ellipsoid.

Occasional in forests in Peninsular India.

Fl. & fr.: February–April.

Local names: *Mal*: Irolimarom, Mungali; *Tam*: Putta thali; *Tel*: Kovangutti.

Trade name: Ray Laurel.

Propagation: by seeds.

Uses: Leaves useful for curing diabetes (Marles and Farnsworth, 1995).

**Adenanthera pavonia** L.

Family: Mimosaceae

Deciduous tree, up to 12m tall, bark grey. Leaves bipinnate, pinnae 4–6 pairs, leaflets 4–8 pairs, elliptic-oblong. Flowers pale yellow and white in spiciform racemes. Fruit pod, brown, linear-flat, falcately curved, seeds 8–14.

Through out India, in deciduous forests, also cultivated.

Sanskrit: Kucandanah, Tamrakah.

Local names: *Hin*: Baragunci; *Kan*: Manjattai; *Mal*: Mancati; *Tam*: Yanai Kuntumani; *Tel*: Bandiguruvinda, mansenikotta.

Trade name: Coral wood tree.

Propagation: by seeds

Uses: Aerial parts useful for curing diabetes (Marles and Farnswarth, 1995).

**Adenostemma lavenia** (L. ) O. Kuntze

Syn: *Verbesina lavenia* L.

Family: Asteraceae

Annual erect herb, up to 1m tall. Leaves elliptic-lanceolate. Flowers white in terminal homogamous heads. Fruit achene.

Fl. & Fr.: October–January.

Uses: Whole plant useful in the treatment of dibetes.

**Adhatoda zeylanica** Medik.

Syn; *Adhatoda vasica* Nees
*Justcia adhatoda* L.

Family: Acanthaceae

Erect shrub, up to 1.5m tall, branchlets pubescent. Leaves oblanceolate. Flowers creamish white in dense, axillary spikes. Fruit capsule, beaked, seeds 4, orbicular, rugose.

Common in plains and submontane regions through out India.

Fl. & Fr.: November–March.

Sanskrit: Vasa,Vasaka.

Local names: *Ben*: Basak; *Guj*: Aradugi; *Hin*: Arusa, Bansa; *Ori*: Arusa, Basung;

*Kan*: Aadusouge; *Mal*: Ayalotakam; *Tam*: Totai, Vacakam; *Tel*: Addasaramu.

Trade name: Vasaka.

Uses: Root and leaf used for curing diabetes

**Adiantum capillus-veneris** L.

Family: Adiantaceae.

Rhizomatous erect herb, up to 30cm tall, rhizome densely scaly. Fronds (leaves) 2–3-pinnate, the lowest pinna slightly branched again, pinnula glabrous, outer margins incised. Sori elliptic or linear, arranged in roundish sinuses one to each lobe.

Occasional along the streams in Punjab, Bihar, Maharashtra and South India.

Local names: *Guj*: Hanspadi; *Hin*: Hansraj, Mubaraka; *Kan*: Hansraj.

Trade name: The Maidenhair Fern.

Uses: Whole plant useful for curing diabetes (Marles and Farnswarth, 1995).

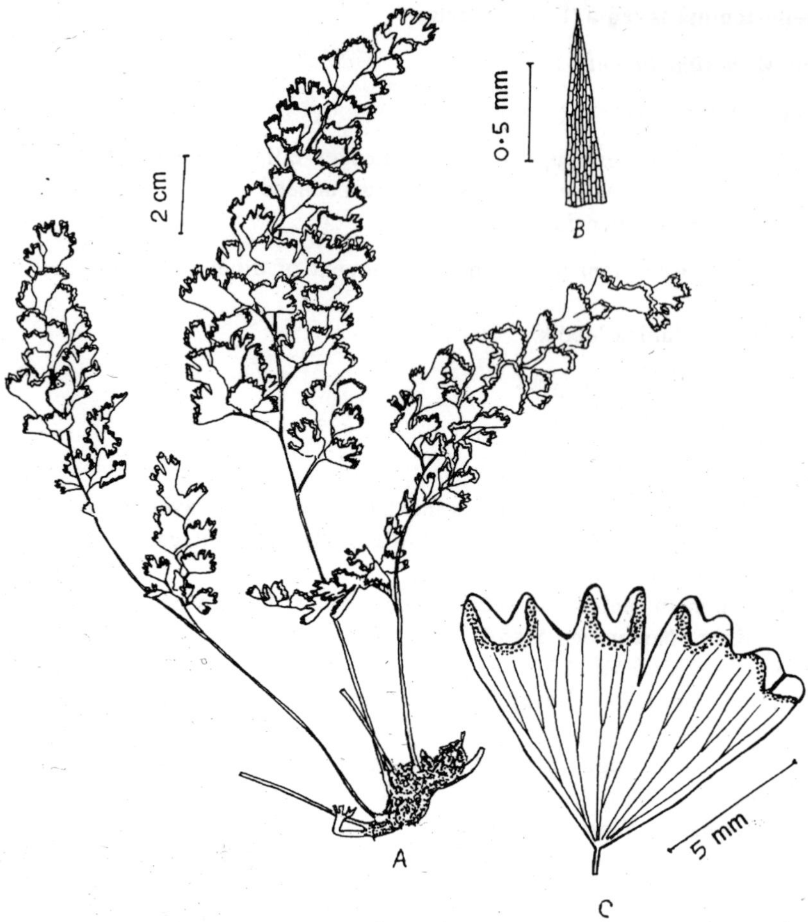


Fig. 7: *Adiantum capillus-veneris* L.
A. Habit; B. Rhizome scale; C. Pinnule enlarged showing venation and sori.

**Aegiceros corniculatum** (L.) Blanco

Syn: *Aegiceros majus* Gaertn.

Family: Myrsinaceae

Evergreen mangrove tree, up to 5m tall. Leaves obovate or lanceolate. Flowers white or pink in axillary and terminal umbels. Fruit follicles.

Found in mangroves of sea coast of India.

Local names: *Ben*: Khalsi, Koilsha, Kulsi; *Hin*: Halsi; *Kan*: Sule; *Mal*: Pukantal; *Mar*: Kanjala; *Ori*: Teluni; *Tam*: Narikandam, Vishnukandal; *Tel*: Dudumarra, Guggilam.

Trade name: Black mangrove, Goat's Horn mangrove.

Uses: Aerial parts useful for treatment of diabetes.

**Aeginetia indica** L.

Family: Orobanchaceae

Parasitic leafless herb of a purplish red colour. Flowers solitary or corymbose. Fruit capsule.

Fl. & Fr.: July–December.

Found throughout India.

Uses: Plant useful for the treatment of diabetes.

**Aegle marmelos** (L.) Correa

Syn: *Crateva marmelos L.*

Family: Rutaceae

Moderate sized, slender, aromatic, armed tree, 6 to 7.5m tall. Bark grey, exfoliating with longitudinal irregular flakes. Leaves 3(5)-foliolate, leaflets ovate-elliptic. Flowers greenish-white in axillary panicles, sweet scented. Fruit ovoid-globose, greenish white, rind woody, seeds-numerous embedded in aromatic pulp.

Common in deciduous forests all over India.

Fl. & Fr.: March–May. Ripen the following year.

Sanskrit: Bilva, Sriphal.

Local names: *Ben, Hin & Mar*: Bael, Sirphal; *Guj*: Bil; *Kan*: Bilvapatre, Byaalada hannu; *Mal & Tam*: Vilvam, Bilva patra; *Mar*: Bili; *Tel*: Maredu, Bilva

Trade name: Holy fruit tree, Bael fruit tree.

Uses: Leaves are useful in treating diabetes. One tea spoon of leaf powder is to be given to the patient's empty stomach daily for seven days (Batra et al., 2002). Leaves of *Aegle* (7), fruit of black pepper (7), seeds of almond (7), seeds of barley (2 table spoon) are soaked in water and kept for two hours. These are then grinded and thus prepared drink is given to the patients daily for 7–10 days (Batra et al., 2002). Clinical trials of unripe fruits also showed hypoglycemic activity.

Active principle: Tannins, Saccharides, Furocoumarins, Furowuinolin alkaloids, N-β-hydroxy-p-methoxyphenylethylcinnamide.

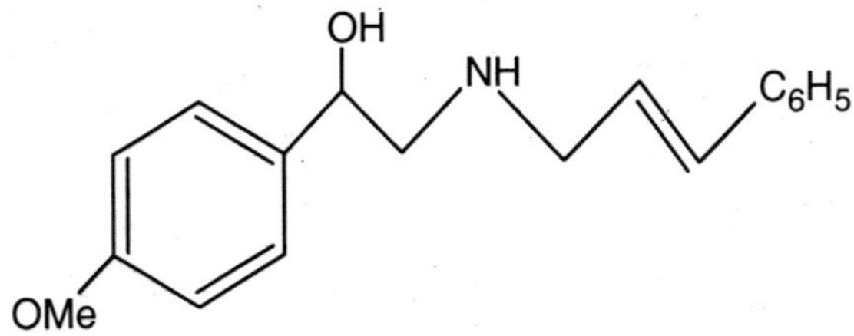


N-β-hydroxy-p-methoxyphenylethylcinnamide

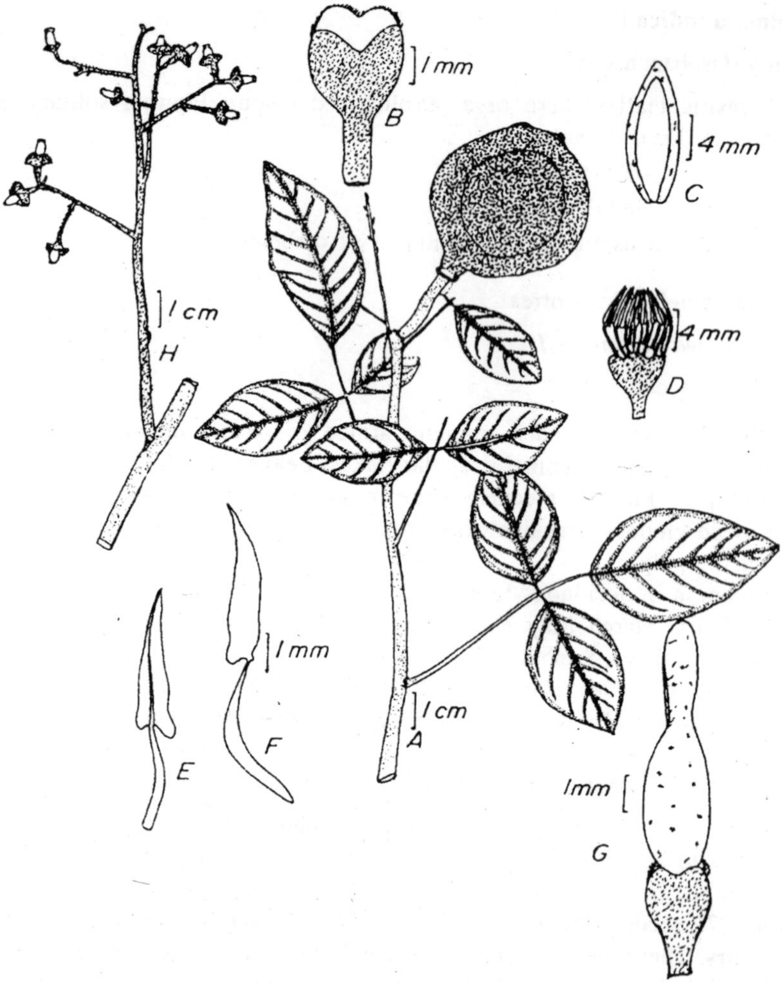


Fig. 8: *Aegle marmelos* (L.) Correa
A. Twig; B. Calyx; C. Petal; D. Androecium; E & F. Stamens; G. Pistil; H. Flowering twig.

**Aerva lanata** (L.) A.L. Juss.

Syn: *Achyranthes lanata* L.

Family: Amaranthaceae.

Annual erect or suberect herb, up to 75cm tall. Leaves alternate to subopposite, ovate, pubescent above, white woolly beneath. Flowers greenish-white in dense axillary spikes. Seeds annular, testa shiny, black.

Occasional weed in cultivated fields, waste lands and hedges throughout tropical India.

Fl. & Fr.: Through out the year.
Sanskrit: Pashanabheda, Bhadra.
Local names: *Ben*: Chaya; *Guj*: Gorakha ganjo; *Hin*: Kapuri jadi; *Kan*: Bilihindi soppu; *Mal*: Cherupula; *Mar*: Kapur-madhura, *Ori*: Paunsia; *Tam*: Sirupoolai; *Tel*: Konda pindi, Pindikura
Propagation: By seeds.

Uses: Plant useful for curing diabetes (Marles and Farnsworth, 1995).

**Aerva sanguinolenta** Blume

Syn: *Aerva scandens* Wall.

Family: Amaranthaceae

Erect or rambling perennial herb or undershrub, up to 1.2m tall.
Found throughout India.

Uses: Whole plant is used to treat Diabetes mellitus.

**Aeschynomene indica** L.

Family: Fabaceae (Papilionaceae)

Annual erect herb, up to 1m tall. Leaves imparipinnate, leaflets numerous, linear-oblong. Flowers pale yellow with maroon streaks on the standard petal, in axillary racemes. Fruit lomentum, 6–8-jointed.
Fl. & Fr.: July–November.
Throughout India.

Uses: Whole plant useful in treatment of diabetes.

**Agapetes sikkimensis** Airyshaw

Family: Ericaceae

Shrub

Found in Sikkim.

Uses: The ethanolic extract (50%) of aerial parts possesses hypoglycemic activity (Asolkar et al., 1992.).

**Ageratum conyzoides** L.

Family: Asteraceae (Compositae).

Annual erect pubescent herb, up to 75cm tall. Leaves ovate. Florets pale blue in terminal homogamous heads; Fruit achene, black.
A common weed of irrigated fields, streams and moist localities throughout India.

Fl. & Fr.: July–January.
Sanskrit: Visamustih.
Local names: *Ben*: Dochunty, Uchunti; *Guj*: Ajagandha, Dholi sadodee; *Kan*: Uralgidda; *Mal*: Appa, Murayampacha; *Mar*: Ghaneraosadi; *Ori*: Boksunga, Poksunga; *Tam*: Pumpillu, Sinnapoompillu; *Tel*: Pumullu.
Trade name: Goat weed, White weed.
Propagation: by seeds.

Uses: Plant useful in the treatment of diabetes.

**Agrimonia eupatoria** L.

Syn: *Agrimonia pilosa* Hook.f.

Family: Rosaceae

Erect, perennial herb. Leaves elliptic-ovate or obovate. Flowers yellow in terminal racemes. Fruit achene.
Found in temperate Himalayas from Kashmir to North Bengal.
Trade name: Agrimony, stickle wort

Uses: Leaves useful in the treatment of diabetes.

**Ailanthus excelsa** Roxb.

Family: Simaroubaceae

Large trees, up to 25m tall with rough bark and soft white wood, branchlets with persistent leaf-scars. Leaves imparipinnate, leaflets 8–14 pairs, subopposite, oblong-lanceolate, inequilateral at base. Flowers large, polygamous, in axillary and terminal panicles. Fruit samara, oblong, coppery red.
Occasional in forests throughout India.
Fl.: January–March. Fr.: March–May.
Sanskrit: Madala, Mahaniba.
Local names: *Guj*: Andusa, Arduri, Moto-arduso; *Hin*: Maharuk, Maharukha; *Kan*: Doddamara, Hemaraheera mara; *Mal*: Matti pongilyam; *Mar*: Mahruk; *Ori*: Mahala, Mahanim; *Tam*: Perru, Perumaruttu; *Tel*: Peddamanu, Peddavepamanu.
Trade name: Tree of Heaven.
Propagation: by root cuttings and seeds.

Uses: The bark is bitter. It has antidiabetic properties (Marles and Farnsworth, 1995).

**Ajuga bracteosa** Wall. ex Benth.

Family: Lamiaceae (Labiatae)

Annual, diffusely branched herb. Leaves ovate, oblanceolate or sub-spathulate. Flowers purplish in axillary whorls.
In North-West India.
Sanskrit: Nilakanthi.
Local names: *Pun*: Khurbanti
Propagation: by division and by seeds.

Uses: The herb has been in use since ancient times and is mentioned in Ayurvedic literature. It is credited with diabetic properties (Marles and Farnsworth, 1995).

**Alangium salvifolium** (L.f.) Wang.

Syn: *Alangium lamarckii* Thw.
*Grewia salvifolia* L.f.

Family: Alangiaceae

Deciduous stragglers, shrubs or trees, up to 20m tall, branchlets at times spinescent. Leaves ovate-oblong to elliptic-lanceolate, chartaceous. Flowers white-cream, fragrant, densely rusty tomentose, often in clusters. Fruit berry, red when ripe.
Common in most states in forests.
Sanskrit: Ankolah, Ankodah.
Local names: *Ben*: Akar-kanta, *Guj & Hin*: Ankol; *Kan*: Ankolimara, Ansaroli, Arinjil, Lucki; *Mal*: Ankolam, Azhinni; *Ori*: Ankula; *Tam*: Alangi; *Tel*: Udaga, Ankolam, Urgu.
Trade name: Sage leaved alangium.
Propagation: by seeds.

Uses: Leaves useful for curing diabetes (Marles and Farnsworth, 1995).

**Albizia julibrissin** Durazz.

Family: Mimosaceae

Medium sized tree.
Found in outer Himalayas from the India east wards towards Sikkim.

Uses: Aerial parts used to treat diabetes.

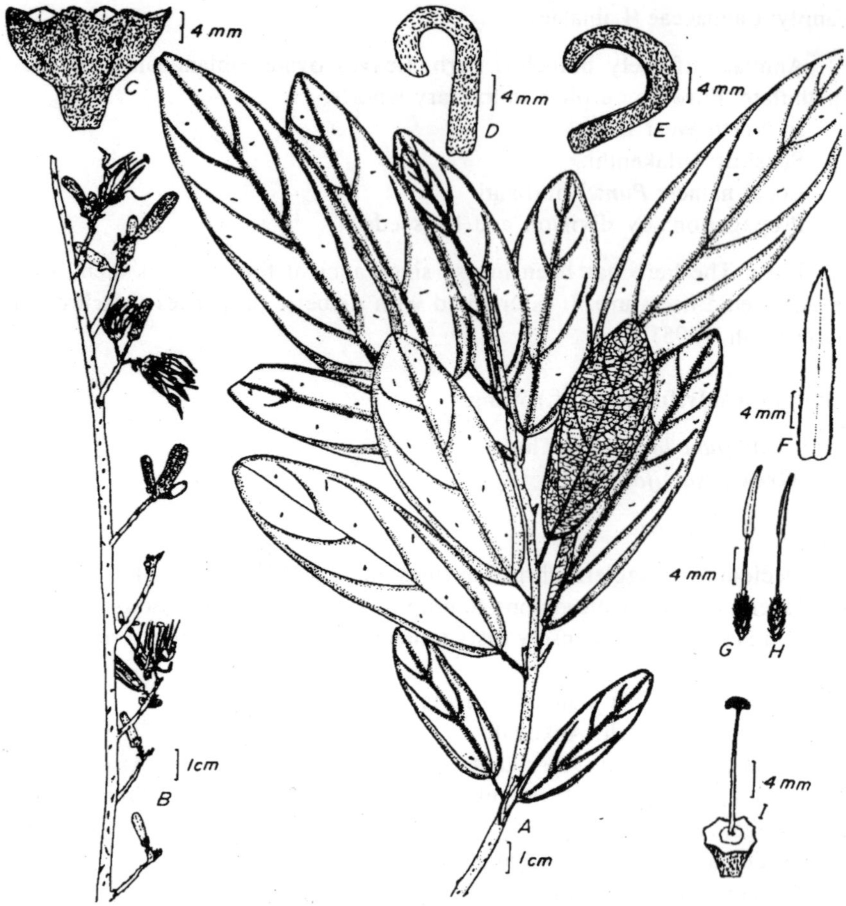


Fig. 9: *Alangiam salvifolium* (L.f) Wang.
A. Twig; B. Inflorescence branch; C. Calyx; D., E. & F. Petals; G. & H. Stamens; I. Pistil.

**Albizia lebbeck** (L.) Benth.

Syn: *Mimosa lebbeck* L.

Family: Mimosaceae

Large deciduous tree, bark brownish-grey. Leaves bipinnate, pinnae 2–4 pairs, leaflets 4–8 pairs, oblong-ovate. Flowers greenish yellow in heads, fragrant. Fruit pod, pale yellow, linear-oblong, strap-shaped. Seeds 2–12, pale brown, flattened.

Common in most forests and plains throughout India. Widely planted along road sides.

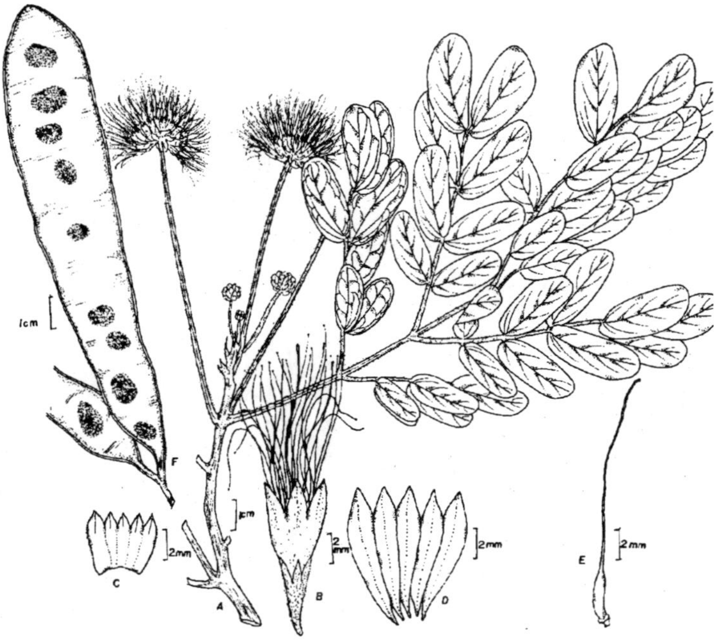


Fig. 10: *Albizia lebbeck* (L.) Willd.
A. Twig; B. Flower; C. Calyx split open; D. corolla split open; E. Pistil; F. Pod.

Fl: March–June. Fr.: June and remains on the tree till the following March.

Sanskrit: Sirish, Bhandi.

Local names: *Ben*: Sirish; *Guj*: Pilosarshio; *Hin*: Siris, Sissa; *Kan*: Bagemara, Kalabaghi; *Mal*: Vagai; *Mar*: Chekola, Sankeswar, Sirisha; *Tam*: Vagei; *Tel*: Dirisana, Sirisamu.

Trade name: Siris tree.

Propagation: By seeds.

Uses: Fruit, root and stem bark have antidiabetic properties.

**Albizia odoratissima** (L.f.) Benth.

Syn: *Mimosa odoratissima* L.

Family: Mimosaceae

Large deciduous tree, 15–25m tall. Bark dark grey. Leaves bipinnate, pinnae 2–5 pairs, leaflets 4–15 pairs, obliquely oblong. Flowers pale yellowish white, fragrant in terminal heads. Fruit oblong pod, reddish brown at maturity.

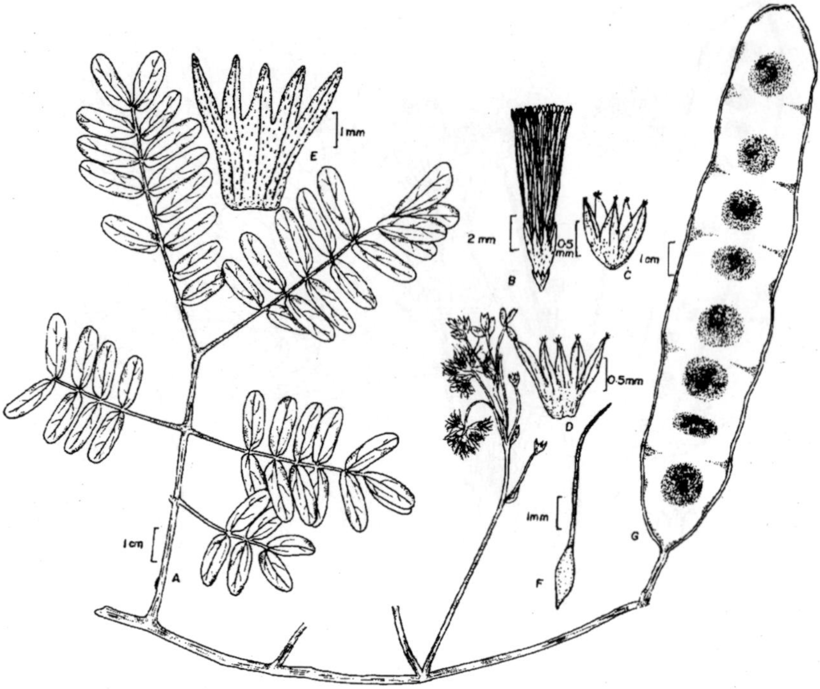


Fig. 11: *Albizia odoratissima* (L.f.) Benth.
A. Twig; B. Flower; C. Calyx entire; D. Corolla entire; E. Corolla split open; F. Pistil; G. Pod.

Common in deciduous forests in most states of India.

Fl. April–June; Fr: June–Dec.

Sanskrit: Bhusirisah.

Local names: *Ass*: Jailoroi; *Guj*: Kalo sarasio, Siris; *Hin*: Bansa, Bas, Bassein, Bersa, kaliasiris; *Kan*: Bassari, Bettassujjalu, Bilivara, Golanchu; *Mal*: Kiriutaakura, Karuvaka, Nellivaka, Pulivaga, Selanui; *Mar*: Chinchawala, Chichonda, Ramsara; *Ori*: Banosirisi, Sirocho, Tinuya; *Pun*: Karmaru, Lasrin,Polach; *Tam*: Kalihurunjil, Kasuvageii, Purusalai, Siltalaivaya; *Tel*: Chinduga, Bandisiduga, Konda chigara.

Trade name: Black siris, kala siris.

Propagation: by seeds

Uses: The bark is used for curing diabetes.

**Albizia procera** (Roxb.) Benth.

Syn: *Mimosa procera* Roxb.

Family: Mimosaceae.

Very large deciduous tree, up to 30m tall. Leaves pinnately compound, pinnae usually 3 pairs, leaflets 6–12 pairs, oblique ovate. Flowers in globose heads. Fruit pod, orange-brown, seeds 10–12, yellow.

Occasional in deciduous forests along river banks.

Fl. & Fr.: April–December.

Local names: *Ben*: Koroi; *Hin*: Gurar, Kurha, safed Siris; *Kan*: Bellate, Chikul, Salvagai, Adhanji; *Mal*: Karunthagara; *Mar*: Kinhai; *Tam*: Konda vagaei, Vet vagai; *Tel*: Tella Chinduga, Tella-chinta.

Trade name: White siris.

Propagation: By seeds.

Uses: Aerial parts useful in the treatment of diabetes.

**Alhagi pseudoalhagi** (Bieb.) Desv.

Syn: *Alhagi camelorum* Fisch.
*Alhagi maurorum* Medic.

Family: Fabaceae (Papilionaceae)

Armed shrub, up to 60cm tall. Leaves oblong. Flowers red in few-flowered axillary racemes, forming panicles at the end of branches. Fruit pod, falcate or straight.

In Maharastra, Gujarat, Punjab, Rajasthan, Bihar and Kashmir.

Local names: *Ben*: Dulal labha, Javasha; *Guj & Mar*: Jawaso; *Hin*: Bharbharra; Jawasa; *Kan*: Billiduruva, durlava; *Tel*: Girikarmika; Tellaginiya chettu.

Trade name: Jawara.

Uses: Whole plant useful in the treatment of diabetes.

**Alisma plantago-aquatica** L.

Syn: *Alisma plantago* L.

Family: Alismataceae

Erect, stout, scapigerous, perennial herb. Leaves linear to ovate-lanceolate. Flowers white or pink with a pale yellow base. Fruit achene, compressed

Found in Himalayas from Kashmir to North Bengal.

Trade name: Mad Dog weed, Water plantain.

Uses: Rhizome used for treatment of diabetes.

**Allamanda cathartica** L.

Family: Apocynaceae

Erect evergreen shrub, up to 4m tall. Leaves whorled, ovate to oblong-lanceolate. Flowers large, showy, bright golden yellow, in terminal cymose panicles. Fruit prickly capsule, many-seeded.

Cultivated, naturalised in southern, central and eastern India.

Local names: *Ben*: Harkakra; *Kan*: Allamandagide, Haladilu; *Mal*: Kolambi; *Tel*: Allamandatige.

Uses: Aerial parts useful in the treatment of diabetes.

**Allium ascalonicum** L.

Family: Liliaceae

Bulbous, perennial herb, bulb white. Leaves basal. Flowers greenish white or purplish white in many-flowered, globose heads on a fistular scape.

Cultivated.

Local names: *Ben*: Gundhun; *Pun*: Gandana, Gandhan.

Trade name: The shallot.

Uses: Bulbs useful in the treatment of diabetes.

**Allium cepa** L.

Family: Liliaceae.

Perennial or biennial with globose bulb. Leaves tubular, blue green. Inflorecence stalk (scape) hollow, up to 50cm long. Flowers greenish white in umbels. Fruit thin skinned capsule, seeds black and angular.

Cultivated throughout India.

Sanskrit: Palanduh, Raktakanda.

Local Names: *Ben & Hin*: Piyaz; *Guj*: Dungari; *Kan*: Nirulli; *Mal*: Chuvannulli; *Mar*: Kanda; *Tam*: Vengayam; *Tel*: Ulligadda, Erragadda

Trade name: Onion.

Propagation: By seeds and bulbs.

Uses: Juice of the bulb lowers the blood glucose level. Regular use of onion in the diet is suggested for diabetics.

**Allium sativum** L.

Family: Liliaceae

Perennial herb, 25–70 cm tall, stem erect, leafy in the middle. Leaves flat, 4–25cm long. Garlic bulb is usually a compound bulb, oval in shape, the skin colour of the bulb is silky white. Flowers reddish or greenish white, in cluster.

Cultivated all over India.

Sanskrit: Arishtha, Shuklakanda.

Local names: *Ben*: Lashan, Lashun, Rasun; *Guj*: Lasan; *Hin*: Lahsan; *Kan*: Belluli, *Mal*, Velluli, Velutha ulli; *Mar*: Lasunas; *Tel*: Vellulli, Tellagadda.

Trade name: Garlic.

Propagation: By seeds.

Uses: Regular use of garlic is useful in the treatment of diabetes.

**Allium tuberosum** Rottl. ex Spreng.

Family: Liliaceae.

Small herb with elongated bulbs. Leaves flat. Flowers in many–flowered umbels.

Found in Eastern India and Western Himalayas.

Trade name: Chinese chives.

Uses: Leaves useful in treatment of diabetes.

**Alocasia macrorrhiza** (L.) Don

Syn: *Alocasia indica* Spach.
*Arum macrorrhizon* L.

Family: Araceae

Stout rhizomatous herb. Leaves ovate. Flowers in spadix enclosed in a pale yellow green spathe, fragrant. Fruit berry.

Cultivated in South India, Maharashtra, Assam and West Bengal.

Sanskrit: Hastikarni.

Local names: *Ben*: Mankachu, *Hin*: Mankanda; *Kan*: Maanaka, Marasani; *Mal*: Marambu, Seem chembu, Venal chembu, *Mar*: Alu; *Tam*: Merukankilangu; *Tel*: Charakanda, Sarachema.

Uses: Rhizome useful in the treatment of diabetes.

**Aloe vera** (L.) Burm. f.

Syn: *Aloe barbadensis* Mill.

Family: Liliaceae

A stoloniferous herb. Leaves dense, aggregated, succulent, ensiform, pale green with distant horny prickles on the margins. Scape 60–90cm long, simple. Raceme dense, flowers reddish-yellow, bisexual. Fruit capsule, ellipsoid.

Common in drier parts of India. It is cultivated in hedge rows.

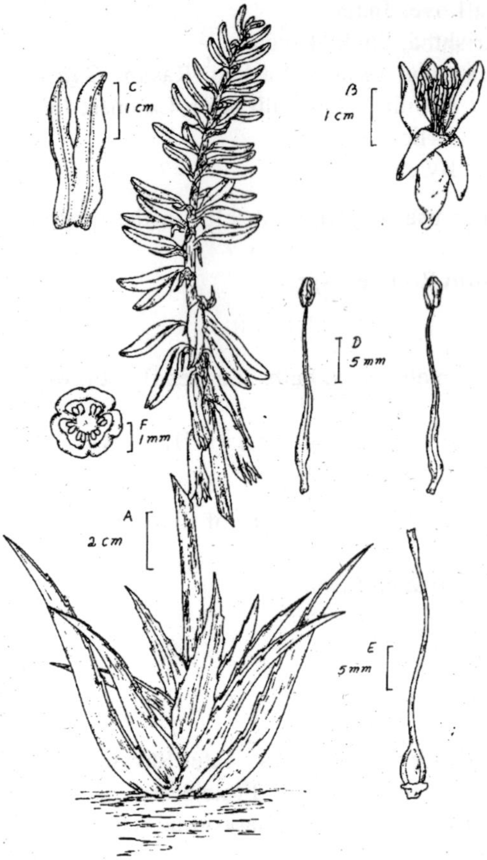


Fig. 12: *Aloe vera* (L.) Burm. f.
A. Habit; B. Flower; C. Perianth lobes (outer and inner); D. Stamens; E. Pistil; F. T.S. of ovary,

Sanskrit: Kumari.

Local names: *Ben*: Ghrita-kumari; *Guj*: Kumarapathu; *Hin*: Gheekunvar; *Kan*: Loli Sara; *Mal*: Kattar vazha, Kumari; *Mar*: Korphad; *Tam*: Kilimukan, Katarezhai, Chirukuttali; *Tel*: Chinna Kalabanda.

Trade name: Indian Aloe.

Propagation: By suckers.

Uses: Leaf powder is in use with hot water, twice per day in treating diabetes.

**Alpinia galanga** (L.) Sw.

Syn: *Maranta galanga* L.
*Languas galanga* (L.) Stuntz.

*Alpinia rheedii* Wight

Family: Zingiberaceae.

Large herb, over 2m tall, rhizome large, hard, woody, aromatic. Leaves large, oblong-lanceolate. Flowers greenish white in terminal panicles. Fruit globose capsule, orange red.

In dense evergreen forests of Assam, Meghalaya, Maharashtra, Tamil Nadu, Karnataka and Andaman & Nicobar islands.

Sanskrit: Sugandhamula, Rasna, Elaparni.

Local names: *Hin*: Bara kalisan; *Kan*: Dhumarasmi, Raasmi; *Mal*: Aratta, Cittaratta; *Mar*: Citta-ratta, Pera-ratta; *Tam*: Arathai, Perarathai, *Tel:* Dumparastramu.

Trade name: Greater galangal.

Propagation: By rhizomes.

Fl. & Fr.: April–December.

Uses: Rhizome useful in the treatment of diabetes.

**Alstonia macrophylla** Wall. ex A. DC.

Family: Apocynaceae

Moderate-sized or tall tree. Leaves oblanceolate or elliptic-lanceolate, ternately whorled. Flowers fragrant, in corymbose cymes at the ends of twigs among leaves. Fruit follicles.

Planted in Gardens.

Trade name: Matchstick tree.

Uses: Whole plant used to treat Diabetes mellitus.

**Alstonia scholaris** (L.) R.Br.

Syn: *Echites scholaris* L.

Family: Apocynaceae.

Large evergreen tree, base buttressed, bark dark grey, nearly smooth, latex milky. Leaves 4–7 in a whorl, coriaceous, elliptc-oblong or obovate. Flowers greenish-white, sub-capitate at the end of the panicle branches. Follicles pendulous, cylindric, seeds numerous, flattened, hairy.

Widely distributed, often planted.

Fl.: December–March. Fr.: May–September.

Sanskrit: Saptaparnah.

Local names: *Ben*: Chattim, Chatwan; *Hin*: Chatium, Saitan-ka-jhad; *Kan*: Jantaala-mara, Janthalle, Koodale, Maddale, Yedelebale; *Mal*: Arilampila, Daivapala, Ezhilampala, Koda-pala, Mukampala; *Mar*: Saptaparni, Satwin;

*Ori*: Chhatiana, Kumbaro, Soptorposi; *Tam*: Ezhilaippalai, Mukkampalai; *Tel*: Edakulapala, Palagaruda.

Trade name: Dita bark tree, shaitam wood.

Propagation: by seeds.

Uses: Whole plant useful in the treatment of diabetes.

**Althaea officinalis** L.

Family: Malvaceae

Downy perennial herb, up to 1.8m tall. Leaves obovoid. Flowers rosy in axillary clusters. Fruit schizocarp.

Found in the Himalayan region from Kashmir to Punjab.

Local names: *Guj & Mar*: Gulkhair, Khaira. *Hin*: Gulkhairo, Khaira; *Kan*: Seemetuti; *Tam*: Simaitutti.

Uses: Leaves and roots used in the treatment of diabetes.

**Ammi visagna** (L.) Lam.

Syn: *Daucus visagna* L.
*Visagna daucoides*

Family: Apiaceae (Umbelliferae).

Robust herb, up to 1.5m tall. Leaves deltoid, pinnately decompound. Flowers white. Fruit oblong-ovoid.

Cultivated as garden ornamental, often as an escape.

Trade name: Khella, Tooth pick ammi, Tooth pick fruit.

Uses: Plant used to treat Diabetes mellitus.

Active constituent: Dihydrosamidin.

**Amomum aromaticum** Roxb.

Family: Zingiberaceae

Perennial herb, up to 90cm tall. Leaves oblong-lanceolate. Flowers pale yellow, in small globose spikes. Fruit capsule.

In Assam, Meghalaya, Sikkim, Northern Bihar, North Bengal.

Local names: *Ben & Hin*: Morang-elaichi; *Mar*: Veldode.

Uses: Rhizome useful in the treatment of diabetes.

**Amomum subulatum** Roxb.

Family: Zingiberaceae

Perennial herb, with leafy stem up to 2.5m tall, rhizomes creeping, branched. Leaves oblong-lanceolate. Flowers white in globose, shortly peduncled spikes, bracts reddish brown. Fruits densely echinate, globose capsules, reddish brown, seeds many.

In Eastern Himalayas.

Sanskrit: Sthulaila, Bhadraila.

Local names: *Ben*: Bara-elachi, Baro-elach, *Guj*: Moti elaichi; *Hin*: Badi Ilayachy; *Kan*: Doddayelakkai; *Mal*: Perelam; *Mar*: Mote veldode; *Ori*: Bada-alaicha; *Tam*: Periya elam; Kattelam, Perelam; *Tel*: Pedda elakkaya, Adavi elakkaya.

Trade Name: Greater cardamom, Nepal cardamom.

Propagation: by rhizome.

Uses: Rhizome useful in the treatment of diabetes

**Amoora wallichii** King

Syn: *Amoora spectabilis* Hiern non Miq.

Family: Meliaceae

Medium sized tree, up to 35m tall. Leaves pinnately compound, leaflets 11–13 pairs, oblong. Flowers small in branched panicles. Fruit obovoid-pyriform capsule.

Evergreen forests of Sikkim, West Bengal, Assam, Manipur and Andaman.

Local names: *Ben*: Lalee, Lali, Pitraj; *Hin*: Lalchini.

Trade name: Amari

Uses: Stem is used in the treatment of diabetes.

**Anacardium occidentale** L.

Family: Anacardiaceae

Tree, up to 8m tall, branchlets glabrous. Leaves simple, obovate, thick coriaceous. Flowers unisexual or polygamous, yellow streaked with pink in terminal panicles. Fruit nut, seated on a large pyriform fleshy body formed by the enlarged disc, seed reniform, testa membranous.

Cultivated in coastal areas, especially near the sea, but now naturalised.

Fl. & Fr: January–May.

Sanskrit: Kajutaka.

Local name: *Ben*: Hijlibadam; *Hin & Mar*: Kaju; *Kan*: Geru bija; *Mal*: Andi Parupu; *Tam*: Mindiri, Mundiri; *Tel*: Jidi mamidi.

Trade name: Cashew nut.

Propagation: By seeds.

Uses: Cashew bark is used to treat diabetes insipidus.

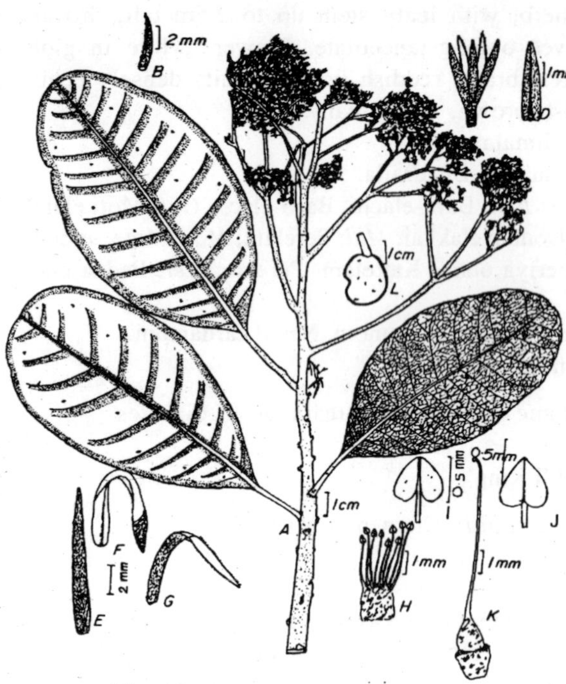


Fig. 13: *Anacardium occidentale* L.
A. Twig; B. Bract; C. Calyx; D. Sepal; E., F. & G. Petals; H. Androecium; I. & J. Stamens; K. Pistil.

**Anamirta cocculus** (L.) Wt. & Arn.

Syn: *Menispermum cocculus* L.

Family: Menispermaceae.

Large climbing shrubs. Leaves ovate-cordate. Flowers greenish in drooping panicles on old wood. Fruit druplets, white.

Rare in forests of Andhra Pradesh, Karnataka, Tamil Nadu, Kerala and Andaman & Nicobar Islands.

Fl. & Fr.: October–April.

Sanskrit: Kakanasika.

Local names: *Ben*: Kakamari; *Guj*: Jarmae, Kakamari, Kakaphula; *Hin*: Jermae, Kakmari; *Kan*: Kaayamari, Kakkesoppugida; *Mal*: Nanjinkura, Pella: *Mar*: Kakaphal, Kakmari, Vatoli; *Ori*: Kalabitinai; *Tam*: Kakkaykolliverai, Nanchenkuru, Paenkottai; *Tel*: Kakamari.

Trade name: Fish berry, Levant nut.

Propagation: By seeds.

Uses: Aerial parts useful for the treatment of diabetes.

**Ananas comosus** (L.) Merr.

Syn: *Ananas sativus* Schult.f.

Family: Bromeliaceae

A perennial herb, up to 1m tall. Leaves rigid, mostly densely tufted in a rosette at the base of the stem, sword-shaped with spiny tip and margins. Flowers in terminal heads. Fruit sorosis formed by an aggregate of fruits, succulent.

Cultivated all over India.

Sanskrit: Anamnasam, Bahunetraphalam

Local names: *Ben*: Ananash; *Guj & Mar*: Ananas; *Hin*: Ananas; *Kan*: Anasahannu; *Mal*: Kaitacchakka, Kappaccakka, Ananas; *Tam*: Annasippalam; *Tel*: Anaasapandu.

Trade name: Pine apple.

Propagation: by suckers

Uses: Plant useful for treatment of diabetes.

**Andrographis paniculata** (Burm.f.) Wall. ex Nees

Syn: *Justicia paniculata* Burm.f.
*Andrographis subspathulata* Clarke

Family: Acanthaceae

Annual erect herb, up to 1.5m tall, stem sharply quadrangular. Leaves lanceolate. Flowers white with maroon streaks on upper lip, in lax spreading axillary and terminal unilateral racemes. Fruit capsule, linear-oblong, acute at both ends, seeds numerous, yellowish brown.

Common weed of plains and open forests all over India.

Fl. & Fr.: July–December.

Sanskrit: Bhuninbah.

Local names: *Ben*: Kalmegh; *Guj*: Kariyatu; *Hin*: Kiryat, Mahatita; *Kan*: Nelabevu, Vayu hullu; *Mal*: Kiriyattu, Kiriyatta; *Mar*: Olenkiryatta; *Ori*: Bhuinimba; *Tam*: Nilavembu; *Tel*: Nelavemu.

English: King of bitters.

Uses: Decoction of whole plant is used 2–3 times a day for the treatment of diabetics.

**Anethum graveolens** L.

Syn: *Peucedanum graveolens* L.
*Anethum sowa* Roxb. ex DC.

Family: Apiaceae (Umbelliferae)

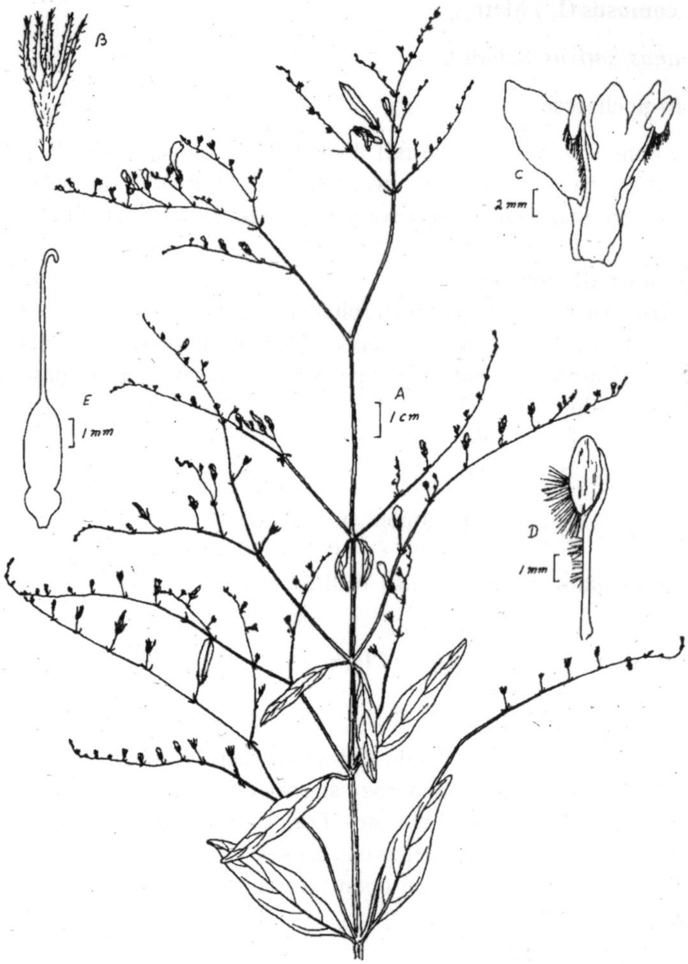


Fig. 14: *Andrographis paniculata* (Burm. f.) Wall ex Nees
A. Twig; B. Calyx; C. Corolla open; D. Stamen; E. Pistil.

Annual, erect, glabrous herb, up to 1m tall. Leaves 2–3-pinnatipartite, segments filiform, Flowers pale yellow in compound umbels. Fruit narrowly winged.

Cultivated in plains throughout India.

Sanskrit: Satapushpa.

Local names: *Hin*: Soya; *Kan*: Sabba-sige; *Mal*: Satakuppa; *Tam*: Satakuppi; *Tel*: Satakuppivittulu.

Trade name: Dill, Garden dill, Anet.

Propagation: By seeds

Uses: Fruit useful in the treatment of diabetes.

**Anethum sowa** Roxb. ex Flem.

Syn: *Peucedanum sowa*

Family: Apiaceae (Umbelliferae)

Annual herb, up to 1.2m tall. Leaves decompound, ultimate segments filiform. Flowers pale yellow in compound umbels. Fruit sub-elliptical, with longitudinal ridges.

Cultivated throughout India.

Sanskrit: Ahichhatra, Shatapushpa.

Local names: *Ben*: Shulupa, Soolpa; *Guj*: Suak, Suva; *Hin*: Sotopha, Sowa; *Kan*: Sabbasige; *Mal*: Chatakuppa; *Mar*: Bantashopa, Shopa; *Tam*: Satakuppi; *Tel*: Shatakuppi-vittulu.

Uses: Plant useful in the treatment of diabetes.

**Angiopteris evecta** (Forst.) Hoff.

Family: Angiopteridaceae (Fern family)

Rhizomatous perennial fern. Stipes up to 150cm × 5cm. Lamina deltoid; up to 230 × 140cm, bipinnate, pinnae subopposite with 3cm long stalk, oblong-lanceolate, pinnules subopposite, shortly stalked, oblong-lanceolate. Sori submarginal and ellipsoidal.

Common along shaded stream banks in thick forests.

Local names: *Tel*: Kalojikanda

Uses: Aerial parts useful in the treatment of diabetes.

**Annona squamosa** L.

Family: Annonaceae

Shrub or small tree, bark grey. Leaves simple, elliptic or oblong-lanceolate, glabrescent. Flowers greenish, solitary, on leaf-opposed peduncles or 2–4 in a cluster. Fruit a fleshy syncarp.

Common in forests of South India, Orissa, Madhya Pradesh, Delhi, Uttar Pradesh, Gujarat, Maharashtra and Assam. Also cultivated for its fruits.

Fl.& Fr.: April–November.

Sanskrit: Sitaphalam, Gandhagathra, Shubha.

Local names: *Ben*: Ata, Seethaphal; *Guj* & *Mar*: Seethaphal; *Hin*: Seethaphal, Sharifa; *Kan*: Seethaphala; *Mal*: Attichakka, Seethapazham; *Ori*: Ato, Seethaphalo; *Tam*: Atta, Seethapazham; *Tel*: Sitaphalamu.

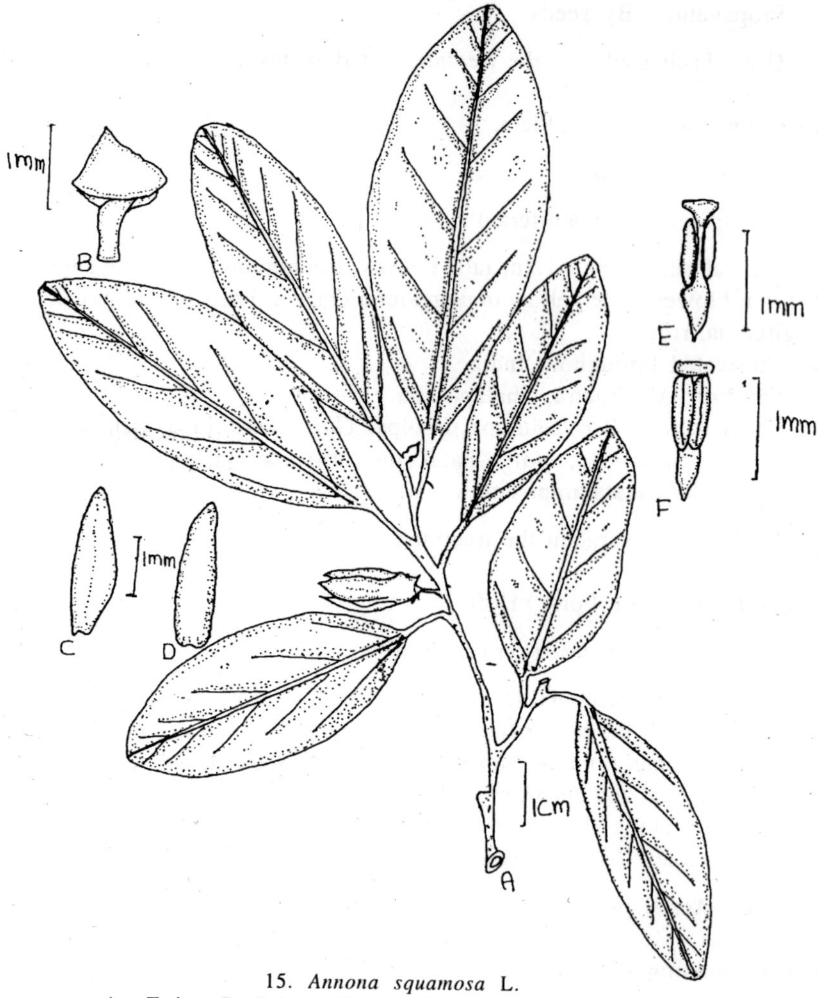


15. *Annona squamosa* L.
A. Twig, B. Calyx, C & D. Petals, E & F. Stamens.

Trade name: Custard apple.
Propagation: by seeds.

Uses: Leaves useful in the treatment of diabetes.

**Anogeissus pendula** Edgew.

Family: Combretaceae

Gregarious bush or a small tree, up to 15m tall. Leaves elliptic-obovate. Flowers in heads. Fruits small, winged, orbicular.

Tropical forests of Rajasthan, Gujarat, Maharashtra, Madhya Pradesh and Haryana.

Local names: *Guj*: Dhan, Dhaumkra.

Uses: Aerial parts used in the treatment of diabetes mellitus.

**Anthocephalus chinensis** (Lam.) A. Rich ex Walp.

Syn: *Cephalanthus chinensis* Lam.
*Anthocephalus cadamba* (Roxb.) Miq.
*Anthocephalus indicus* A.Rich
*Nauclea cadamba* Roxb.

Family: Rubiaceae

Large tree. Leaves elliptic-oblong. Flowers fragrant, greenish yellow, in terminal globular heads. Fruit orange-yellow when ripe.

Fl. & Fr.: February–May.

Uses: Stem bark is used to treat Diabetes.

**Aphanamixis polystachya** (Wall.) Parkes.

Syn: *Aglaia polystachya* Wall.
*Amoora rohituka* (Roxb.) Wight & Arn.

Family: Meliaceae

Large tree, up to 35m tall. Leaves odd pinnate, leaflets 45 pairs, opposite, ovate-oblong. Flowers white in axillary panicles. Fruit capsule, globose.

From U.P to Assam and Western and Eastern Ghats.

Local names: *Ben*: Pittarau; Tikatraj; *Hin*: Harin-hara; *Kan*: Mullumunthala; *Mal*: Chemmaram; *Mar*: Rohada; *Tam*: Malampuluvan; *Tel*: Chaweramnu.

Uses: Stem useful in the treatment of diabetes.

**Apium graveolens** L.

Family: Apiaceae (Umbelliferae).

Annual or biennial, erect herbs, 30cm–1m tall, root is tuberous. Leaves pinnately compound with long stalks. Flowers greenish white in terminal compound umbels. Fruit cremocarp.

In foot hills of Himalayas in Punjab, Himachal Pradesh and Uttar Pradesh; also cultivated.

Sanskrit: Ajmoda, Anthpatrika.

Local names: *Ben*: Cheendani, Chanu, Randhuni; *Hin*: Ajmod, Ajmad,

Bari ajmod; *Kan*: Selerina; *Mar*: Ajmoda; *Tam*: Celery-Keerai.
Trade name: Celery
Propagation: by seeds.

Uses: Leaves have antidiabetic property.

**Aporosa lindleyana** Baill.

Family: Euphorbiaceae

Much branched, ever green glabrous tree, up to 15m tall. Leaves elliptic-oblong, lanceolate. Flowers unisexual, male yellow in catkin like spikes, female pale green in bracteate spikes. Fruit ovoid or globose capsule.

Common all over peninsular India in wet deciduous and evergreen forests.

Sanskrit: Valaka.

Local names: *Kan*: Sali, Salle, Sulla; *Mal*: Ponvetti, Vetti; *Tam*: Vettikan, Vettil.

Medicinal uses: Whole plant used for the treatment of diabetes.

**Arachis hypogaea** L.

Family: Fabaceae

Annual diffuse or erect herb, 25–35cm tall. Leaves pinnate, leaflets 2 pairs, oblong or obovate. Flowers yellow, axillary, fascicled. Fruit pod, ripening underground, hard, indehiscent, inflated, 1–3-seeded, seed with thin reddish brown seed coat and two fleshy white cotyledons.

Cultivated throughout India.

Sanskrit: Bhueanakah, Mandapi.

Local names: *Ben*: Chini-badam; *Guj*: Mugphali; *Hin*: Mungphali; *Kan*: Nilakadali; *Mal*: Kappalandi, Nilakkatala; *Mar*: Bhuimug; *Tam*: Nelakadalai, Verkatalai; *Tel*: Verusanagalu.

Trade name: Ground nut, Peanut
Propagation: By seeds.

Uses: Seeds useful in the treatment of diabetes.

**Arctium lappa** L.

Family: Asteraceae (Compositae)

Erect herb, up to 2.5m tall, roots fusiform. Leaves ovate-cordate. Flowers in sub-corymbose heads. Fruit achene, angled, ribbed.

In Himalayas from Kashmir to Simla.

Trade name: Common Burdock, Great Burdock.

Uses: Root is used to treat Diabetes mellitus.

**Areca catechu** L.

Family: Arecaceae (Palmae)

Tree, trunk slender. Leaves large, leaflets numerous, linear-lanceolate. Flowers small in spadices. Fruit orange or scarlet, ovoid, smooth.

Cultivated in South India.

Sanskrit: Poogiphalum, Gubk.

Local names: *Ben*: Gua, Supari; *Guj*: Soparul; *Hin & Mar*: Supari; *Kan*: Adike; *Mal*: Adakka, Marom; *Pun*: Supari, *Tam*: Paakku maram, Kamugu; *Tel*: Vakka.

Trade name: Areca nut.

Propagation: By seeds.

Uses: Fruit useful in the treatment of diabetes.

**Argemone mexicana** L.

Family: Papaveraceae

Annual prickly herbs, stem greyish-white with yellow latex. Leaves both radical and cauline, white, spiny on margins and veins, sessile, amplexicaul, oblong-ovate, glaucous.

Fruit poricidal capsule, prickly, seeds blackish-brown.

Common weed in open wastelands and cultivated fields and road sides, through out India.

Sanskrit: Swarnakshiri, Bhramadandi.

Local names: *Ben*: Shialkanta; *Guj*: Darudi; *Hin*: Bharbhand; Brahmadundi, Satyanashi; *Kan*: Datturigidda; *Mal*: Bhramadanti; *Mar*: Pilva dhotra, *Ori*: Kantakusham; *Tam*: Kurukkum; *Tel*: Balurakkasi, Brahmadandi, Yerrikusuma*:* *Urdu*: Baramadandi.

Trade name: Prickly poppy, Mexican poppy.

Uses: Flowers useful in the treatment of diabetes.

**Argyreia cuneata** Ker—Gawl.

Syn: *Convolvulus cuneatus* Willd.
*Lettsomia cuneata* Roxb.
*Rivea cuneata* Wight.

Family: Convolvulaceae

Climbing or shrubby plant, up to 1.5m tall. Leaves elliptic or obovate. Flowers deep bright purple in axillary peduncled cymes. Fruit berry, ellipsoid, yellow brown when ripe.

Cultivated in gardens
Local names: *Kan*: Acheegide, Attargidda, *Mar*: Bondwail, Mahalungi.

Uses: The leaves are reported to be effective in diabetes.

**Argyreia nervosa** (Burm.f.) Bojer

Syn: *Argyreia speciosa* Sweet

Family: Convolvulaceae

A very large climbing shrub with stout, white-tomentose stems. Leaves broadly ovate or ovate-cordate, glabrous above, densely white-tomentose beneath. Flowers rose-purple, in axillary clustered cymes. Fruit ovoid berry.

Occasional in open forests throughout India.

Fl. & Fr: July–December.

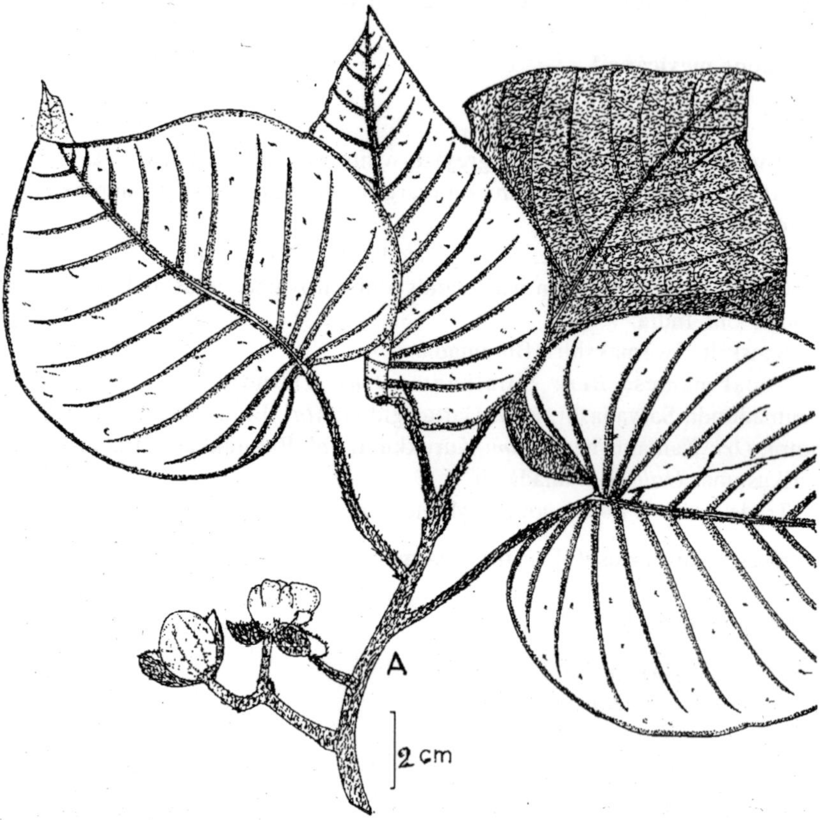


Fig. 16: *Argyreia nervosa* (Burm. f.) Boj.
A. Twig.

Sanskrit: Samudrapalaka.

Local names: *Ben*: Bichtarak; *Guj* & *Mar*: Samudrasoka; *Hin*: Samundar-ka-pat; *Kan* & *Tel*: Samudrapala, Chandrapala; *Mal*: Marikkunni, Marututari, Samudrapacha; *Ori*: Bryddhotareko; *Tam*: Samuddirapaccha; *Tel*: Chandrapada.

Trade name: Elephant creeper.

Uses: Leaves useful in the treatment of diabetes.

**Aristolochia indica** L.

Family: Aristolochiaceae

Twining shrub, stem grooved. Leaves obovate-oblong. Flowers greenish-white, tube with globose inflated base, then bent at right angle and

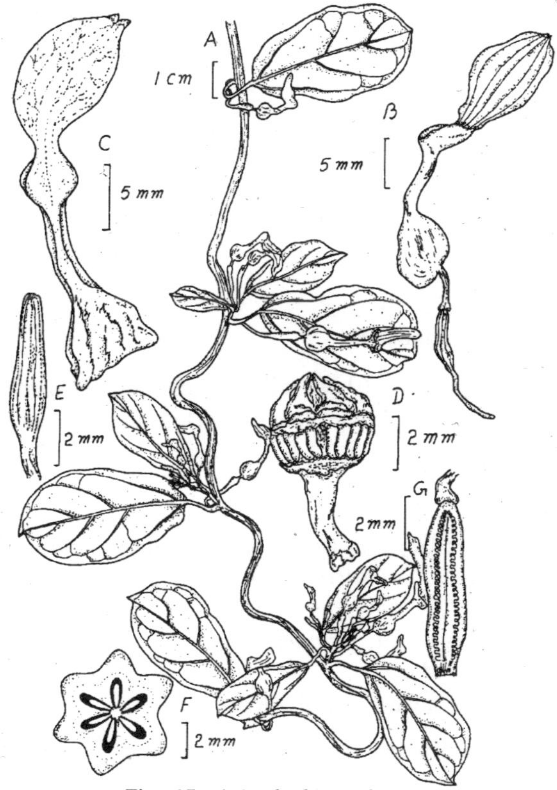


Fig. 17: *Aristolochia indica* L.
A. Twig; B. Flower; C. Perianth; D. Stylar column with stamens; E. Anther; F. T.S of ovary; G. L.S. of ovary.

suddenly narrowed into a cylindric tube. Fruit capsule, oblong, 6-valved, opening from below upwards, seeds many, laterally winged.

Found growing throughout India, in the plains and low hills.

Fl.: & Fr.: September–March.

Sanskrit: Eswari, Sunanda, Arkamula.

Local names: *Ben* & *Hin*: Isarmul, Isharmul; *Guj*: Arkamul, Nirvel, Sapasan; *Kan*: Eashwari-beru; *Mal*: Ishwara-mulli, Karalakam; *Mar*: Kadula; *Tam*: Garuda-kkodi; Paerum kizhagu; *Urdu*: Shapesand. *Tel*: Eswari.

Trade name: Serpent root plant, Indian birth wort.

Uses: Whole plant useful in the treatment of diabetes.

**Armoracia rusticana** Gaertn.

Syn: *Armoracia lapathifolia* Gilib.
*Cochlearia armoracia* L.

Family: Brassicaceae

Perennial herb, up to 90cm tall, root thick, whitish, fleshy. Lower leaves oblong, upper leaves smaller, lanceolate. Flowers white in racemes. Fruit pod, globose, obovoid or ellipsoid.

Grown in hill stations.

Trade name: Horse-radish.

Uses: Root used in the treatment of diabetes.

**Artemisia absinthium** L.

Family: Asteraceae (Compositae)

Herb to semi-shrub, 60–120 cm tall, Leaves long petioled, silky pubescent on both sufaces, the lower leaves abrupt pinnate and upper ones simple. Flowers in capitula, yellow, fruit achene.

Cultivated.

Sanskrit: Indhana, Damar.

Local names: *Ben* & *Guj*: Mastaru; *Hin*: Vilayathi absinthin; *Kan*: Urittige, Uruvala; *Mal*: Nilampala, Tirunitripachcha; *Mar*: Serpana; *Tam*: Machi patri. *Tel*: Machapatri.

Trade name: Worm wood, Madder wood

Propagation: by seeds.

Parts used: Flower heads, aerial shoots, leaves.

Uses: Plant useful for the treatment of diabetes.

**Artemesia dracunculus** L.

Family: Asteraceae

Perennial, erect herb. Leaves linear or linear-oblong. Flower in terminal heads

Found in alpine regions of Kashmir and Western Himalayas.

Trade name: Dragon mugwort, Estragon, Tarragon.

Uses: Aerial part is used to treat diabetes mellitus.

**Artemesia nilagirica** (Clarke) Pamp.

Syn: *Artemesia vulgaris* auct non L.

Family: Asteraceae (Compositae).

More or less slender, hoary pubescent or tomentose herbs, 1–1.5m tall. Leaves large, ovate-elliptic or prominently lobed, or incised, laciniate. Flowers in heads.

Deccan peninsula, Maharashtra, Karnataka, Tamil Nadu and Kerala.

Sanskrit: Barha Grnthika, Vishirnakhya.

Local names: Garhwal: Kunja; *Hin*: Dona, Gathirome, Magtari, Nugduna, Samri; *Mal*: Makkippuvu, Masipatri; *Mar*: Gathona, Surband, Nagdona; *Ori*: Donoya, Gondhoinaro; *Tam*: Mashibattiri, Tirunama; *Tel*: Davanamu, Machipatri.

Trade name: Indian wormwood, Fleabane.

Uses: Whole plant useful in the treatment of diabetes.

**Artocarpus communis** J.R. & G. Forst

Syn: *Artocarpus altilis* (Park.) Fosberg
*Artocarpus incisus* L.f.

Family: Moraceae.

Tall tree, up to 35m tall. Leaves pinnatifid, rhomboid, elliptic or ovate. Flowers unisexual, male in catkins, female in thick club shaped structures. Fruit syncarp, ellipsoid or globose.

Cultivated in South India.

Trade name: The bread fruit.

Uses: Plant useful in treatment of diabetes

**Artocarpus heterophyllus** Lam.

Syn: *Artocarpus integrifolius* auct. non L.f.

Family: Moraceae.

A large evergreen tree, bark black mottled green, smooth. Leaves oblong, coriaceous, dark green. Inflorescence cauliflorous and also from the main branches, tender heads enclosed by glabrous leafy scales which fall off leaving annular scars at base. Fruit very large, elliptic-oblong, covered with spinous projections, seeds smooth, ovoid.

Cultivated throughout hotter parts of india, indigeneous to evergreen forests of Western Ghats.

Fl. & Fr.: January–July.

Sanskrit: Panasah.

Local names: *Ass*, *Ben* & *Hin*: Kanthal; *Guj*: Vanas; *Hin*: Chakki, Kathar, Kotal, Panos, Panasa; *Kan*: Halasina, Halasu, Kantakapha, Kujje, Kuvi, Guffa panash, Tage; *Mal*: Chakka, Palava Itichchakka, Kandakiphala, Pilava, Varikka; *Mar*: Panas, Phanas; *Ori*: Ichdopholo, Kontokalo, Panasa; *Tam*: Murasambalam, Palasu Pagal, Palavu, Panasam, Vasukkou, Varukkai, Pila, Verappala; *Tel*: Panasa; *Urdu*: Katajal.

Trade name: Jack fruit tree.

Uses: Leaves useful in the treatment of diabetes.

**Arundo donax** L.

Family: Poaceae (Gramineae)

Tall, perennial grass, up to 5m tall, rhizomes creeping. Leaves linear-lanceolate. Spikelets in panicles, silky hairy. Fruit oblong.

Throughout plains.

Fl. & Fr.: July–December

Sanskrit: Kadi laka

Local names: *Ben*: Gaha nal; *Hin*: Baranal; *Tam*: Korukkai; *Tel*: Adavikeekasa gaddi

Uses: Aerial parts useful in the treatment of diabetes.

**Asparagus gonocladus** Baker

Family: Liliaceae

Much branched, subscandent, armed undershrub. Cladodes flat. Flowers white in paniculate racemes. Fruit berry, red when ripe.

Peninsular India, Gujarat and Bihar.

Local names: *Ben*: Satmuli; *Guj*: Shatvari; *Hin*: Shakakul; *Kan*: Majjigagadde; *Mal*: Shatavali; *Mar*: Satavarimul; *Tam*: Kilavari; *Tel*: Challagaddalu; Pillipichara.

Uses: Use of tuberous root powder mixing with leaf powder of *Gymnema sylvestre* twice per day lowers blood glucose level.

**Astragalus candolleanus** Royle

Family: Fabaceae (Papilionaceae)

Low, rigid, decumbent, perennial shrub.
Found in the western Himalayas.
Local names: *Hin*: Rudanti, Rudrawanti.

Uses: Whole plant used to treat diabetes.

**Atropa belladonna** L.

Family: Solanaceae

Erect, glandular-pubescent, perennial herb, 60–90cm tall, with creeping root stock. Leaves petiolate, ovate-lanceolate. Flowers large, bell-shaped, pale purple, tinged yellow or green, in axils of leaves, solitary or in pairs. Fruit globose berry, purple-black, surrounded at the base by the enlarged, spreading calyx, many-seeded.

It is found in Kashmir at altitudes of 2000 to 3500m, also cultivated in western Himalayas from Simla to Kashmir between 1800m and 3000m.

Local names: *Ben*: Yebruj; *Hin*: Angurshafa, Sagangur; *Kashmiri*: Sagangur; *Pun*: Suchi.

Trade name: Deadly nightshade, Belladonna.

Propagation: By seeds.

Uses: Leaves have antidiabetic properties.

**Avena fatua** L.

Family: Poaceae

Annual grass, up to 1.5m tall. Leaves scaberulous. Spikelets in panicles, awned.

In Plains and hills of North India, Sikkim and Meghalaya.

Local names: *Hin*: Ganer, Kuljud; *Pun*: Ganer jei, upwa.

Trade name: Wild oat.

Uses: Whole plant useful in the treatment of diabetes.

**Avena sativa** L.

Family: Poaceae

Annual grass. Leaves linear-lanceolate.
Cultivated in hill stations.
Trade name: Oats.

Uses: Seeds useful in the treatment of diabetes.

**Averrhoa carambola** L.

Family: Averrhoaceae

Evergreen tree, up to 8m tall, bark smooth. Leaves imparipinnate, leaflets ovate-oblong, elliptic or lanceolate. Flowers pink or purple in axillary panicles. Fruit berry, yellow or golden-brown, oblong, seeds arillate.

Cultivated in gardens.

Fl. & Fr.: June–November.

Sanskrit: Brihaddala, Dharaphala.

Local names: *Ben*: Kamarak, Kamranga; *Guj*: Kamarakha; *Hin*: Kamaranga, Kamrak, Karmal; *Kan*: Kamarakshi; *Mal*: Chaturpuli, Pulicchi; *Mar*: Kamarakha, Karmare; *Tam*: Tamarathai, Tamratta; *Tel*: Kamarak, Karmel, Tamarts.

Trade name: Carambola apple, Coromandel gooseberry.

Propagation: By seeds

**Azadirachta indica** A.Juss.

Syn: *Melia azadirachta* L.

Family: Meliaceae

Medium sized tree, up to 15m tall, bark brown with vertical furrows. Leaves pinnate, leaflets 6–10 pairs, oblique. Flowers white in axillary panicles. Fruit one-seeded drupe, Yellow when ripe, seeds ellipsoid, cotyledons thick, fleshy, oily.

Common all over India both in plains and forests.

Fl.& Fr.: March–April, Fruits ripen from May–July.

Sanskrit: Picumarda, Nimbah.

Local names: *Ben & Hin*: Nim; *Mal*: Vepa; *Kan*: Bevu, Bevina, Olle Bevu; *Mal*: Veppu, Arya veppu; *Mar & Guj*: Limba, Nimbay; *Tam*: Vembu, Veppam; *Tel*: Vepa, Yapa.

Trade name: Neem Tree, Margosa tree.

Propagation: The plant can be propagated through seeds in all types of soils. It grows best in places with 50–70 cm rainfall and temperature of 20–43$^{o}$ C.

Uses: Leaves and seeds have antidiabetic properties.

**Balanites aegyptiaca** (L.) Del.

Syn: *Balanites roxburghii* Planch.
*Ximenia aegyptiaca* L.

Family: Balanitaceae

Small tree, up to 4m tall. Leaves 2-foliolate, leaflets elliptic-ovate or oblong. Flowers whitish, axillary or supra axillary, pseudoumbels. Fruit drupe, ashy green, elliptic-oblong or ovoid.

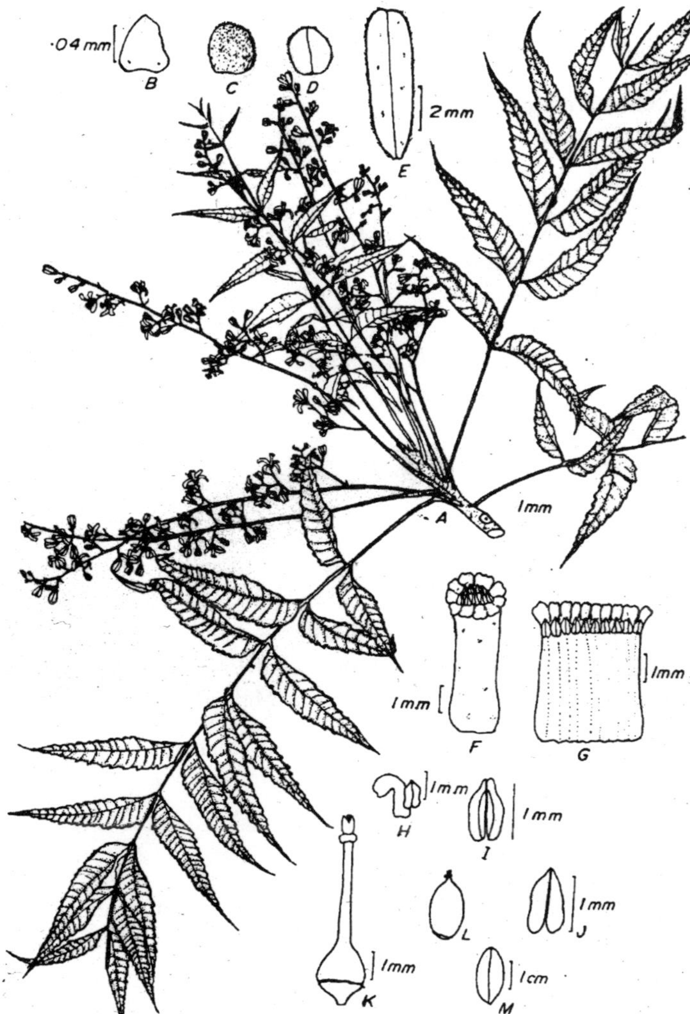


Fig. 18: *Azadirachta indica* A. Juss.
A. Twig; B–D. Sepals; E. Petal; F. & G. Staminal column whole and spread out; H. Staminal column lobe with anther; I. & J. Anthers; K. Pistil; L. Fruit; M. Seed.

Almost throughout India.
Fl. & Fr.: September–July.

Uses: Fruit is used to treat Diabetes.

**Bambusa arundinacea** (Retz.) Willd.

Syn: *Bambos arundinacea* Retz.

*Bambusa bambos* (L.) Voss
*Arundo bambos* L.

Family: Poaceae (Gramineae)

Large thorny shrub, culms thick, erect, 9–30m tall, internodes hollow. Leaf sheaths hairy, blade trigonous, broad. Inflorescence a pseudopanicle of spiklets, clustered in heads, spicate branchlets.

Occasional in forests throughout India.

Fl. & Fr.: Very infrequent

Sanskrit: Vamsah, Tawaksiri.

Local names: *Ben*: Bans, Behar, Katausi; *Guj*: Wans; *Hin*: Kanta Bans; *Kan*: Andebidiru, Habbidiru; *Mal*: Illi, Mulla; *Mar*: Bambu, Mandga; *Ori*: Bendo, Kontobanso; *Tam*: Mullumungil; *Tel*: Veduru.

Trade name: Thorny bamboo.

Uses: Whole plant has antidiabetic properties.

**Bambusa nutans** Wall. ex Munro

Family: Poaceae.

Moderate sized, bamboo, up to 15m tall.

Found from Himachal Pradesh to Arunachal Pradesh and Meghalaya.

Local names: *Ben*: Makla, Nal Bans; *Hin*: Mala Bans;

Uses: Aerial parts useful in the treatment of diabetes.

**Bambusa vulgaris** Schrad. ex Wendl.

Family: Poaceae.

Moderate sized bamboo, up to 18m tall, culms bright green or striped green and yellow. Leaves linear-lanceolate. Spikelets in bracteate cluster.

Found in warmer parts.

Local names: *Ben*: Basini bans; *Mar*: Kalaka; *Ori*: Sundrogai; *Tam*: Ponmungil.

Uses: Leaves useful in the treatment of diabetes.

**Barleria cristata** L.

Family: Acanthaceae.

Undershrub, up to 1m tall. Leaves elliptic–lanceolate. Flowers purplish-pink, violet or white, in axillary or terminal racemes. Fruit capsule.

Found throughout India.

Fl. & Fr.: September–February.

Uses: Whole plant useful in the treatment of diabetes.

**Barleria prionitis** L.

Family: Acanthaceae.

A spinous bushy undershrub, about 1m tall, axillary spines 2–4, white, young shoots pubescent. Leaves elliptic-ovate, glabrescent. Flowers subsessile, solitary or in cymose clusters in lower axils. Fruit capsule, ovoid.

In waste lands and road sides.

Fl. & Fr.: September–January.

Sanskrit: Bindi, Mridukanta, Vajradanti.

Local names: *Ben & Ori*: Kanta jali; *Guj*: Kanta-shelio; *Hin*: Jhinti, Kat Sreya, Jhinti, Piyabasa; *Kan*: Mullu gorante; *Mar*: Pivali koranti: *Ori*: Daskeanta; *Mal & Tam*: Shemmuli; *Tel*: Mullugorinta.

Trade name: Common yellow nail Dye.

Propagation: by seeds

Uses: Whole plant useful in the treatment of diabetes.

**Barringtonia acutangula** (L.) Gaertn.

Syn: *Eugenia acutangula* L.

Family: Barringtoniaceae-Lecythidaceae.

Evergreen tree, up to 10m tall, trunk short, bark thick, dark grey, distinctly furrowed on old trees, branchlets densely pubescent. Leaves thin-coriaceous, oblanceolate-ovate. Flowers pale pink or red in axillary, pendulous, spicate racemes. Fruit berry, ovoid with persistent calyx tube. Seed solitary, ovoid.

Common in plains along streams and swamp forests.

Fl.: April–June, Fr.: December–January.

Sanskrit: Hinjar.

Local names: *Ass*: Kanapa; *Ben*: Hijal, Kumia; *Guj*: Samudraphal; *Hin*: Hijal Hyal, Hyar, Hifful, Sanebdar phal; *Kan*: Holekauva, Mavikubia; *Mal*:Attampu attupera *Mar*: Dattaphal; *Ori*: Hinjal, Hijal; *Tam*: Kadappay, Adampai, Samuthiraphal; *Tel*: Kanapa, Kurpa.

Trade name: Indian oak, Small Indian Oak.

Uses: Root useful in the treatment of diabetes.

**Bauhinia purpurea** L.

Syn: *Phanera purpurea* (L.) Benth.

Family: Caesalpiniaceae.

Densely foliaceous tree, up to 12m tall, bark grey to brown. Leaves oblong or suborbicular, leaflets connate about half-way up. Flowers large, purple or white. Fruit pod, linear-oblong.

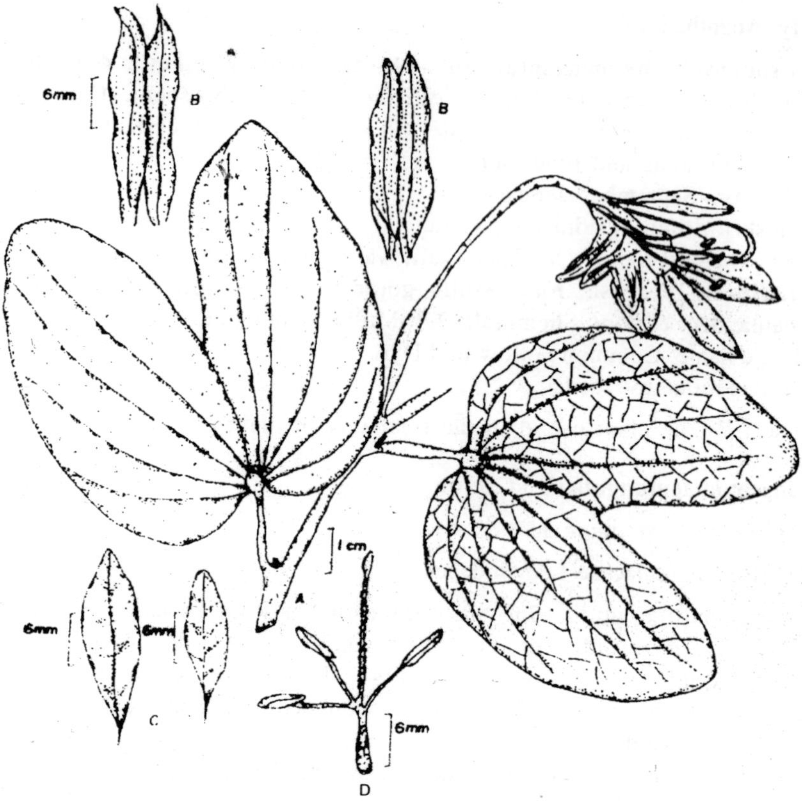


Fig. 19: *Bauhinia purpurea* L.
A. Twig; B. Sepals; C. Petals; D. Pistil with stamens.

Throughout India, often cultivated.

Fl. & Fr.: October–March.

Local names: *Ben*: Deva–Kanchan, Rakta kanchan; *Hin*: Khairwal; *Kan*: Baswonapada, sarul; *Mal*: Chuvanna-mandaram; *Mar*: Atmatti; *Tam*: Mandari, Segappumandari, *Tel*: Kanchanam.

Propagation: By seeds.

Uses: Leaves useful in the treatment of diabetes.

**Bauhinia semla** Wunderlin.

Syn: *Bauhinia retusa* Ham. ex Roxb.

Family: Caesalpiniaceae

Deciduous tree. Leaves broader than long. Leaves with two leaflets, palmately nerved. Flowers yellow with purple streaks in terminal panicles. Fruit pod, flattened.

Found in greater part of India.

Fl. & Fr.: September–February.

Uses: Seeds used for treating diabetes.

**Bauhinia variegata** L.

Family: Caesalpiniaceae

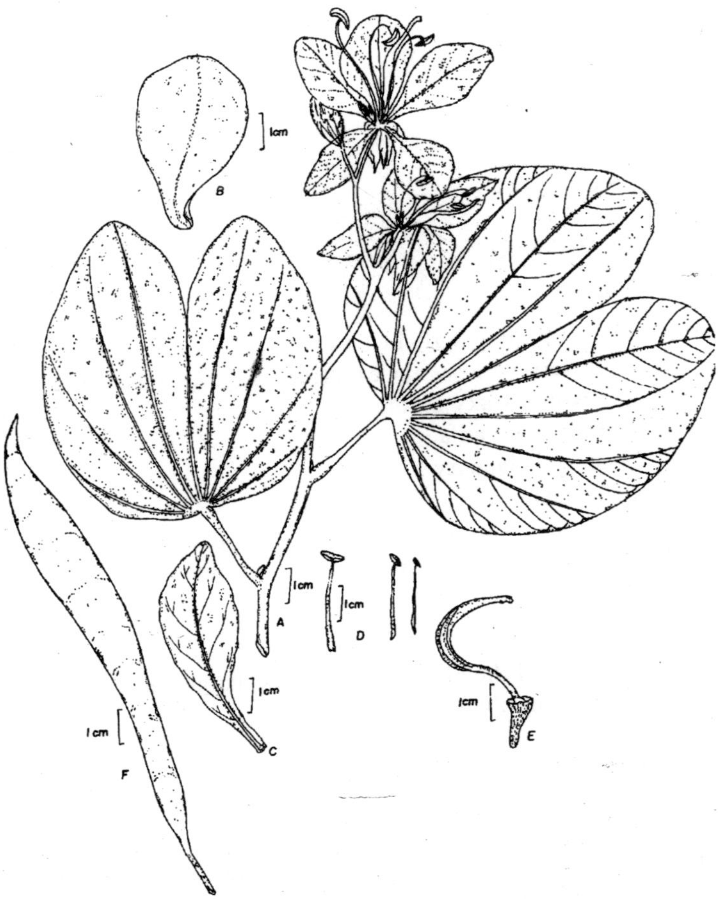


Fig. 20: *Bauhinia variegata* L.
A. Twig; B. Sepal; C. Petal; D. Stamens; E. Pistil; F. Pod.

Deciduous tree, up to 13m tall, bark grey, longitudinally cracked. Leaves ovate, leaves bilobed, leaflets connate about two thirds, thin coriaceous. Flowers large, white or pink or purple with one petal variegated yellow in short racemes. Fruit linear-oblong pod, brown, flat, dehiscent.

Occasional in forests, often cultivated.

Fl. & Fr.: February–May.

Sanskrit: Kavidara.

Local names: *Ben*: Rakta Kanchan; *Hin*: Barial, Gurial, Gwiar, Kachnar, Kandan, Kaniar, Khairwal, Koliar, Kural, Poarinana; *Kan*: Arsinantige, Ayata, Bilikanjival, Irkubalitu, Kanchavala; *Mal*: Kovidaram, Chuvannamandaram, Unna; *Mar*: Kanchan, Rakta Kanchan, Kanraj, Kavidara, Thur; *Ori*: Boroda, Kosonara, Kanjonu, Rongakonjonu; *Tam*: Mandarai, Segappumandarai, Segappu manchori, Vellaippuvatti; *Tel*: Devakanchanamu, Kanjaramu, Madapaku; *Urdu*: Kachnal.

Trade name: Mountain Ebony.

Propagation: By seeds.

Uses: Floweres useful in treating diabetes.

**Benincasa hispida** (Thunb.) Cogn.

Syn: *Benincasa cerifera* Savi

Family: Cucurbitaceae

Large climbing or trailing herb. Leaves large, 5–7-lobed, reniform-rotund, hispid beneath. Flowers yellow, unisexual, axillary, solitary. Fruit broadly cylindric, covered with a waxy bloom.

Cultivated throughout India

Fl. & Fr.: Decemebr–January.

Sanskrit: Kusmandah

Local names: *Ben*: Chalkumra; *Guj*: Bhurukohlu; *Hin*: Kumbra, Panikumhra, Petha; *Kan*: Budikumbala; *Mal*: Kum palam; *Mar*: Kohala; *Tam*: Pusanikkai; *Tel*: Budida gummadi

Propagation: By seeds

Uses: Various parts of the plant are valued in indigenous medicine. The fruits are useful in curing diabeties.

**Berberis aristata** DC.

Family: Berberidaceae

Armed shrubs, 1–3m tall, spines solitary towards apex, 2–3-fid at base. Leaves obovate to elliptic-obovate. Flowers in racemes. Fruit ovoid or oblong-ovoid berry, bright red.

In Garhwal Himalayas in Uttaranchal.

Sanskrit: Daruharidra

Local names: *Ben*: Dfar haldi; *Hin*: Chitra, Darhald, Rasaut; *Mar*: Daruhald.

Trade name: Indian barberry.

Uses: Root useful in the treatment of diabetes.

**Berberis vulgaris** L

Syn: *Berberis callibotrys* Aitch. ex Koehne

Family: Berberidaceae

Shrub, up to 3m tall, stem red brown to pale brown. Leaves simple, oblong-obovate, spinose. Flowers yellow. Friuit globose to obovoid berry, black.

Cultivated.

Trade name: Europaen barberry.

Propagation: By seeds and by layering

Uses: Stem bark useful in the treatment of diabetes.

**Bergenia stracheyi** (Hook.f. & Thoms.) Engl.

Syn: *Saxifraga stracheyi* Hook.f. & Thoms.
*Saxifraga ciliata* Lindl.

Family: Saxifragaceae

Perennial herb. Leaves obovate. Flowers many, fragrant, white with a pink tinge or purple in compact inflorescence.

Found from Kashmir to Uttaranchal.

Uses: Root is used in the treatment of diabetes.

**Beta vulgaris** L.

Family: Chenopodiaceae.

Annual or biennial tuberous herb with condensed stem. Leaves simple in rosette, ovate. Flowers 2–3 in a cluster on long slender spike, appearing in the second year.

Cultivated in many parts of India.

Sanskrit: Palakya.

Local names: *Ben*: Bitepalang; *Hin*: Palak, Chukkandar, *Kan*: Biturutu; *Mal*: Bittruttu, Neycira, *Tam*: Cenciral; *Tel*: Bitrutu.

Trade name: Beet root.

Propagation: By seeds.

Uses: Aerial parts and root useful in the treatment of diabetes.

**Bidens pilosa** L.

Family: Asteraceae (Compositae)

Annual erect herb, up to 50cm tall. Leaves trifoliolate, segments ovate-lanceolate. Flowers yellow in terminal heads. Fruit achene, black.
Occasional through out India in Hills.
Fl. & Fr.: November–February
Propagation: By seeds.

Uses: Plant showed hypoglycemic activity.

**Biophytum nervifolium** Thw.

Syn: *Biophytum sensitivum* DC.

Family: Oxalidaceae

Annual unbranched herb. Leaves radical, paripinnate, leaflets 8–10 pairs, oblong, glabrous. Flowers red, orange, yellow in terminal umbels. Fruit capsule, oblong-ovoid. Seeds prominently ridged.
Common weed in waste lands, cultivated fields, rare in forests throughout the tropical regions of India.
Fl. & Fr.: September–December.
Sanskrit: Lajjalu, Jalapushpa.
Local names: *Ben*: Jhalai; *Guj*: Jharera; *Hin*: Lajalu, Laksmana; *Kan*: Haramuni, Jalapushpa; *Mal*: Mukkutti; Nilaccurunki, Tintanali; *Mar*: Ladjou, Lahanamulki; *Tel*: Pulichinta.

Uses: Plant useful in the treatment of diabetes.

**Bixa orellana** L.

Family: Bixaceae.

Evergreen tree, up to 5m tall, young branches densely, dark silky. Leaves cordate, coriaceous, glabrous on both surfaces. Flowers purplish, large in terminal panicles, showy, fragrant. Fruit reddish brown capsule, ovoid, soft bristly, seeds trigonous.
Cultivated for its dye.
Sanskrit: Sinduri.
Local names: *Ass*: Jarat, Jolandar; *Ben*: Latkan, Watkanna; *Guj*: Sinduri; *Hin*: Latkan, Latkhar, Vatkhana, Sindhuria; *Kan*: Arnattu, Kesari, Bangrakayi, Rangmalle, Sannjabhale; *Mal*: Kuppamannal; *Mar*: Kisri, Sendri; *Ori*: Gulbas, Guliabha, Japhoran, Latkons; *Tam*: Amudadaram, Avam, Varagumanjal; *Tel*: Jaffra.

Trade name: Annotto.
Propagation: By seeds.

Uses: Aerial parts and seeds useful in the treatment of diabetes.

**Boenninghausenia albiflora** Reichb. ex Meissn.

Syn: *Ruta albiflora* Hook.

Family: Rutaceae

Slender, erect, perennial herb, up to 60cm tall. Leaves 3–4-pinnate, leaflets obovate or obcordate. Flowers white in terminal, leafy cymose panicles. Seeds black.

Found in Himalayas form Kashmir to Arunachal Pradesh, Meghalaya and Mizoram.

Uses: Whole plant useful in the treatment of diabetes.

**Bombax ceiba** L.

Syn: *Bombax malabaricum* DC.
*Salmalia malabarica* (DC.) Schott.& Endl.

Family: Bombacaceae.

Tall decidous tree, up to 30m tall, armed with prickles, bark greyish, smooth. Leaves crowded at the ends of branches, digitately 5–7-foliolate, glabrous. Flowers large, solitary or paired, bright crimson. Fruit capsule, oblong. Seeds many, enveloped by dense white silky floss.

Along streams in deciduous forests, often cultivated.

Fl.: February–April, Fr.: ripen from March to May.

Sanskrit: Nirgandha pushpi, Panchaparni.

Local names: *Ben*: Pagun, Roktosimul, Simul; *Guj*: Sawar, Shimalo; *Hin*: Semul, Ragatsemal; *Kan*: Elava, Booruga; *Mal*: Elavu, Mullilavu; *Mar*: Kantesavar, Savar; *Ori*: Simuli nuagarh; *Tam*: Mulilavu, Ilavu; *Tel*; Buruga.

Trade name: Red silk cotton Tree.

Propagation: By seeds.

Uses: Flowers and stem bark useful in the treatment of diabetes.

**Borassus flabellifer** Murr.

Syn: *Borassus flabelliformis* Murr.

Family: Arecaceae (Palmae).

A tree with tall stem, up to 40m tall. Leaves simple, palmately fan shaped, plicate, petiole stout, spinous. Flowers unisexual, dioecious (male and female plants separate). Fruit a large subglobose drupe, yellow when ripe with 1–3 fibrous pyrenes.

Common in coastal regions, occasional inland.

Fl. & Fr.: February–April.

Sanskrit: Tala, Tadarumah.

Local names: *Ben*: Tal, Talgacchi; *Guj*: Tad; *Hin*: Tal, Tar; *Kan*: Tale, Pane; *Mal*: Karimapana, Pana; *Mar*: Tad, Tamas; *Ori*: Talo, Tanlo, Trinorajo; *Tam*: Etakam; *Tel*: Tadichettu.

Trade name: Palmyra palm.

Propagation: By seeds.

Uses: Sap useful in the treatment of diabetes.

**Borreria verticillata** (L.) G.F.W.Mey

Family: Rubiaceae

Much branched perennial, up to 75cm tall. Leaves oblong-lanceolate. Flowers white in subterminal heads.

Introduced from Tropical America and now fairly common on waste lands in the Western Ghats of Karnataka.

Uses: Plant useful in the treatment of diabetes.

**Boswellia serrata** Roxb. ex Colebr.

Syn: *Boswellia glabra* Roxb.

Family: Burseraceae.

Large tree, up to 15m tall. Leaves apically clustered, imparipinnate, leaflets oblong to lanceolate. Flowers pale pink or white, in axillary panicles. Fruit drupe, greenish-yellow when ripe, 1-seeded.

North-West, Central and Peninsular India.

Fl. & Fr.: March–August.

Uses: Fruits, stem and gum useful in the treatment of diabetes.

**Bougainvillea spectabilis** Willd.

Family: Nyctaginaceae

Woody scandent or straggling shrub with stout spines. Leaves ovate. Bracts purple, pink or brick red. Flowers small, yellow, clustered at the ends of branches.

Often cultivated for its showy flowers throughout India.

Uses: Use of leaf paste twice per day helps in lowering blood glucose. Oral administration of the leaf juice (1 ml of juice = 1 gm of leaves) at the rate of 1g/kg/day for 14 days or more significantly reduced the hyperglycemic response in alloxan induced diabetes in rabbits.

**Brassica oleracea** L.

Family: Brassicaceae

Cultivated.

Uses: Leaf is used to treat diabetis mellitus

**Brassica rapa**

Family: Brassicaceae

Cultivated.

Uses: Root is useful in the treatment of diabetes.

**Bruguiera gymnorhiza** (L.) Lam.

Syn: *Bruguiera conjugata* Merr.
*Bruguiera eriopetala* Hemsl. *p.p.*

Family: Rhizophoraceae

Large ever green, buttressed tree, up to 36m tall. Leaves elliptic or elliptic-oblong, coriaceous. Flowers solitary, axillary. Fruit obconic, scarlet.

In Estuarine forests along coasts of India.

Uses: Aerial parts useful in the treatment of diabetes.

**Buchanania lanzan** Spreng.

Syn: *Buchanania latifolia* Roxb.

Family: Anacardiaceae.

Evergreen tree, up to 10m tall, bark dark grey, fissured. Leaves broadly oblong-ovate, glabrescent above, slightly villous beneath. Flowers creamish in axillary and terminal villous panicles. Fruit globose drupe, black, seeds 1 or 2.

Occasional in deciduous forests.

Fl. & Fr.: January–May.

Sanskrit: Tapasya-priya.

Local names: *Ben*: Pival, Chironji; *Hin*: Piyar, Achar; *Kan*: Murkial, Morave; *Mal*: Mural, Munnapelu Mungapera; *Guj & Mar*: Chironji, Charoli; *Ori*: Charee; *Tam*: Morala, Modama; *Tel*: Sarapappu, Morli, Chinna morli.

Tarde name: Almondette tree, Cheronjee.

Propagation: by seeds.

Uses: Powder of leaf or seed helps in controlling glucose levels at early stage of diabetes.

**Buddleja officinalis** Maxin.

Family: Buddlejaceae; Loganiaceae

Evergreen tree or semideciduous shrub, up to 10m tall. Leaves long, entire or fine-toothed. Flowers lilac in panicles, fragrant.

Reported to occur in Bihar.

Uses: Plant used to treat diabetes.

**Bupleurum falcatum** L.

Family: Apiaceae.

Erect, variable, perennial herb, up to 1.2m tall. Leaves linear to oblong-lanceolate or spathulate. Flowers yellow. Fruit oblong, brown.

In Himalayas from Kashmir to Bhutan.

Trade name: Hare's ear.

Uses: Root is used to treat Diabetes mellitus.

**Butea monosperma** (Lam.) Taub.

Syn: *Erythrina monosperma* Lam.
*Butea frondosa* Koen.ex Roxb.

Family: Fabaceae (Papilionaceae).

Small to medium sized deciduous tree, trunk crooked and irregular, bark grey or dark brown, rough, branchlets tawny tomentose. Leaves trifoliolate, lateral leaflets rhomboid, terminal leaflet ovate. Flowers flame coloured or scarlet. The tree is leafless when flowering. Fruit pod, velvety brown, base wing like, indehiscent with out seeds. Seeds compressed, brownish.

Throughout India except Jammu & Kashmir and Arunachal Pradesh.

Sanskrit: Palasah.

Local names: *Ben*: Palas; *Guj*: Khakra; *Hin*: Chinchra, Desuka jhad, Dhak, Kakria; *Kan*: Muttala, Mutthuga; *Mal*: Brahmabriksham, Kinshukam, Puppulas, Shamata; *Mar*: Palas, Parasa; *Tel*: Moduga; Palashpapra.

Trade name: Flame of the forest, Bengal king.

Uses: Leaves useful in the treatment of diabetes.

**Caesalpinia bonduc** (L.) Roxb.

Syn: *Guilandinia bonduc* L.
*Caesalpinia crista* L.
*Caesalpinia bonducella* Flem.

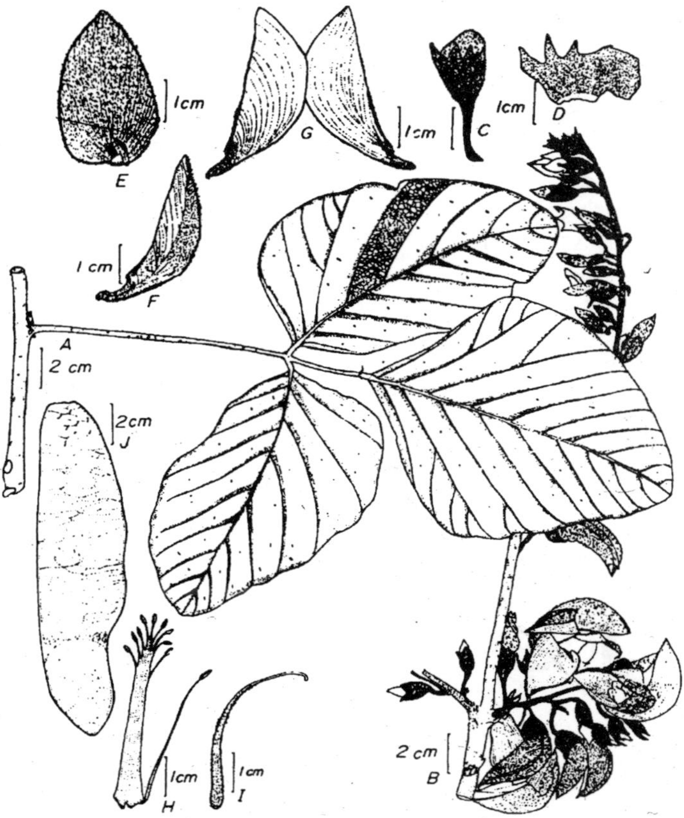


Fig. 21: *Butea monosperma* (Lam.) Taub.
A. Vegetative twig; B. Flowering twig; C. Calyx; D. Calyx split open; E. Standard petal; F. Wing petal; G. Keel petal; H. Staminal column split open; I. Pistil; J. Pod.

Family: Caesalpiniaceae

Armed straggler, prickles recurved, branchlets densely pubescent. Leaves bipinnate, pinnae 6–7 pairs, leaflets 6–8 pairs per pinna, elliptic-oblong. Flowers in axillary racemes, yellow. Fruit pod, oblong, strongly prickled, 1–2-seeded. Seed subglobose.

Occasional in plains in hedges and waste lands.

Fl. & Fr.: June–November.

Sanskrit: Kuberakshi.

Local names: *Ben*: Nata; *Hin*: Kanja, Karanju; *Kan*: Gajagakayi; *Mal*: Kazhan chikkuru; *Mar*: Gajaga, Sagargoto; *Tam*: Avil, Gujju; *Tel*: Gacchakaya.

Trade name: Fever nut, Bonduc nut.

Uses: Plant useful in the treatment of diabetes.

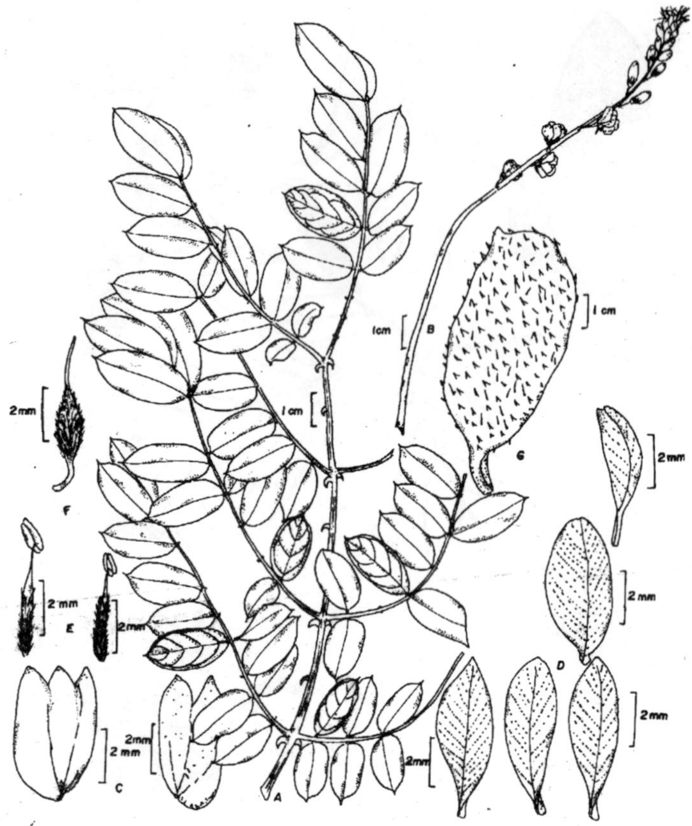


Fig. 22: *Caesalpinia bonduc* L.
A. Twig; B. Inflorescence; C. Sepals; D. Petals; E. Stamens; F. Pistil; G. Pod.

**Caesalpinia coriaria** (Jacq.) Willd.

Family: Caesalpiniaceae

Unarmed tree, up to 15m tall. Leaves pinnate, pinnae 3–9 pairs, leaflets about 20 pairs, oblong. Flowers greenish yellow in terminal panicles. Fruit pod, twisted.

Cultivated and naturalized.

Fl.: May–June; Fr: August–Novemeber.

Trade name: American sumac.

Local names: *Kan*: Vilayatialdekayi; *Tam*: Konapali in Kimaram; *Tel*: Divi divi.

Uses: Aerial parts used in the treatment of diabetes.

**Caesalpinia cucullata** Roxb.

Family: Caesalpiniaceae

Large, woody, prickly, climbing shrub. Leaves bipinnate, pinnae 2–5 pairs, leaflets 3–5 pairs, ovate-elliptic. Flowers bright yellow or orange in terminal or axillary panicles. Fruit pod, flat.

Almost throughout India.

Local names: *Kan*: Mulloduballi; *Mal*: Kakakalingivalli; *Tam*: Indumatticcingai; *Tel*: Gabbusikaya.

Uses: Aerial parts used in the treatment of diabetes.

**Caesalpinia digyna** Rottl.

Family: Caesalpiniaceae

Much branched prickly climbing shrubs. Leaves bipinnate, pinnae 8–10 pairs, leaflets 8–10 pairs. Flowers pale yellow with red streaks in supra axillary racemes. Fruit pod, torulose.

East Himalayas, Assam, Bihar, Tripura, West Bengal, Orissa, Andhra Pradesh and Tamil Nadu.

Fl. & Fr.: August–March.

Local names: *Ben*: Amal kochi, Umul Kuchi; *Hin & Mar*: Vakerimul; *Tel*: Nanigatcha. *Ori*: Gilo.

Trade name: Teri pods.

Uses: Root used in the treatment of diabetes mellitus.

**Cajanus cajan** (L.) Millsp.

Syn: *Cajanus indicus* Speng.
*Cytisus cajan* L.

Family: Fabaceae (Papilionaceae)

Erect, much branched bushy shrub, up to 3m tall. Leaves 3-foliolate, leaflets elliptic-oblong, soft pubescent. Flowers yellow in terminal panicles. Fruit pod, compressed between seeds, pubescent, seeds 3–5, red to brown.

Cultivated throughout India.

Fl. & Fr.: October–March.

Sanskrit: Adhaki, Tuvari

Local names: *Ben, Hin & Mar*: Arhar, Tuvar; *Kan*: Togari, *Mal*: Tuvara, Tuvarapparippu, *Tam*: Tuvarai; *Tel*: Kandulu.

Trade name: Red gram, Pigeon pea, Arhar.

Propagation: By seeds.

Uses: Seeds useful in the treatment of diabetes.

**Cajanus crassus** (Prain & King) Van der Maesen

Syn: *Atylosia crassus* Prain & King
*Atylosia mollis* Benth.
*Atylosia volubilis* (Blanco) Gamble

Family: Fabaceae (Papilionaceae)

Suffruticose climber, up to 5m long. Leaves 3-foliolate, leaflets rhomboid-ovate. Flowers yellow, in axillary panicled racemes. Fruit pod, depressed between seeds.

Western Himalaya, Terai region, peninsula, central and Eastern India, Andaman Islands.

Uses: Aerial parts used to treat diabetes.

**Calamintha umbrosa** Fisch & Mey.

Family: Lamiaceae( Labiatae)

Profusely branched, slender herb. Leaves ovate or ovate-lanceolate. Flowers light pink with purple streaks, sometimes white in dense whorls. Fruit nutlet.

Temperate Himalayas from Kashmir to Bhutan and hills of Kerala, Tamil Nadu and Karnataka.

Uses: Whole plant used in the treatment of diabetes.

**Calendula officinlis** L.

Family: Asteraceae (Compositae)

Aromatic, erect, annual herb, up to 60 cm tall. Leaves lower spathulate, upper lanceolate. Flowers bright orange-yellow in terminal heterogamous heads. Fruit achene.

Cultivated in India

Local names: *Hin*: Zergul; *Tam*: Thulukka samanthi.

Trade name: Calendula, Pot marigold.

Propagation: By seeds.

Uses: Plant useful in the treatment of diabetes.

**Calotropis gigantea** (L.) R.Br.

Syn: *Asclepias gigantea* L.

Family: Asclepiadaceae.

Soft white woolly shrubs, up to 2m tall, latex milky. Leaves decussate, obovate-oblong, sparsely pubescent. Flowers purplish in axillary and terminal umbellate cymes. Fruits paired follicles, oblong, inflated. Seeds oblong with white silky coma.

Common weed of wastelands and cultivated fields all over India in plains.

Fl. & Fr.: Through out the year.

Sanskrit: Arkah, Aditya.

Local names: *Ben*: Akand, Gurtakand, Swetakand; *Guj*: Akado; *Hin*: Ag, Ak, Akand, Ark, Madar; *Kan*: Arka, Lekkedagide; *Mal*: Erukku, Vellerukku; *Mar*: Akand, Lal akra, Lal madar; *Ori*: Akondo, Kotuki; *Tam*: Erukkam, Verukku; *Tel*: Thella jilledu.

Trade name: Gigantic swallow wort.

Propagation: By seeds.

Uses: Roots are used to treat diabetes.

**Caltha palustris** L.

Syn: *Caltha govaniana* Wall.

Family: Ranunculaceae.

Perennial erect herb, up to 60cm tall. Leaves deltoid, reniform. Flowers bright yellow in corymbs. Fruit of follicles, seeds many, black.

Himalayas in damp places.

Fl. & Fr.: June–September.

Uses: Whole plant is used to treat diabetes.

**Calystegia hederacea** Wall.

Syn: *Calystegia japonica* (Thunb.) Miq.
*Convolvulus wallichianus* Spreng.

Family: Convolvulaceae

Annual or perennial herb, prostrate or climbing, up to 1.8m long. Leaves cordate or sagittate. Flowers solitary, axillary, pinkish purple. Fruit capsule, ovoid.

Found in plains of North India from Punjab to West Bengal.

Trade name: Japanese Bindweed.

Uses: Plant used in the treatment of diabetes.

**Camellia sinensis** (L.) O. Kuntze

Syn: *Camellia theifera* Griff.
*Thea sinensis* L.

Family: Theaceae

Evergreen shrub or tree, 9–15m tall (60–150 cm tall owing to pruning in cultivation). Leaves alternate, elliptic-ovate or lanceolate. Flowers white, fragrant, solitary or 2–4 together. Fruit depressed capsule, 3-seeded.

Cultivated in hilly regions in Assam, Darjeeling and South India.

Sanskrit: Syamaparni, Chaha.

Local names: *Ben & Hin*: Chay, Cha; *Guj*: Cha; *Kan*: Teyaku; *Mal*: Theyila; *Mar*: Chaha; *Ori*: Cha; *Tam*: Teyila; *Tel*: Teyaku.

Trade name: Tea plant.

Medicinal uses: Leaves useful in the treatment of diabetes.

**Campsis grandiflora** (Thunb.) K. Schum.

Syn: *Campsis chinensis* Voss.
*Tecoma grandiflora* Loises

Family: Bignoniaceae

Extensive creeping shrub, up to 9m long. Leaves compound, leaflets 7–9, oblong-lanceolate. Flowers large, scarlet.

Grown in gardens as ornamental.

Trade name: Chinese trumpet creeper.

Uses: The flowers are reported to be used in the treatment of diabetes.

**Canavalia gladiata** (Jacq.) DC.

Syn: *Dolichos gladiatus* Jacq.
*Canavalia ensiformis* auct.

Family: Fabaceae (Papilionaceae.)

Stout woody perennial or biennial twining shrubs, branches terete. Flowers purplish in axillary racemes. Fruit legume, thickened along both sutures, seeds 8–20, pink or red.

Two varieties, one wild (not edible) and another cultivated (edible) occur in India.

Fl.& Fr.: September–March.

Sanskrit: Maha-Shibee.

Local names: *Ben*: Makhan shim; *Guj*: Talavardi, Tarvardi; *Hin*: Lal kadsumbal; *Kan*: Shembi avare, Tumakai; *Mal*: Vaalamara, Vaal avara; *Mar*: Abai; *Tam*: Segappu thambattai; *Tel*: Thamba, Thamma.

Trade name: Jack Bean, Sword Bean.

Propagation: By seeds.

Uses: Seeds useful in the treatment of diabetes.

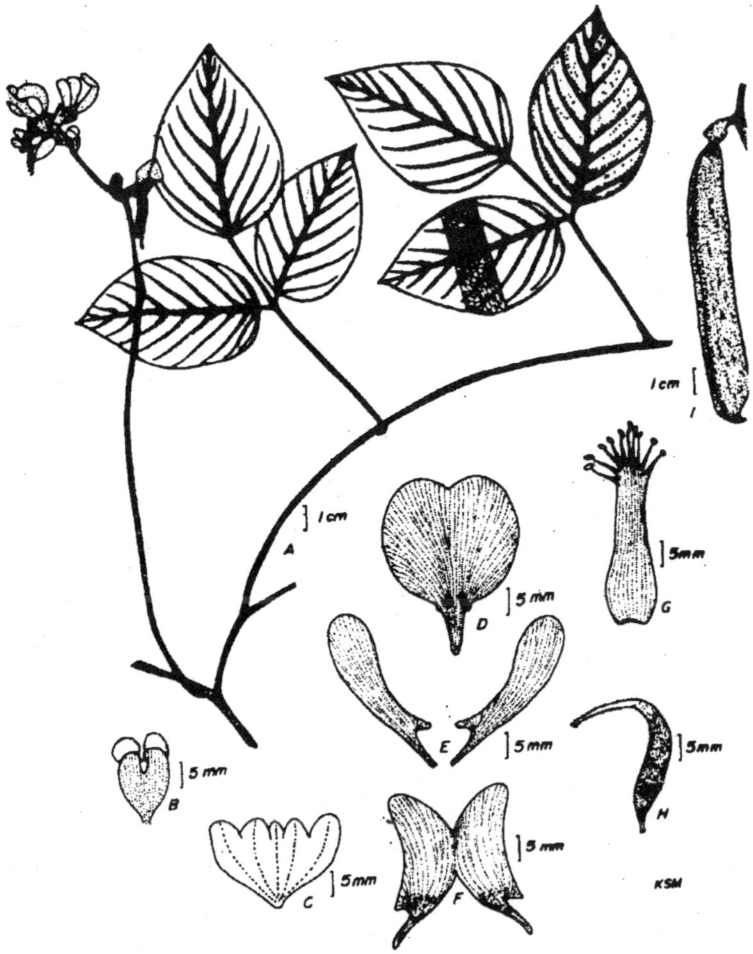


Fig. 23: *Canavalia gladiata* (Jacq.) DC.
A. Twig; B. Calyx; C. Calyx split open; D. Standard petal; E. Wing petals; F. Keel petals; G. Staminal column; H. Pistil, I. Pod.

**Canna indica** L.

Syn: *Canna orientalis* Roscoe

Family: Cannaceae

Perennial erect herb, to 1.5m tall. Leaves elliptic-lanceolate, glabrous. Flowers scarlet, orange or yellow in terminal spikes. Fruit globose or ellipsoid capsule.

Grown as an ornamental.

Fl. & Fr.: Round the year.

Sanskrit: Devakuli.

Local names: *Ben*: Sarbajaya; *Hin*: Sabba jaya; *Kan*: Kadu bale, kakale, kalahu; *Mal*: Kandamanivazha, Kattuvazha; *Tam*: Kalvaazhal, Poovaazhai; *Tel*: Krishna Tamara.

Trade name: Indian Reed, Flowering reed.

Propagation: By Rhizomes.

Uses: Aerial parts useful in the treatment of diabetes.

**Cannabis sativa** L.

Family: Cannabinaceae

Annual herb, 1–2m tall. Leaves opposite below, alternate above, 7–9-fid below, 3–5-fid above. Flowers unisexual, dioecious. Fruit globose achene.

Ciltivated rarely.

Sanskrit: Bhang.

Local names: *Ass., Ben., Guj., Hin. & Mar.*: Bhang, Charas, Ganja; *Kan*: Bhang, *Mal*: Kanchanchottai; *Ori.*: Ganjee; *Tam.*: Bhangi, Ganja; *Tel*: Ganjayi

Trade name: True Hemp, Bhang, Ganja, Charas.

Uses: Flowers, leaves and resin useful in the treatment of diabetes.

**Canscora decussata** Roem.& Schult.

Family: Gentianaceae.

Annual erect herb, up to 30cm tall, stem 4-winged. Leaves elliptic-lanceolate, 3-nerved. Flowers white or pale pink in axillary or terminal dichasial cymes. Fruit obscurely 2-valved capsule. Seeds angular.

Occasional in moist places throughout India.

Fl. & Fr.: November–March.

Sanskrit: Sankhapushpi.

Local names: *Ben*: Dhankuni; *Hin*: Shankaphuli; *Mar*: Sankhvel, Titavi.

Uses: Plant useful in the treatment of diabetes.

**Capparis spinosa** L.

Family: Capparaceae

Evergreen shrub, low trailing or prostrate. Flowers white.

Found in Punjab, Rajasthan and north-western India.

Fl. & Fr.: December–March

Trade name: Capers.

Uses: Plant useful in the treatmnet of diabetes.

**Capsicum annuum** L.

Family: Solanaceae.

Annual or slightly perennial, erect bushy herb, glabrous. Leaves simple, ovate–lanceolate. Flowers solitary or in pairs, long-pediceled. Fruit berry, 1.5–5cm long, varies in form, red at maturity.

Commonly cultivated all over India for its fruit.

Sanskrit: Katuirah, Rakta Maricha.

Local names: *Ben*: Lanka-morich, Lalmorich; *Hin*: Lalmirch, Gachmarich; *Kan*: Kempu-menasu, Mensina kai; *Mal*: Mulaku; *Tam*: Milagay; *Tel*: Mirapakaya.

Trade name: Chillies, Red chillies.

Uses: Fruits useful in the treatment of diabetes.

Active constituent: Capsaicin.

**Capsicum frutescens** L.

Family: Solanaceae.

A perennial shrub, up to 2m tall. Leaves elliptic-ovate. Flowers greenish-white, 2–5 in terminal bunches. Fruit elongate berry, red when ripe, many-seeded, seeds circular, compressed.

Rare in waste lands.

Fl. & Fr.: Round the year.

Sanskrit: Katuvirah.

Local names: *Ben*: Gachmarich, Lalmarich, Lal lankamarich; *Kan*: Lodademenisinakayee, Phirangimenisinakayee; *Mal*: Kappalmulaka; Parankimulaka; *Mar*: Lavangi mirchi, Mirchi, Tambuda-mirchi; *Ori*: Dhangehh, Dhanlankmirich; *Tam*: Mullagay, Cosimilahai; *Tel*: Golkonda Mirapa.

Trade name: Golkonda Chillies.

Propagation: By seeds.

Uses: Aerial parts and seeds useful in the treatment of diabetes.

**Caragana brevispina** Royle ex Benth.

Family: Fabaceae (Papilionaceae)

Erect shrub. Leaves pinnately compound, leaflets oblong, stipules spiny. Flowers pale yellow. Fruit flattened pod.

Temperate and alpine regions of Western Himalayas.

Local names: *Pun*: Nyamzo

Uses: Aerial parts used to treat diabetes.

**Carica papaya** L.

Family: Caricaceae.

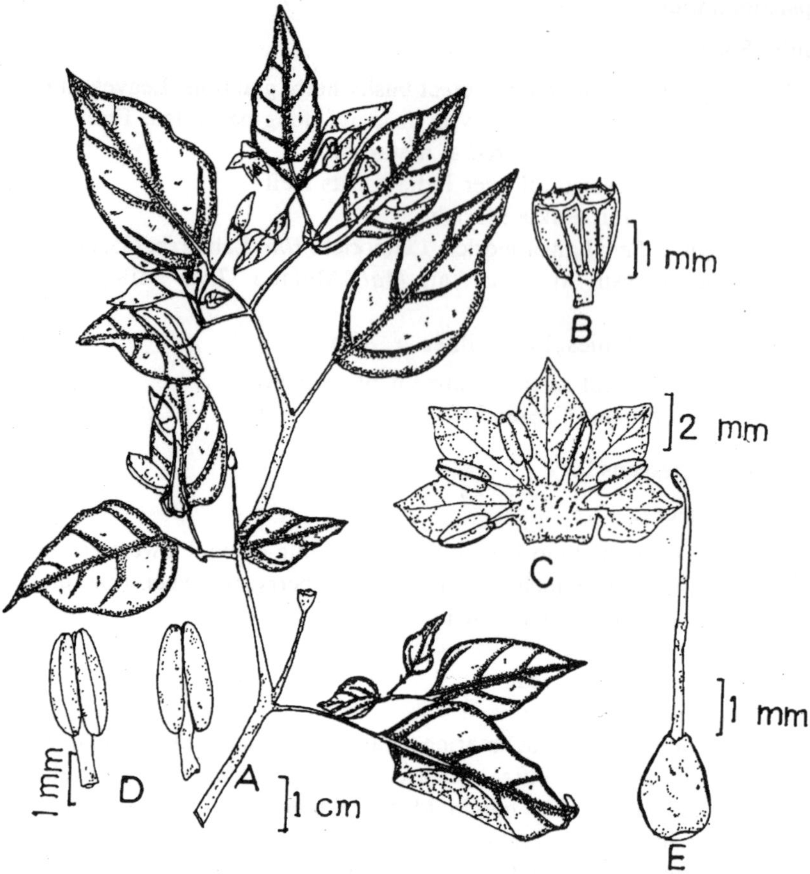


Fig. 24: *Capsicum frutescens* L.
A. Twig; B. Calyx; C. Corolla split open with stamens; D. Stamens; E. Pistil.

Soft wooded, unbranched tree, trunk hollow. Leaves long petioled, very large, palmately 5–7-lobed. Flowers creamish, polygamous. Fruit berry, yellow at maturity, seeds numerous, black.

Cultivated all over India.

Sanskrit: Brahmairandah, Eranda, Karkati.

Local names: *Ben*: Papeya, Pappaiya; *Guj*: Papayi, Popaiyun; *Hin*: Papeeta; *Kan*: Paringimara; *Mal*: Kappalam, Pappayam; *Mar*: Papaya; *Tam*: Pappali; *Tel*: Boppay, Boppasi.

Trade name: Papaya.

Propagation: By seeds.

Uses: Use of fruit juice every morning on empty stomach for 3 weeks helps in reducing glucose level.

**Carthamus tinctorius** L.

Family: Asteraceae (Compositae)

Annual erect herb, up to 1m tall. Leaves alternate, oblong, spiny. Flowers orange yellow in terminal heads. Fruit white, shiny.

Cultivated in black soils in dry lands.

Sanskrit: Kusumbha.

Local names: *Ben*: Kusum, Kusumphu; *Guj*: Kusumbho; *Hin*: Kusum, Kameh; *Kan*: Kusume, Kusumbhe; *Mar*: Kardai, Kurdi; *Tam*: Sendrakam; *Tel*: Kusuma.

Trade name: Safflower.

Propagation: By seeds.

Uses: Seeds useful in the treatment of diabetes.

**Carvia callosa** (Nees) Bremek.

Syn: *Strobilanthes callosus* Nees

Family: Acanthaceae

Aromatic shrub. Leaves elliptic-lanceolate. Flowers light purple or deep blue, in axillary, strobiliform spikes. Fruit ovoid capsule.

Found in Western Ghats, Western and Central India.

Local names: *Guj*: Pandadi; *Mar*: Garvi.

Uses: Aerial pars useful in the treatment of diabetes.

**Casearia esculenta** Roxb.

Family: Flacourtiaceae

Shrub or tree, up to 6m tall. Leaves elliptic-lanceolate. Flowers light yellow in axillary clusters. Fruit capsule.

Eastern and Western Ghats and hills of North–Eastern India.

Local names: *Hin*: Chilla, Pimpri; *Kan*: Doddahanise; *Mal*: Malampavatta, Panimurangam; *Mar*: Kulkulta, Mori; *Tam*: Kakkaipilai, Kirari, *Tel*: Konda junguru.

Uses: Root and stem bark used in the treatment of diabetes.

**Cassia alata** L.

Family: Caesalpiniaceae

Shrubs, up to 2m tall, branchlets glabrescent. Leaves pinnately compound, leaflets 8–12 pairs, oblong, inequilateral, thin coriaceous, glabrous, rachis narrowly winged. Flowers yellow in terminal dense racemes, bract spathaceous. Fruit pod, oblong, thin, straight, seeds 50 or more.

Cultivated, sometimes run wild in West Bengal, Bihar, Orissa, Arunachal Pradesh, Assam, Meghalaya, Manipur, Mizoram, Nagaland, Tripura, Andhra Pradesh, Karnataka, Tamil Nadu and Kerala.

Sanskrit: Dadhrugna, Dvipagsti.

Local names: *Ass*: Dadulhou, Daudpata; *Ben*: Dadmardan, Dadmari; *Hin*: Dadmurdan, Datkapat; *Kan*: Doddasagate, Simyagase; *Mal*: Elakajam, Simayakatti; *Mar*: Dadamardan; *Ori*: Dadumaardano, Jadumari; *Tam*: Anjali, Simalyagatti, Vanduglolli; *Tel*: Sima avise.

Trade name: Ringworm cassia.

Uses: Aerial parts and leaves useful in the treatment of diabetes.

**Cassia auriculata** L.

Family: Caesalpiniaceae

Erect bushy undershrubs, 1.5–2.5m tall, stipules large, foliaceous, reniform, persistent. Leaves pinnately compound, leaflets 7–12 pairs,

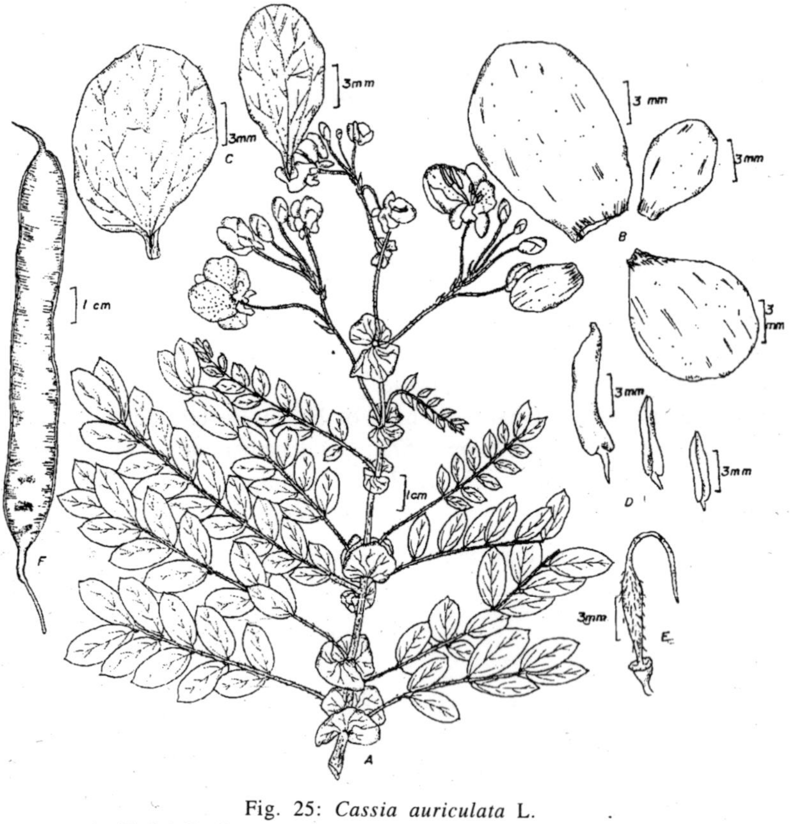


Fig. 25: *Cassia auriculata* L.
A. Twig; B. Sepals; C. Petals; D. Stamens; E. Pistil; F. Pod.

oblong-obovate, thin coriaceous. Flowers yellow with orange veins, in axillary and terminal corymbs. Fruit pod, linear, flattened, torulose, seeds 10–15, laterally compressed.

Common in waste lands in Jammu & Kashmir, Punjab, Haryana, U.P., Bihar, West Bengal, Orissa, M.P., Rajasthan, Gujarat, Maharashtra, Goa, Andhra Pradesh, Karnataka, Tamil Nadu and Kerala.

Fl. & Fr.: Round the year.

Sanskrit: Charmaranga, Mayahari.

Local names: *Guj*: Aval, Awal; *Hin*: Taroda, Tarval, Tarvar, Tarwar; *Kan*: Avarika, Ollatangedi, Sakusina, Tangadi, Tangedu; *Mal*: Avara, Aviram, Ponnaviram; *Mar*: Taravada, Taroda; *Ori*: Mayahari, Tarwad; *Tam*: Avarai, Avaram, Sadurguli; *Tel*: Tangedu.

Trade name: Tanner's Cassia.

Uses: Flowers, leaves and seeds useful in the treatment of diabetes.

**Cassia fistula** L.

Syn: *Cassia rhombifolia* Roxb.

Family: Caesalpiniaceae

Small or medium sized deciduous tree. Leaves compound, leaflets 4–8 pairs, opposite, broadly ovate, thick coriaceous. Flowers bright to golden yellow in lax, pendent, branched raceme. Fruit 40–50cm long pod, cylindric, dark blackish-brown.

Common in deciduous forests through out the country.

Fl. March–May Fr.: May–December.

Sanskrit: Aragvadha, Suvarnaka.

Local names: *Ass*: Sonaru, Sunalu; *Ben*: Amultas, Bandarlati; *Guj*: Balla, Garmala; *Hin*: Amaltas, Bandarlauri, Girimalah; *Kan*: Aragina, aragvadha, Arevata, Kakkai; *Mal*: Konna, Kriitamalam, Saturangulam; *Mar*: Bhavabaya, Bahava, Bawa, Chimkani, Garmala; *Ori*: Souturongulo, Sunari; *Pun*: Karangal Alash, Ali, Kaniar; *Tam*: Appai, Aragoram, Arkkuvadam, Irali, Sarakkandai; *Tel*: Rela; *Urdu*: Amaltash.

Trade name: Rela.

Propagation: By seeds.

Uses: Flowers, seeds and stem bark useful in the treatment of diabetes.

**Cassia javanica** L.

Family: Caesalpiniaceae

Medium-sized tree. Leaves imparipinnate, leaflets 8–14 pairs, oblong. Flowers bright rose or pink. Fruit pod, cylindrical, dark brown.

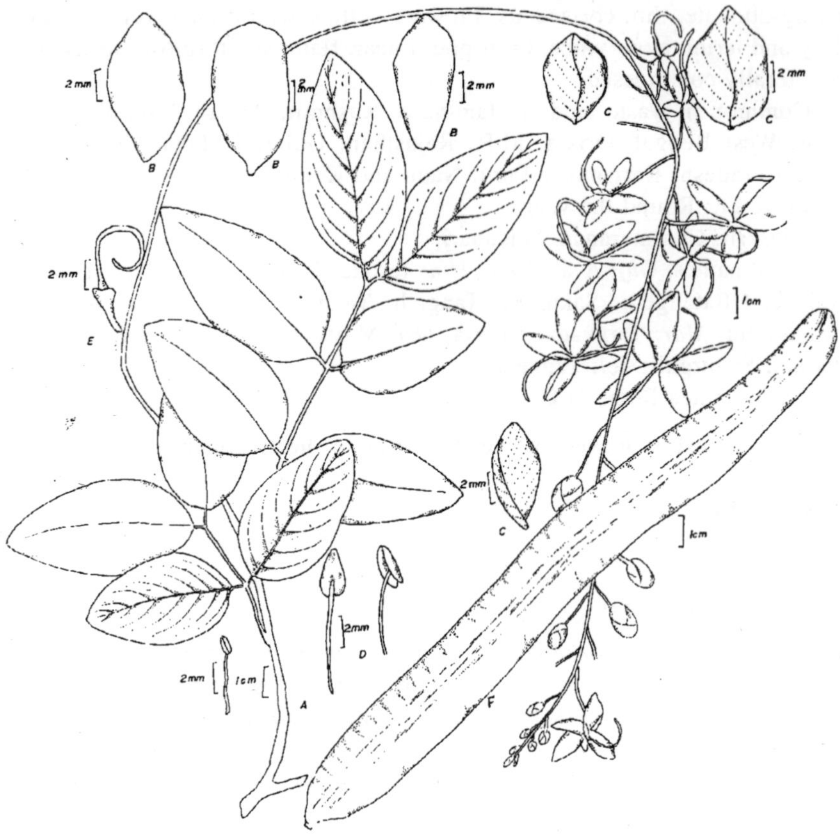


Fig. 26: *Cassia fistula* L.
A. Twig; B. Sepals; C. Petals; D. Stamens; E. Pistil; F. Pod.

Native to Java, introduced into the Indian gardens.
Trade name: Apple-blosson senna, Javanese cassia.

Uses: Aerial parts used to treat diabetes.

**Cassia occidentalis** L.

Syn: *Senna occidentalis* Roxb.

Family: Caesalpiniaceae

Erect, glabrous undershrus, up to 3m tall, branchlets glabrous. Leaves 10–15cm long, paripinnate, leaflets 3–5 pairs, elliptic-ovate, membranous, glabrous above, thinly hairy beneath. Flowers bright reddish yellow in axillary and terminal corymbose racemes. Fruit pod, brown with yellow margins, seeds 20–25, greenish brown.

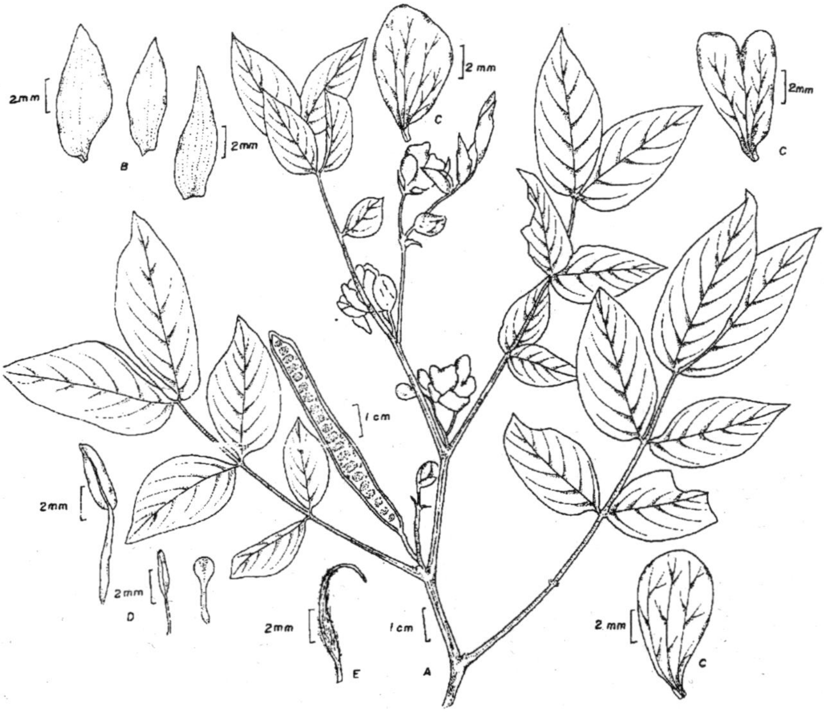


Fig. 27: *Cassia occidentalis* L.
A. Twig; B. Sepals; C. Petals; D. Stamens; E. Pistil.

Common on road sides and wastelands all over India.

Fl. & Fr.: Through out the year.

Sanskrit: Kasam arda, Kanaka.

Local names: *Ass*: Hant-tenga, Naguni, Jhanjani-gach, Eski, Kalalabanda; *Ben*: Kalkashundu; *Guj*: Nanichimad, Kasodari, Kasundari, Chamediyan; *Hin*: Banbhates, Bari-kasondi, Kasondi; *Kan*: Anecogate, Doddatagase, Nelatagase; *Mal*: Ponnaviram, Karinthakara, Natram-takara; *Mar*: Hikal, Rankasvinda, Kashoda; *Ori*: Kasundiri; *Pun*: Kasundi; *Tam*: Nattam-takarai; *Tel*: Kasinda, *Urdu*: Kasonji.

Uses: Leaves useful in the treatment of diabetes.

**Cassia senna** L.

Syn: *Cassia angustifolia* Vahl

Family: Caesalpiniaceae

Herb, up to 1.5m tall. Leaves alternate, pinnately compound, leaflets 4–7 pairs, linear-lanceolate. Flowers greenish–yellow in terminal or axillary racemes. Fruit pod, greenish black when ripe.

Fl. & Fr.: July–September.

Uses: Plant useful in the treatment of diabetes.

**Cassia sophera** L.

Family: Caesalpiniaceae

Diffuse undershrubs, up to 3m tall. Leaves 10–15cm long, leaflets 6–10 pairs, oblong-lanceolate, glaucous. Flowers yellow in terminal and axillary racemes. Fruit pod, linear-oblong, septate, seed ovoid, flat, dark brown.

Common in all plains districts, by road sides and on waste lands through out India.

Fl. & Fr.: July–January.

Sanskrit: Kasamanda, Suvarnamayaheri.

Local names: *Ass*: Lkalkasand, Chhota-eski, Kashinda; *Ben*: Kalkasunda; *Guj*: Jambli, Kasundari, Kuwadice, Sundari; *Hin*: Chakwar, Kasundari, Kesundi, Banar; *Kan*: Kashamard, Kulakashinda; *Mal*: Ponnantagara; *Mar*: Kasodi,

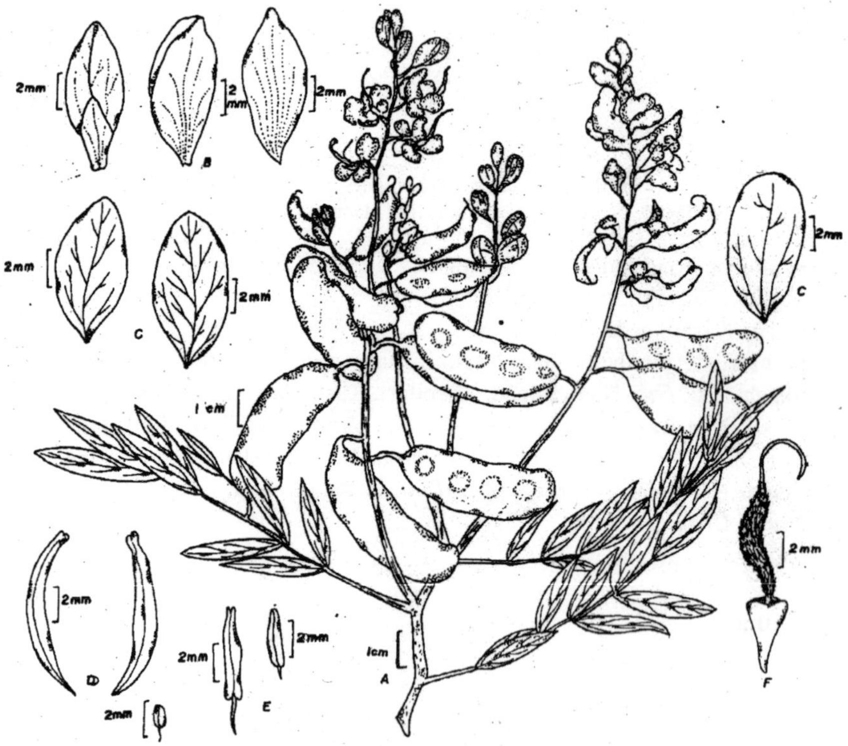


Fig. 28: *Cassia senna* L.
A. Twig; B. Sepals; C. Petals; D. Staminodes; E. Stamens; F. Pistil.

Rantankala; *Ori*: Kolakasund, Kasundiri; *Tam*: Nalal, Peraviral, Sulari, Ponnavirai; *Tel*: Kondakasinda, Pyditangedu; *Urdu*: Kala-kashanji.

Trade name: Senna sophera, Kasa marda.

Uses: Seeds and stem bark useful in the treatment of diabetes.

**Cassia surattensis** Burm.f.

Syn: *Cassia glauca* Lam.

Family: Caesalpiniaceae

Shrub or small tree, up to 9m tall. Leaves bipinnate, leaflets 4–6 pairs, elliptic-oblong. Flowers yellow, in axillary racemes. Fruit pod, flat.

Throughout India, often cultivated.

Fl. & Fr.: August–December.

Local names: *Kan*: Adavitangedi, Betadevare; *Mal*: Takara, Vellatakara; *Mar*: Mothatharvad; *Tam*: Kovalai, Vellarai; *Tel*: Metta tangedu.

Trade name: Glaucous cassia

Uses: Aerial parts used in the treatment of diabetes mellitus.

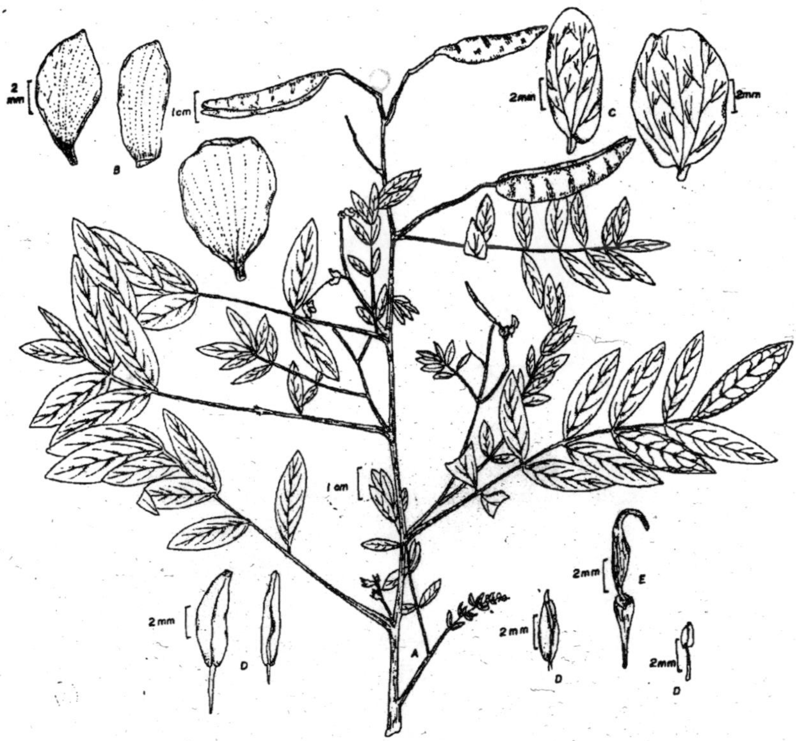


Fig. 29: *Cassia sophera* L.
A. Twig; B. Sepals; C. Petals; D. Stamens; E. Pistil.

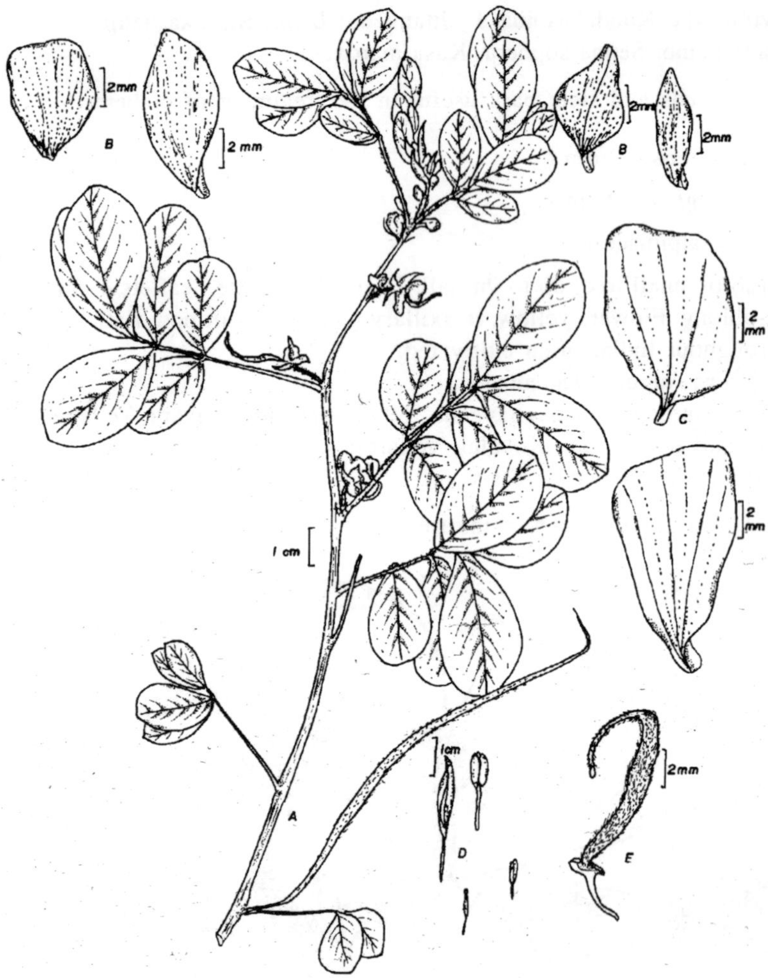


Fig. 30: *Cassia tora* L.
A. Twig; B. Sepals; C. Petals; D. Stamens; E. Pistil.

**Cassia tora** L.

Family: Caesalpiniaceae

Annual herbs, up to 20cm tall, crisped hairy in young branches. Leaves 6–8cm long, pinnately compound, leaflets 3–5 pairs, sessile, obovate-oblong, thin coriaceous. Flowers golden yellow or with reddish tinge, solitary or geminate, axillary. Fruit pod, linear, puberulous, 10–15 × 0.3cm, seeds about 20, faintly tetragonal.

Common on waysides and waste places and fallow lands through out India.

Fl. & Fr.: September–December.

Sanskrit: Chakramardah, Prapunnatah, Prisnaparni, Dodamari.

Local names: *Ass*: Gol-eski, Daridiga, Tewitnyansyrang, Bomnedelua; *Ben*: Panevar, Chakunda; *Guj*: Pochandio, Kanariya, Kawario; *Hin*: Chakunda, Panevar, Pawad, Chakavat; *Kan*: Gandutogache, Taragasi, Cagace; *Mal*: Chakramardrakam, Takara; *Mar*: Tankli, Tarota, Takala; *Ori*: Chakund, Chakor; *Pun*: Pawas, Panwar; *Tam*: Senavu, Vindu, Tagarai; *Tel*: Tantmu, Tagirisa, Tellakashinda.

Trade name: Foetid Cassia.

Uses: Seeds useful in the treatment of diabetes.

**Castanospermum australe** A. Cunn. & C. Fraser ex Hook.

Family: Fabaceae (Papilionaceae)

Evergreen tree, up to 30m tall. Leaves imparipinnate, leaflets 11–17, ovate-elliptic or broadly oblong. Flowers yellow, orange to red in racemes. Fruit pod, seeds black.

Native to Australia, cultivated in India for shade and ornament.

Uses: Isolate was found to have hypoglycemic activity.

**Casuarina equisetifolia** L.

Family: Casuarinaceae.

Tall, leafless tree, up to 15m tall, branchlets arising from the axils of scales. Leaves scaly, alternating with ribs of the upper node. Flowers unisexual. Male flowers in terminal catkins, female in globose-ovoid cone like heads. Fruit nutlets, compressed, winged.

Widely planted along the coast.

Fl. & Fr.: February–August.

Local names: *Ben*: Jau; *Guj*: Vilaya saru; *Hin*: Jangli saru, Jangli-jhau, Sarrosh-phar; *Kan*: Sarve mara, Chabaku, Kasrike; *Mal*: Chavukku; *Mar*: Suru; *Tam*: Savukku, Civa varni; *Tel*: Sarugudu.

Trade name: Beef wood.

Propagation: by seeds.

Uses: Aerial parts useful in the treatment of diabetes.

**Catha edulis** (Vahl) Forsk. ex Endl.

Family: Celastraceae

Shrub or small tree, up to 7m tall. Leaves ovate-lanceolate to elliptic. Flowers small, white, in short cymes. Fruit capsule, woody, oblong, seeds brown.

Grown in gardens in Gujarat, Maharashtra and Karnataka.

Trade name: Abyssinian tea, African tea, cafta, Khat.

Uses: Leaf and stem used in the treatment of diabetes mellitus.

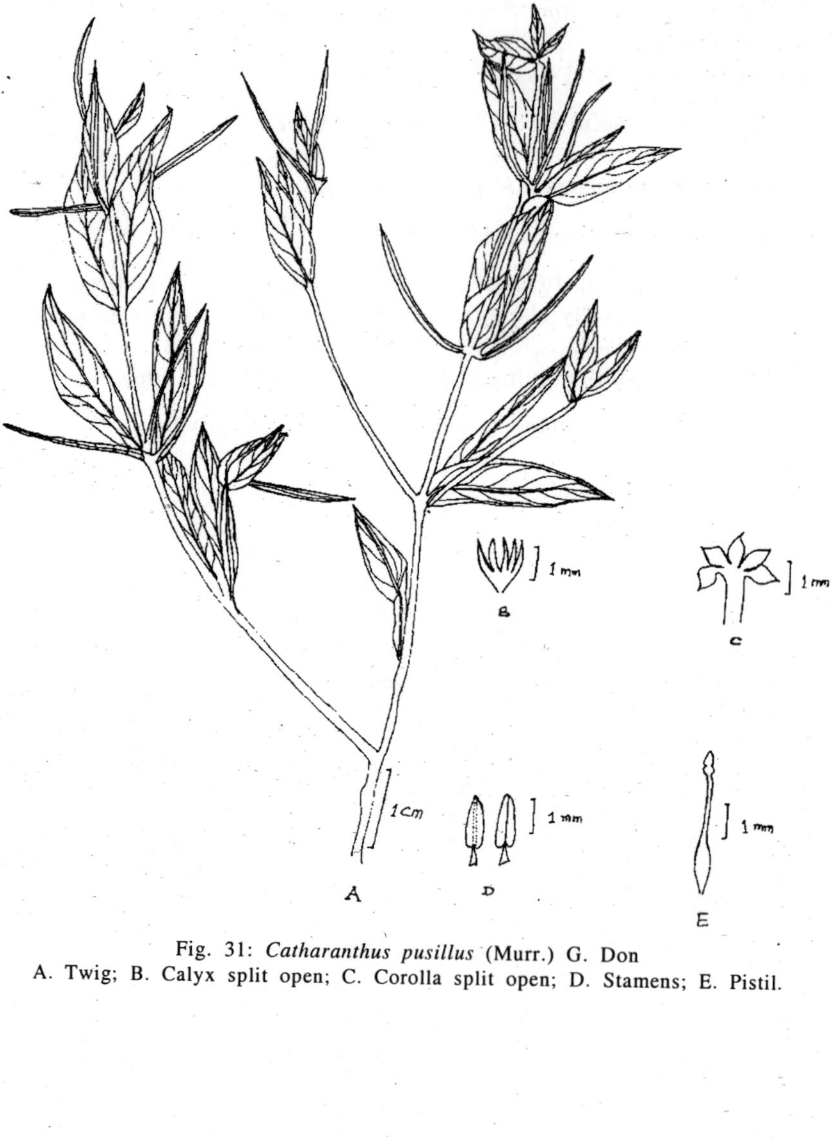


Fig. 31: *Catharanthus pusillus* (Murr.) G. Don
A. Twig; B. Calyx split open; C. Corolla split open; D. Stamens; E. Pistil.

**Catharanthus pusillus** (Murr.) G.Don

Syn: *Vinca pusilla* Murr.
*Lochnera pusilla* (Murr.) K.Schum.

Family: Apocynaceae.

Annual erect herb, to 30 cm tall, branchlets terete below, quadragular above. Leaves lanceolate, glabrous. Flowers white in terminal or axillary 5–7-flowered corymbs. Fruit capsule, seeds black.

Occasional weed in cultivated fields throughout the greater part of India.

Fl. & Fr.: July–December.

Sanskrit: Sangki.

Local names: *Kan*: Vishakanegale soppu; *Mal*: Kapavila; *Tam*: Milagaipoondu; *Tel*: Errimirapa, Kondamirapa.

Propagation: By seeds.

Uses: Plant useful in the treatment of diabetes.

**Catharanthus roseus** (L.) G.Don

Syn: *Vinca rosea* L.
*Lochnera rosea* (L.) Reichnb.

Family: Apocynaceae.

A perennial undershrub, up to 50cm tall. Leaves elliptic obovate to oblong, opposite decussate. Flowers pink or white, solitary or paired, axillary. Fruit a pair of follicles, many-seeded.

Cultivated all over India, mainly as an ornamental, some times for medicine.

Fl. & Fr.: Round the year.

Sanskrit: Nityakalyani, Shanthapushpa.

Local names: *Ben*: Gulferinghi, Nayantara; *Guj*: Barmasi; *Hin*: Sadabahar, Sadasuhagan; *Kan*: Kempukasi kanegale; *Mal*: Usham alari; *Mar*: Sadaphul; *Ori*: Ainskati; *Tam*: Sudukadu mallikai; *Tel*: Billa ganneru.

Trade name: Madagascar periwinkle.

Propagation: It is propagated by seeds.

Uses: The whole plant is hypoglycemic.

Active Principles: Alkaloids 16-Epi-19S-Vindoline, Gomaline, Vinceapusine, 16-Epi-Z-isositsirikine, Fluorocarpamine N-oxide, Pericyclinine, Catharanthamine, Vinblastine, Vindoline, Ajmalacine, Tetrahydro alstonine, Catharanthine and Leurosine

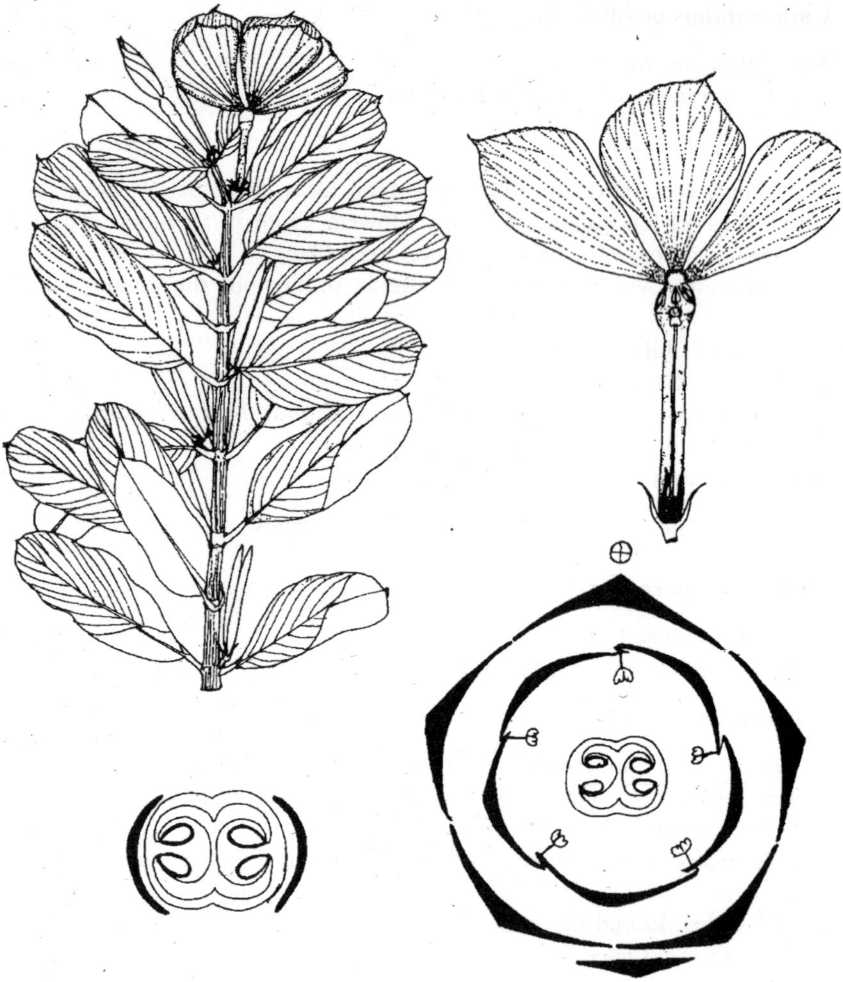

Fig. 32: *Catharanthus roseus* (L.) G. Don.
A. Twig; B. L.s. Flower; C. T.s. of voary; D. Floral diagram.

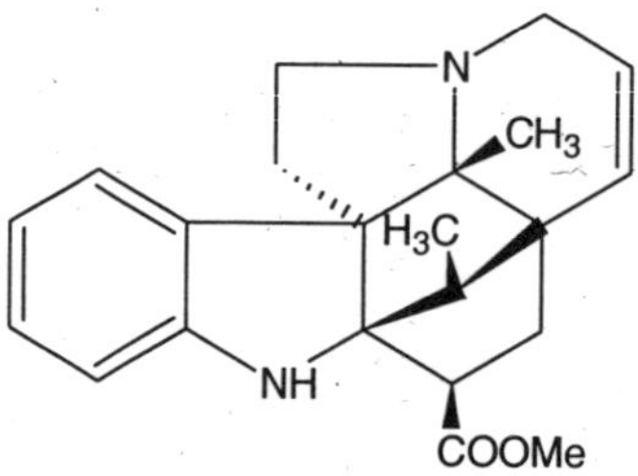


1--16-Epi-19S-Vindolinine

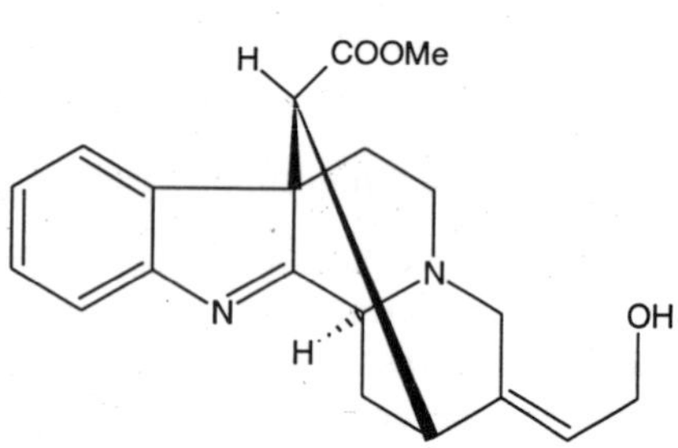


2--Gomaline

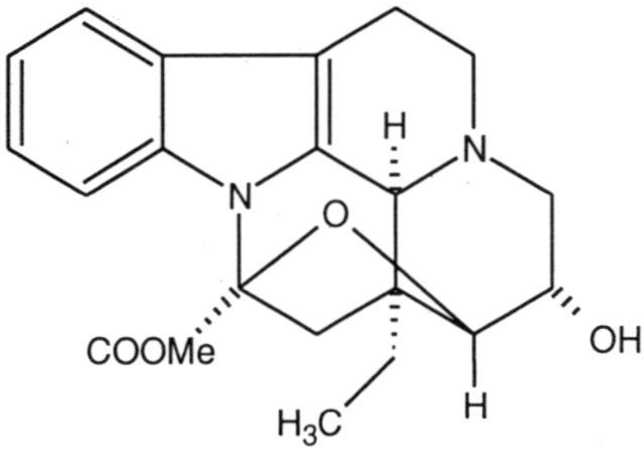


3--Vinceapusine

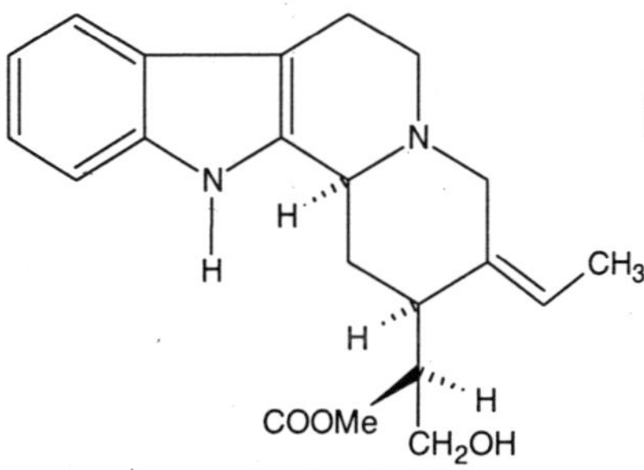


4--16-Epi-Z-isositsirikine

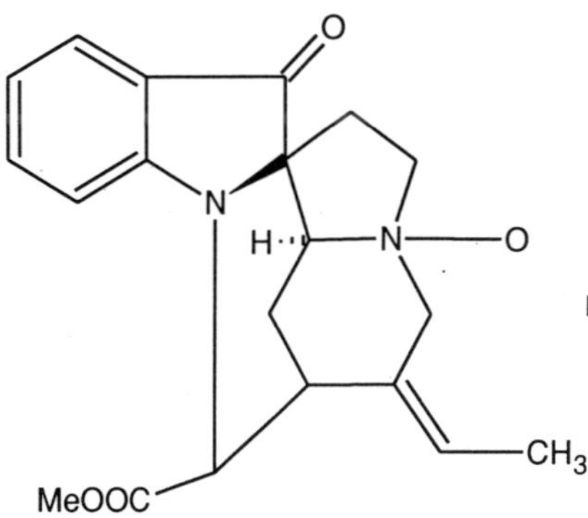


5--Flurocarpamine N-oxide

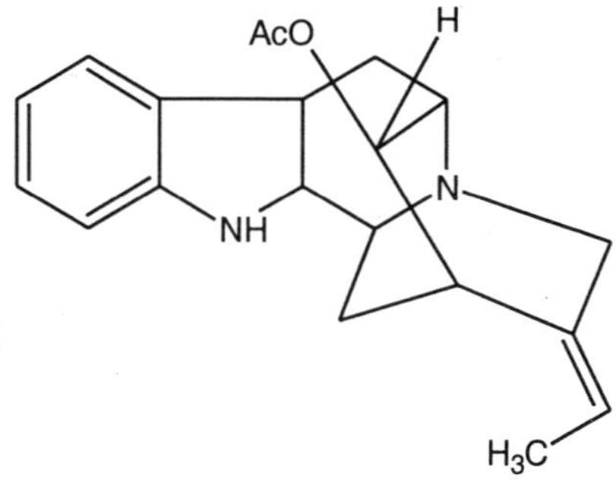


6--Pericyclinine

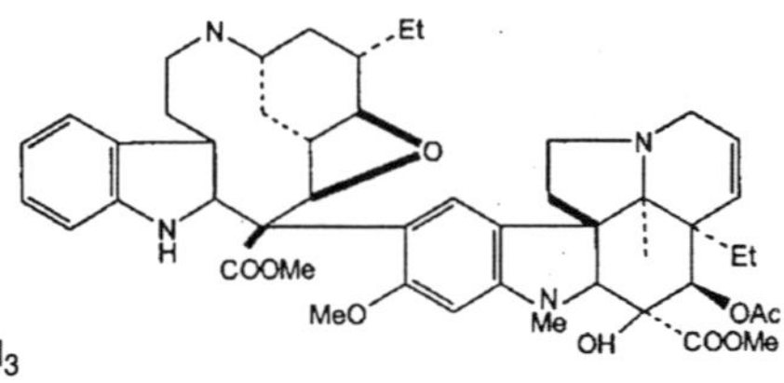


7--Catharanthamine

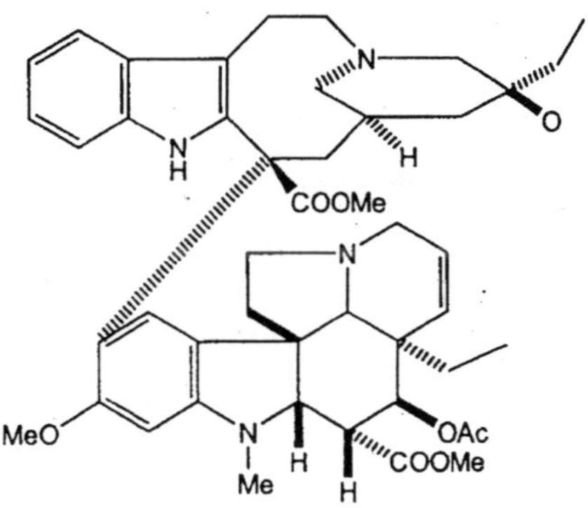


8--Vinblastine

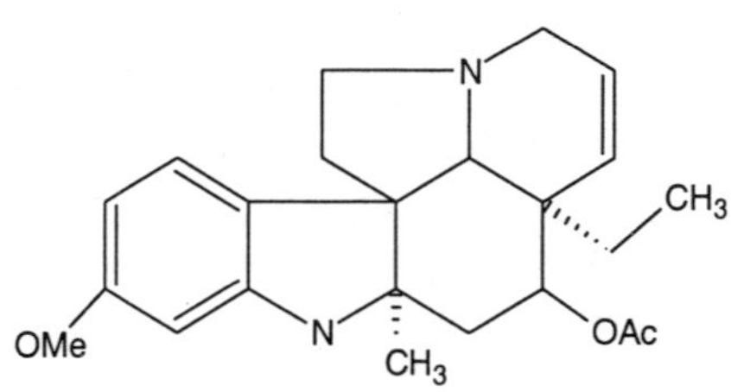


9--Vindoline

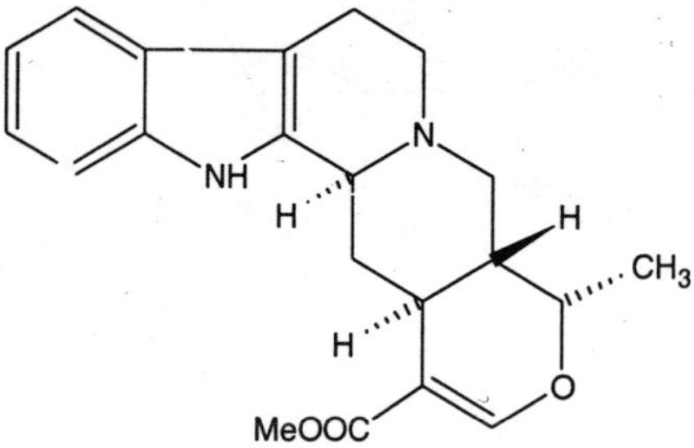


10--Ajmalicine

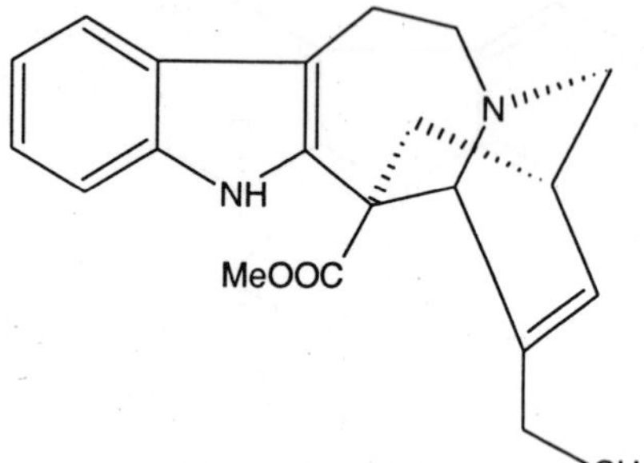


12--Catharanthine

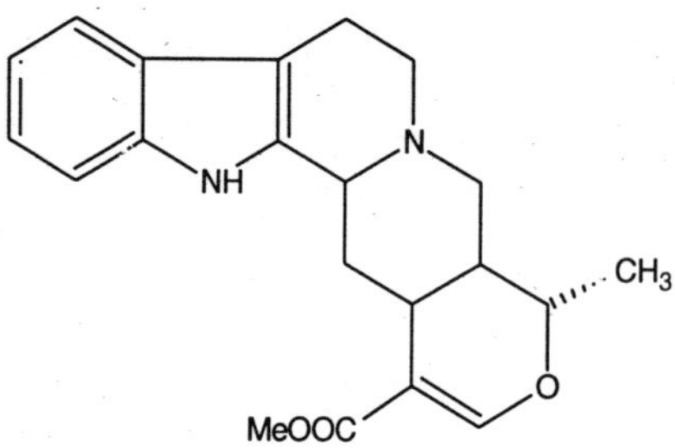


11--Tetrahydroalstonine

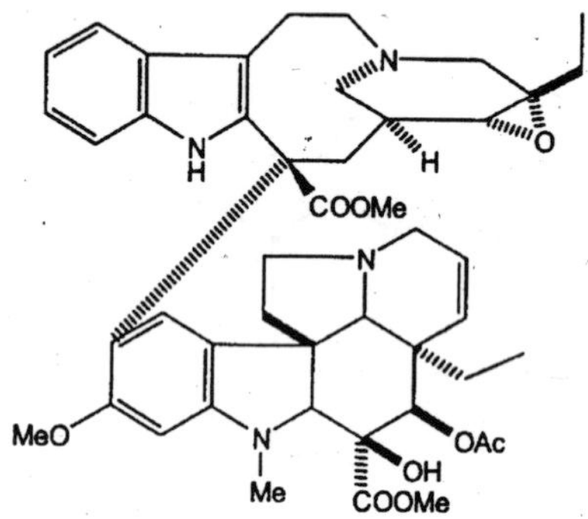


13--Leurosine

**Catunaregam spinosa** (Thunb.) Tirv.

Syn: *Gardenia spinosa* Thunb.
*Randia dumetorum* (Retz.) Poir.
*Gardenia dumetorum* Retz.
*Randia brandisii* Gamble

Family: Rubiaceae

A small armed shrub. Leaves elliptic lanceolate or obovate, sparsely pubescent above, densely pubescent below. Flowers in axillary corymbs, greenish white. Fruit globose berry.

Common in scrub jungles through out India.

Fl. & Fr.: February–June.

Sanskrit: Madana, Shalya.

Local names: *Hin*: Mainphal, Manmyol, Karhar; *Ori*: Mohan, Salara, Pativa; *Kan*: Kare, Banegar, Mangri; *Mal*: Kara; *Mar*: Chela, Peralu, Wagatta, Mindhal; *Pun*: Arara; *Tam*: Marykkallamkayman kari; *Tel*: Manga.

Trade name: Emetic nut.

Propagation: by seeds.

Uses: Fruits and stem bark useful in the treatment of diabetes.

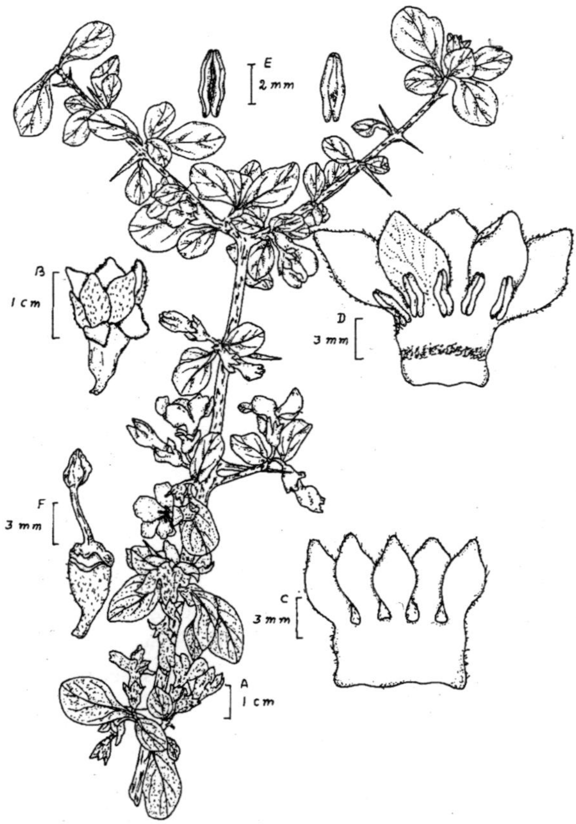


Fig. 33: *Catunaregum spinosa* (Thunb.) Tirveng.
A. Twig; B. Flower; C. Calyx; D. Corolla; E. Stamen-ventral view and dorsal view; F. Pistil.

**Ceiba pentandra** (L.) Gaertn.

Syn: *Eriodendron anfructuosum* DC.

Family: Bombacaceae.

Tall trees, trunk straight, prickly when young, up to 30m tall, branches horizontal.

Leaves 6–9-foliolate, leaflets oblanceolate or elliptic or oblong. Flowers clustered at the ends of branches, white or yellowish. Fruit ellipsoidal capsule, seeds many.

Often cultivated.

Sanskrit: Swetha Salmali.

Local names: *Ben*: Schetsimul; *Hin*: Hattian, Katun, safed simul; *Kan*: Bili-buraga; *Mal*: Ilavu, Mullilavu; *Mar*: Pandhari, Salmali; *Tam*: Ilavum; *Tel*: Burugu, Tellaburugu.

Trade name: White silk cotton tree.
Propagation: by seeds.

Uses: Roots and stem bark useful in the treatment of diabetes.

**Centaurea melitensis** L.

Family: Asteraceae

Annual, erect herb. Radical leaves lyrate pinnatifid, cauline leaves linear. Flowers yellow in heads.
In Nilgiris.
Trade name: Nappa–thistle., Reyless Centaury.

Uses: Flowers used to treat diabetes mellitus.

**Centella asiatica** (L.) Urban.

Syn: *Hydrocotyle asiatica* L.

Family: Apiaceae (Umbelliferae).

A perennial prostrate herb, creeping with long stolons, rooting at nodes. Leaves simple, orbicular-reniform, puberulous. Flowers pink or red in axillary fasciculate umbels, central flowers sessile, laterals pedicellate. Fruit ovoid, mericarp 7–9-ribbed, prominently reticulate.
Common in wet places all over India.
Fl. & Fr.: Through out the year.
Sanskrit: Mandukaparni.
Local names: *Ben*: Thankuni, Tholkuri; *Guj*: Moti brahmi; *Hin*: Brahmi, Kulakudi; *Kan*: Thambooli soppu; *Mal*: Muttil, Kutanni; *Mar*: Karinga, Karivana; *Ori*: Thalkudi; *Tam*: Vallarai, Cilukki; *Tel*: Saraswathi aku.
Trade name: Indian penny wort.
Propagation: Rooted stem cuttings and by seeds.

Uses: Whole plant useful in the treatment of diabetes.

**Centipeda minima** (L.) A.Br. & Aescher

Syn: *Centipeda orbicularis* Lour.

Family: Asteraceae

Prostrate herb. Leaves obovate-oblong. Flowers yellow, in solitary, axillary heads. Fruit oblong achene.
Throughout India in damp places.
Sanskrit: Chikkani
Local names: *Ben*: Mechitta; *Hin*: Nagdowam, Nakk-dikni; *Mar*: Nakashikani

Trade name: Sneezewort.

Uses: Whole plant used to treat diabetes mellitus.

**Ceratonia siliqua** L.

Family: Caesalpiniaceae

Small tree, up to 15m tall. Leaves paripinnate, leaflets 3–5 pairs. Flowers unisexual, in axillary racemes, white, yellow–green or red. Fruit pod, curved.

Introduced and naturalized in Punjab and Karnataka.

Trade name: The Carob–bean tree, Locust bean.

Uses: Seeds used to treat diabetes.

**Ceriops decandra** (Griff.) Ding Hou

Syn: *Ceriops roxburghiana* Arn.

Family: Rhizophoraceae

Shrub or small tree, up to 6m tall. Leaves obovate or elliptic-oblong. Flowers greenish white in axillary condensed capitate inflorescences. Fruit ovoid.

Found in Mangroves of East coast.

Local names: *Ben*: Bara goran; *Hin*: Goran; *Ori*: Gartah; *Tam*: Chiru, Kandel; *Tel*: Gatharu, Goran.

Uses: Aerial parts useful in the treatment of diabetes.

**Ceriops tagal** (Perr.) Robins.

Syn: *Rhizophora tagal* Perr.
*Ceriops candolleana* Arn.

Family: Rhizophoraceae

Glabrous shrubs or small trees up to 90cm tall. Leaves obovate-oblong or spathulate. Flowers white, in axillary clustered cymes.

Found along coastal forests of Peninsular India, Sundarbans and Andaman and Nicobar Islands.

Fl. & Fr.: June–July

Local names: *Ben*: Goran: *Mal*: Ann. Kandal., *Mar*: Chauri; *Ori*: Gartah; *Tam*: Chira, Kandal; *Tel*: Gadara

Uses: Stem bark useful in the treatment of diabetes.

**Chromolaena odorata** (L.) King & Robins.

Syn: *Eupatorium odoratum* L.

Family: Asteraceae

Erect herb to subshrub, up to 2m tall. Leaves ovate. Flowers pink in terminal homogamous heads. Fruit achene, 5-ribbed.

Naturalised in Eastern and Southern India

Fl. & Fr.: December–May.

Local names: *Ben*: Assam-lota.

Propagation: By seeds.

Uses: Plant useful in the treatment of diabetes.

**Chrysanthemum indicum** L.

Family: Asteraceae.

Perennial herb, up to 90cm tall. Leaves ovate to oblong-ovate, pinnately cleft. Flowers yellow in terminal heads.

Commonly grown in gardens.

Uses: Flowers used in the treatment of diabetes mellitus.

**Chrysanthemum leucanthemum** L.

Family: Asteraceae.

Perennial herb, rootstock rhizomatous, stems erect. Basal and lower leaves round to obovate-spathulate, upper leaves ovate-oblanceolate or lanceolate-oblong, toothed to pinnatifid.

Cultivated in U.P., Himachal Pradesh and Kashmir.

Trade name: Field–Daisy, Marguriete, Moon daisy herb, Ox-eye daisy.

Uses: Plant used in the treatment of diabetes mellitus.

**Chrysopogon aciculatus** (Retz.) Trin.

Syn: *Andropogon aciculatus* Retz.

Family: Poaceae.

Perennial tufted grass, up to 60cm tall, geniculately ascending. Leaves oblong. Spikelets in panicle. Fruit caryopsis, linear.

Throughout India

Local names: *Ben*: Chorkanta; *Hin*: Lampa, Surwala; *Kan*: Ganjigarikehallu; *Tam*: Tuttiri; *Tel*: Putti gaddi.

Trade name: Lesser spear-grass; Love-grass, Spear–grass.

Uses: Whole plant used for the treatment of diabetes.

**Cicer arietinum** L.

Family: Fabaceae

Annual erect, much branched, glandular pubescent herb. Leaves imparipinnately compound, leaflets ovate. Flowers pink, axillary, solitary. Fruit turgid pod, seeds reddish brown with a beak.

Cultivated throughout India

Fl. & Fr.: November–February

Sanskrit: Canakah

Local names: *Ben*: But, chola, *Guj*: Chana; *Hin*: But, Chana, Chole, *Kan*: Kadale; *Mal*: Katala; *Mar*: Harbara; *Tam*: Katalai; *Tel*: Sanagalu.

Trade name: Bengal gram, Chick pea.

Uses: Seeds useful in the treatment of diabetes. Experiments have shown that the intake of water extract of Bengal gram enhances the utilization of glucose in both diabetic and normal persons. Tests were conducted at the Central Food Technological Research Institute in Mysore on a chronic diabetes patient whose insulin requirement was of the order of forty units a day. When kept on a diet which included liberal supplements of Bengal gram extract, the condition of the patient improved considerably and his insulin requirement was reduced to about twenty units per day. Diabetes patients who are on a prescribed diet which does not severely restrict the intake of carbohydrates, but include liberal amounts of Bengal gram extract, have shown considerable improvement in their fasting blood sugar levels, glucose tolerance, urinary excretion of sugar and general condition.

Active principle: Garbenzol.

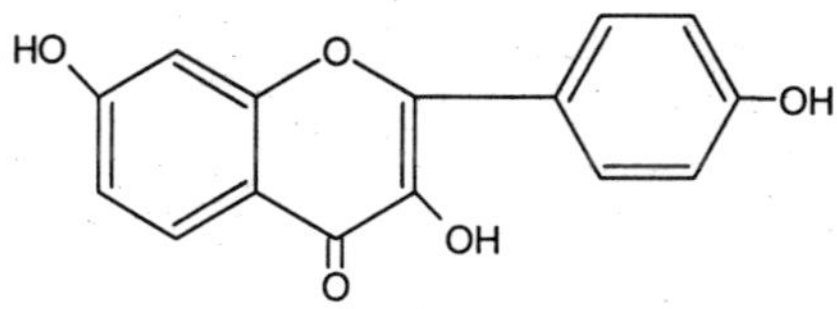


Garbenzol

**Cichorium endivia** L.

Family: Asteraceae (Compositae).

Annual decumbent herb, up to 1m tall. Leaves lanceolate, runcinate or pinnatifid, semiamplexicaul. Flowers in axillary and terminal compound heads. Fruit achene, obcompressed.

Rarely found as a weed in cultivated fields in Uttar Pradesh, Maharashtra, Rajasthan, Kerala and Tamil Nadu.

Sanskrit: Kasani.

Local names: *Ben*: Kassin

Trade name: Garden Endive, Endive.

Propagation: By seeds

Uses: Leaves useful in the treatment of diabetes.

**Cichorium intybus** L.

Family: Asteraceae (Compositae).

Erect, perennial, herb with milky latex, up to 90cm tall, taproot fleshy. Leaves broadly oblong, oblanceolate or lanceolate forming rosette, upper leaves cordate-amplexicaul. Flowers bright blue in ligulate heads, terminal or axillary. Fruit angled achene, crowned with a ring of pappus scales.

Cultivated throughout India. Wild in Punjab.

Sanskrit: Kasani.

Local names: *Ben*: Kasni, *Guj*: Kasni; *Hin*: Hinduba, Kasni; *Kan*: Kachani; *Mal*: Chikkari; *Tam*: Chikkari, Kasini; *Tel*: Chikori; Kasini vittulu.

Trade name: Chickory, Endive

Propagation: By seeds.

Uses: Leaves and roots used to treat diabetes.

**Cinchona officinalis** L.

Family: Rubiaceae

Slender tree, up to 9m tall. Leaves lanceolate or ovate-lanceolate, glabrous. Flowers pink or purple coloured in short corymbiform terminal and axillary compound cymes. Fruit ovoid-oblong capsule.

Cultivated in Nilgiris at an elevation of 1800–2000m.

Sanskrit: Sinkona, Kunayanah.

Local names: *Hin*: Kunain; *Kan*: Sinchona; *Mal*: Sinkona; *Tam*: Cinkona; *Tel*: Cinchona

Trade name: Quinine bark, Peruvian bark.

Propagation: By seeds, grafting.

Uses: Stem bark used in the treatment of diabetes.

**Cinnamomum aromaticum** Nees

Syn: *Cinnamomum cassia* Blume

Family: Lauraceae

Evergreen aromatic tree, up to 18m tall. Leaves oblong-elliptic, dark shiny green. Flowers small in lax, spreading terminal and axillary panicles. Fruit drupe, black when ripe.

Wild in Mizoram, cultivated in Tamil Nadu.

Trade name: Chinese Cinnamon, chinese cassia

Uses: Stem bark used in the treatment of diabeties.

**Cinnamomum camphora** (L.) Presl.

Family: Lauraceae

Medium sized tree with an enlarged base, up to 10m tall. Leaves ovate, whitish beneath. Flowers yellow in panicles.

Cultivated in Nilgiris.

Sanskrit: Karpurah.

Local names: *Hin*: Kapur; *Kan*: Karpura; *Mal*: Cutakkarpuram̀; *Tam*: Karpuram; *Tel*: Karpuramu, Paccha karpuramu.

Trade name: Camphor tree.

Propagation: By seeds.

Uses: Aerial parts useful in the treatment of diabetes.

**Cinnamomum sulphureum** Nees

Family: Lauraceae

Medium sized trees, bark smooth, reddish brown outside, dull red inside. Leaves sub-coriaceous, ovate-lanceolate or elliptic-oblong, glaucous beneath. Flowers greenish-yellow in terminal and axillary panicles. Fruit oblong berry.

Common in Western Ghats of Karnataka, Kerala and Tamil Nadu.

Local names: *Kan*: Matta dalchini, Pinga dalchini.

Propagation: by seeds and through stem cuttings

Uses: Leaves and stem bark useful in the treatment of diabetes.

**Cinnamomum tamala** (Buch–Ham.) Nees

Family: Lauraceae

Moderate sized evergreen tree, up to 7m tall. Leaves ovate-lanceolate or ovate-oblong, three nerved. Flowers yellowish white in axillary and terminal, lax puberulous panicles. Fruit black drupe.

In Himalayan region of West Bengal, Assam and Garhwal.

Sanskrit: Tamalapatram

Local names: *Hin*: Tejpatt; *Kan*: Kadu lavanga patte; *Mal*: Paccila; *Tam*: Tamalapattri; *Tel*: Talisa patri, Adavi lavanga patri.

Uses: Stem bark and root useful in the treatment of diabetes.

**Cissampelos pareira** L.

Family: Menispermaceae

Slender climbers with hairy branches. Leaves reniform, orbicular or cordate. Flowers unisexual, greenish yellow, minute, male in panicles, female

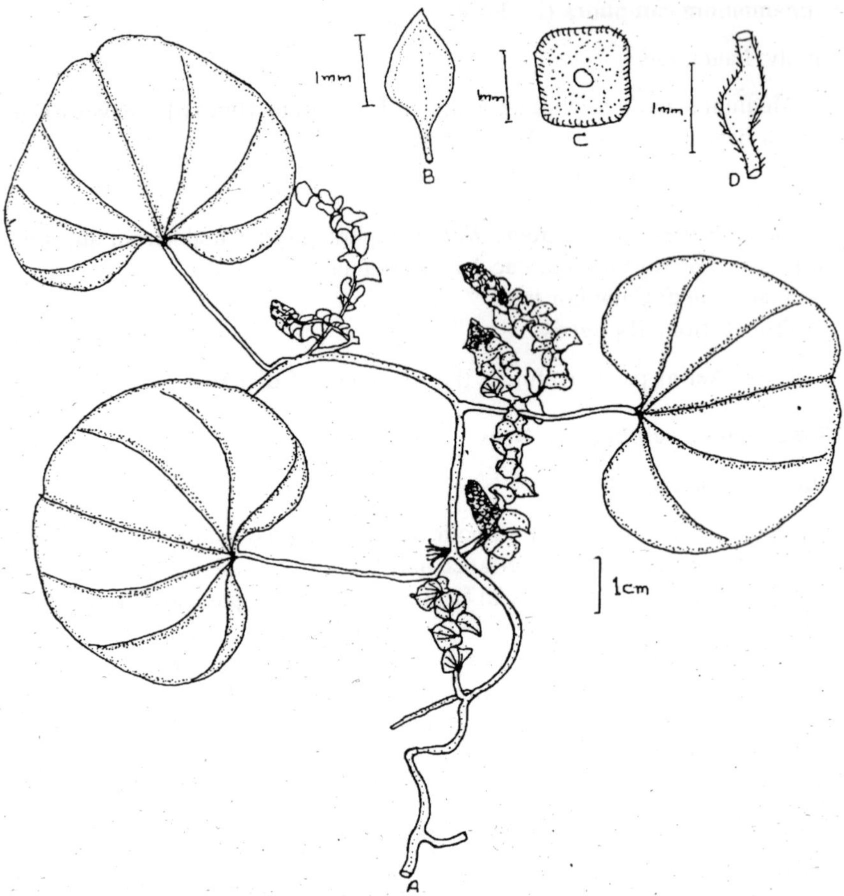


Fig. 34: *Cissampelos pareira*
A. Female Twig; B. Sepal; C. Petal; D. Pistil.

in pendulous racemes in axils of conspicuous bracts. Fruit ovoid drupe, scarlet.

Common through out India from plains to 1700m.

Fl. & Fr.: April–October.

Sanskrit: Patha, Vriddhakarnika, Ambastha, Laghupatha.

Local names: *Ben*: Akaleja, Akandi; *Guj*: Karandhiva; *Kan*: Kodupalli, Pariraaberu; *Mal*: Kattuvalli, Malathangi; *Mar*: Pahadmul; *Ori*: Akarnamini, Okanabindu; *Tam*: Appatta, Panumushtie; *Tel*: Adavibankateega, Vishaboddi.

Trade name: Velvet-leaf pareira, False pareira brava or root.

Uses: Plant useful in the treatment of diabetes.

**Cissus repens** Lam.

Syn: *Vitis repens* (Lam.) Wight & Arn.

Family: Vitaceae

Slender trailing shrub, tendrils leaf-opposed, forked. Leaves ovate. Flowers in compound umbellate cymes. Fruit globose berry, usually 1-seeded.

South India, Himalaya, North-East India.

Fl. & Fr.: August–November.

Uses: Whole plant useful for the treatment of diabetes.

**Citherexylum subserratum** Sw.

Family: Verbenaceae

Small trees, up to 5m tall. Leaves elliptic-ovate, chartaceous. Flowers white in terminal drooping racemes.

Fl. & Fr.: May–October.

Uses: Aerial parts useful for the treatment of diabetes.

**Citrullus colocynthis** (L.) Schrad.

Syn: *Colocynthis vulgaris* Schrad.

Family: Cucurbitaceae.

Trailing scabrid herbs, tendrils slender, simple or 2–3-fid. Leaves ovate or narrowly triangular, deeply 3–7-lobed, lobes pinnatifid, densely villous. Flowers unisexual, solitary. Fruit globose, striped green and white when young, yellow when ripe, seeds yellowish-brown.

Found wild in the warm, arid and sandy parts throughout India up to 1500m

Fl. & Fr.: June–December.

Sanskrit: Chitraphala, Indravarooni.

Local names: *Ben* & *Hin*: Indrayan, Makal; *Guj*: Indrak, Indravana, Indrayan; *Kan*: Pavamekkakayi; Tumtikayi; *Mal*: Peykomutti; *Mar*: Indrayan, Kadu vrindavana; *Tel*: Etipuccha, Verripuccha, *Urdu*: Indrayan.

Trade name: Colocynth, Bitter apple.

Uses: Whole plant useful in the treatment of diabetes.

**Citrullus lanatus** (Thunb.) Matsumura & Nakai

Syn: *Citrullus vulgaris* Schrad.

Family: Cucurbitaceae

Trailing, hispid, annual herb. Leaves ovate to obovate, lobes bipinnatifid, scabrous. Flowers yellow, solitary, or paired, unisexual, monoecious. Fruit globose or oblong, rind green mottled or striped with longitudinal irregular bands, flesh soft, spongy, juicy, reddish pink, sweet, seeds compressed, black.

Cultivated throughout India.

Local names: *Ben, Guj, Hin, Mar, Ori & Urdu*: Kalingad, Tarbuch, Tarbuz, Tarmz; *Kan*: Kalangadi balli, Kargunje; *Mal*: Thannimatham; *Tam*: Poiychaviral, Tharbuzapalam; *Tel*: Karumboja, Pucchakayi.

Propagation: By seeds.

Uses: Plant useful in the treatment of diabetes.

**Citrus aurantifolia** (Christm.) Swingle

Family: Rutaceae.

Armed shrub or small tree, 2–3m tall. Leaves elliptic-ovate, petiole winged. Flowers white or pink in lax axillary racemes. Fruit round to oval, greenish yellow when ripe, rind very thin.

Wild in the warm valleys of Himalayas, cultivated elsewhere for its fruit.

Sanskrit: Nimbuka. Bribat Jambhira.

Local names: *Ben*: Kaghzilebu, Patilebu; *Guj*: Khata limbu; *Hin*: Kaghzi nimbu; *Kan*: Limbe, Nimbe; *Mal*: Chernnaragam, Erumichinarakam; *Tam*: Elu michai; *Tel*: Nimma.

Trade name: Acid lime, Sour lime, Bitter lime.

Propagation: By seeds.

Uses: Aerial parts useful in the treatment of diabetes.

**Citrus aurantium** L.

Family: Rutaceae.

Armed trees, up to 8m tall with a rounded crown and smooth greyish-brown bark. Leaves ovate, petioles are broadly winged, tapering to a wingless base. Flowers white in axillary cymes, sweet scented. Fruit subglobose, loose skinned, orange when ripe, with hollow core when ripe.

Rarely cultivated.

Local names: *Hin*: Khatta; *Kan*: Heralay; *Mal*: Karna; *Tam*: Nurangam, Narattai; *Tel*: Mallikanaragi.

Trade name: Bitter orange, Sour orange or seville orange.

Propagation: By seeds, cuttings, budding and grafting.

Uses: Fruit useful in the treatment of diabetes.

**Citrus limon** (L.) Burm.f.

Family: Rutaceae

Much branched thorny shrub. Leaves ovate, petiole slightly winged. Flowers white, axillary, solitary or clustered. Fruit oblong, or ovoid, bright yellow with terminal nipple, pericarp thick, seeds many.

Cultivated in plains and hills throughout India.

Sanskrit: Jam birah.

Local names: *Ben*: Baranebu, Goranebu; *Guj*: Motulimbu; *Mar*: Idalimbu, Thoralimbu. *Hin*: Jamiri nimbu, *Kan*: Limbe, *Mal*: Cerunarakam; *Tam*: Elumiccai; *Tel*: Peddanimma, Nimma

Trade name: Lime.

Uses: Plant useful in the treatment of diabetes.

**Clausena pentaphylla** (Roxb.) DC

Family: Rutaceae

Strongly aromatic shrub.

Distributed in sub-Himalayan tract from Garhwal to Sikkim.

Local names: *Hin*: Ratanjote

Uses: Aerial parts useful in treatment of diabetes.

**Clematis barbellata** Edgew.

Syn: *Clematis napaulensis* auct. non DC.

Family: Ranunculaceae

Large woody climber. Leaves 3-foliolate, leaflets ovate or ovate-lanceolate. Flowers dull purple in axillary fascicles. Fruit achene.

In forests of North-West Himalayas.

Fl: Feb–Aug; Fr: June–October.

Uses: Aerial parts are used to treat diabetes.

**Clematis montana** Buch–Ham. ex DC.

Family: Ranunculaceae

Robust woody climbers. Leaves ternately 3-foliolate, leaflets ovate or ovate-lanceolate. Flowers white, cream-yellow or purplish outside in axillary fascicles. Fruit achene.

In Temperate and subtropical forests in Himalayas.

Fl: May–July; Fr: May–September.

Uses: Aerial parts are used to treat diabetes.

**Clerodendrum phlomides** L.

Family: Verbenaceae.

A shrub, up to 3m tall, branchlets pubescent. Leaves deltoid-ovoid. Flowers cream in axillary or terminal panicles. Fruit obovoid drupe.

Common in hedges near villages in many parts of India.

Fl. & Fr.: February–May.

Sanskrit: Arani, Vijaya, Agnimantha, Agnimanthini.

Local names: *Guj, Hin & Mar*: Arni; *Kan*: Taggi; *Mal*: Tirutali; *Tam*: Takkari, Taludalai; *Tel*: Thakkalaku, Thakkalomni.

Trade name: Wind killer, Glory tree.

Uses: Whole plant useful for the treatmentt of diabetes

**Clerodendrum serratum** (L.) Moon.

Family: Verbenaceae.

Erect shrubs, up to 2m tall, stem quadrangular. Leaves obovate or elliptic-oblong, glabrescent above, pubescent below. Flowers violet or lilac in terminal panicles. Fruit drupe, 4-lobed, black when ripe.

Widely distributed in India.

Fl. & Fr.: August–December.

Propagation: by seeds.

Sanskrit: Bhriguja, Angaravallari, Bharangi.

Local names: *Guj & Mar*: Bharungi; *Hin*: Bharangi; *Kan*: Gantubarangi; *Mal*: Cherutekku, Kankabharni; *Tam*: Sirutekku; *Tel*: Gantubarangi.

Uses: Whole plant useful for the treatment of diabetes.

**Clerodendrum viscosum** Vent.

Syn: *Clerodendrum infortunatum* auct non L.

Family: Verbenaceae

Shrub, up to 2m tall, branches 4-gonous. Leaves ovate or almost orbicular. Flowers in terminal cymose panicles, pinkish white. Fruit drupe, subglobose, black when ripe.

Throughout India, as under growth in forests up to 1800m and as weed in wastelands.

Fl. & Fr.: November–March.

Sanskrit: Bhandirah.

Local names: *Ben & Hin*: Bhant; *Kan*: Basavanapada, Ibbane; *Mal*: Peruku, Peruvellam; *Tam*: Karukanni; *Tel*: Gurrapukattiyaku.

Uses: Whole plant useful for the treatment of diabetes.

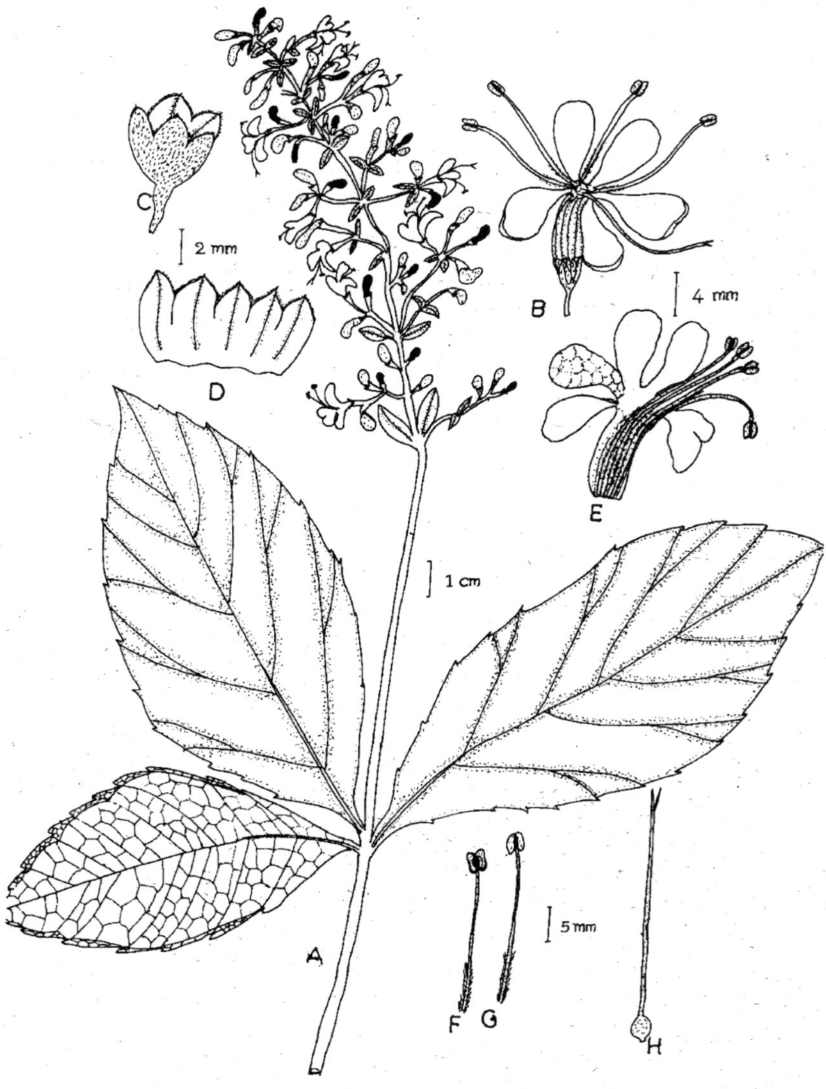


Fig. 35: *Clerodendrun serratum* (L.) Moon
A. Twig; B. Flower; C. Calyx; D. Calyx split open; E. Corolla split open; F & G. Stamens, H. Pistil.

**Coccinia indica** Wight & Arn.

Syn: *Coccinia grandis* (L.) Voigt

Family: Cucurbitaceae.

Perennial herbaceous tendrillar climbers, tendrils slender, simple. Leaves entire or palmately lobed, glabrous. Flowers unisexual, white, solitary or subcymose, female flowers white, solitary. Fruit ovoid berry, red when ripe, many-seeded, seeds ovoid-oblong, compressed.

Common on hedges and bushes all over India.

Fl. & Fr.: Through out the year.

Sanskrit: Bimbi, Bimbika.

Local names: *Ben*: Telakucha; *Guj*: Ghobe, Gluru; *Hin*: Kunduri; *Kan*: Todekai; *Mar*: Bimbi, Tendli; *Tam*: Kovai kai; *Tel*: Dondakaya.

Trade name: Ivy Gourd.

Uses: Powder of leaves and roots is used 3 times a day for the treatment of diabetes.

**Cocculus hirsutus** (L.) Diels

Syn: *Menispermum hirsutum* L.
*Cocculus villosus* (Lam.) DC.
*Menispermum villosum* Lam.

Family: Menispermaceae

Climbing evergreen shrub. Leaves ovate-cordate, pubescent above, velvety-tomentose below. Flowers in axillary panicles. Fruit drupelets, globose, black purple.

Common in forests.

Flnames: *Ben*: Huyer; *Guj*: Vevati; *Hin*: Jamtikibel; *Kan*: Soggadi-valli, Dusari balli; *Mar*: Vasan Vel; *Tam*: Kattukkodi; *Tel*: Dusaritige.

Uses: Aerial parts useful for the treatment of diabetes.

**Cochlearia armoracia** L.

Syn: *Armoracia lapathifolia* Gilib.

Family: Brassicaceae (Cruciferae)

Root is tuberous and cylindrical.

Grown in Gardens both in North India and in the hill stations in South India.

Trade name: Horse radish.

Propagation: From pieces of fresh root.

Uses: Plant useful in the treatment of diabetes.

**Cocos nucifera** L.

Family: Arecaceae (Palmae)

Tall, unbranched tree. Leaves pinnatisect, 2–6m long, rachis stout, leaflets numerous, reduplicate. Flowers unisexual, enclosed in a spathe, drooping spikes bearing few female flowers at their base and many male flowers in the upper portion. Fruit obtusely trigonous drupe, greenish yellow.

Through out India, frequent in coastal areas.

Sanskrit: Narikelavrksah.

Local names: *Ben*: Dab, Narikel; *Hin*: Nariyal, Nariyal-ka-ped; *Kan*: Tengu; *Mal*: Tennu, Nalikeram; *Mar*: Narel; *Tam*: Tenkai-maram, Tennai-maram; *Tel*: Kobbari chettu, Tenkaya (fruit).

Trade name: Coconut

Uses: Fruit and leaves useful for the treatment of diabetes.

**Coffea arabica** L.

Family: Rubiaceae.

Small ever green tree, up to 5m tall. Leaves oblong-elliptic, opposite, glossy, pointed at the tip. Flowers showy, fragrant, white, clustered in the leaf axils. Fruit round, mucilaginous, red when ripe. Seeds oval, grey green, enclosed in a silvery testa.

Cultivated in Karnataka, Kerala, Tamil Nadu and Andhra Pradesh.

Sanskrit: Rajpiluh.

Local names: *Ben, Guj, Hin, Kan, Mal, Mar, Tam & Tel*: Kaphi, Coffee.

Fl. & Fr.: March–October

Trade name: Coffee.

Propagation: by seeds.

Uses: Seeds useful for the treatment of diabetes

**Coix lacryma–jobi** L.

Family: Poaceae (Gramineae).

Tall, perennial, erect grass, up to 1.5m tall, rooting at lower nodes. Leaf sheaths 4–6cm long, blades linear-lanceolate. Racemes nodding or drooping from long peducles, carrying male and female spikelets. Female spikelet enclosed in a hardened polished involucre. Fruit subglobose or ellipsoid.

In moist localities through out India.

Fl. & Fr.: October–February

Sanskrit: Gavedhukah

Local names: *Hin*: Gurlu; Samkru; *Kan*: Manjutti; *Mal*: Kattugotampu, Kakkappalunku; *Tam*: Kattukuntumani; *Tel*: Adavi guruginja.

Trade name: Job's Tears.

Uses: Aerial parts and seeds useful for the treatment of diabetes.

**Colchicum luteum** Baker

Family: Liliaceae

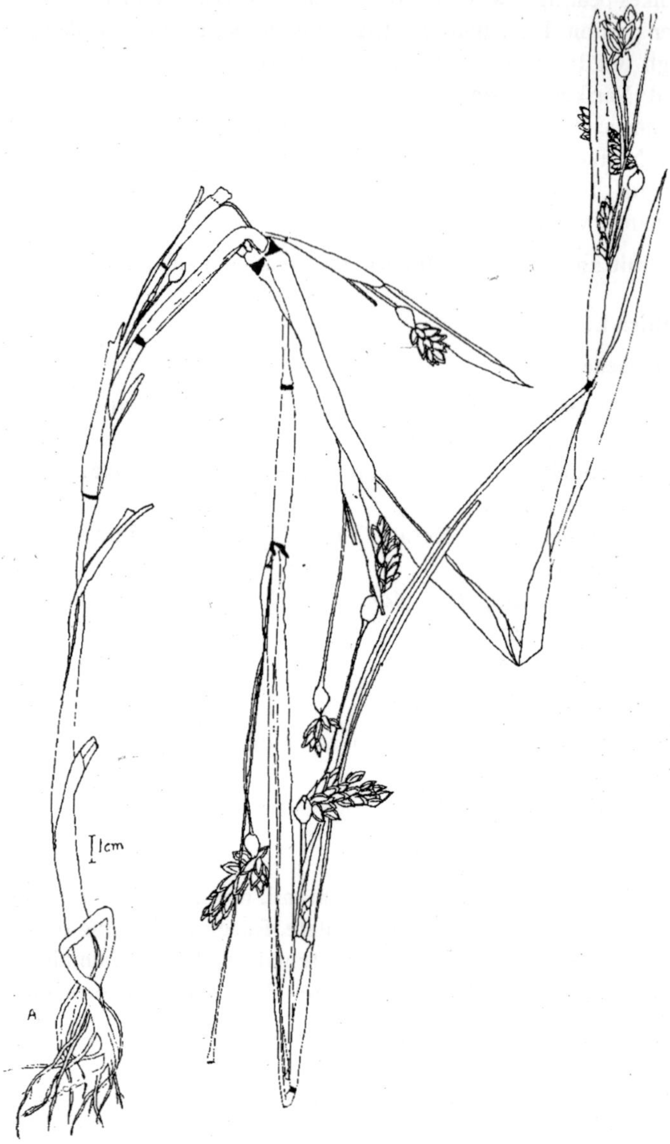


Fig. 36: *Coix lacryma-jobi* L.
A. Twig

Annual herbs, corms conical in shape, brownish. Leaves narrow. Flowers yellow. Fruit to 4cm long, beaks recurved.

Found in north-western Himalayas between 700 and 2800m in open grassy places.

Sanskrit: Hiranytuth

Local names: *Hin*: Hirantutiya; *Kashmiri*: Irkim, Moond; *Pun*: Suranjam-Karvi.

Uses: Corm useful for the treatment of diabetes.

Threatened medicinal plant

**Commiphora myrrha** (Nees) Engl.

Syn: *Balsamodendron myrrha* Nees

Family: Burseraceae

A small tree.

Indigenous to north-east Africa especially Somaliland. Collected in Saudi Arabia, Iran, Thailand and sold in Indian Bazars.

Sanskrit: Bolah, Rasagandhah.

Local names: *Hin*: Bol, Hirabol; *Kan*: Bola; *Mal*: Narumpasamaram, Narumpasa; *Tam*: Vellaippapolam; *Tel*: Balinthra, Polam.

Uses: Gum useful for the treatment of diabetes.

**Commiphora wightii** (Arn.) Bhandari

Syn: *Commiphora mukul* Engl.
*Balsamodendron mukul* Hook. ex Stocks.

Family: Burseraceae

A much branched shrub., up to 4m tall. The branches end in sharp spines. Bark corky. Leaves 3-foliolate, highly aromatic, glabrous. Flowers small, brownish. Fruit ovoid drupe, red when ripe.

Grows wild in arid zones of India, especially in Rajasthan.

Sanskrit: Guggulu, Kanshika.

Local names: *Hin*: Guggul, Gugul; *Kan*: Guggula; *Mal*:Guggulu, Mahisksagulgulu; *Mar*: Gugulu, Mahisaksagulgulu; *Tam*: Gukkulu, Kukkil; *Tel*: Maisakshi, Gugul.

Uses: The Guggul of commerce is the pale yellow or brown aromatic gum resin obtained from the bark. Guggul is a complex mixture of steroids, diterpenoids, aliphatic esters, carbohydrates and varieties of organic ions. Guggul has antilipidaemic activity. Guggul is used in the treatment of diabetes.

**Convolvulus pluricaulis** Choisy

Syn: *Convolvulus prostratus* Forsk

*Convolvulus microphyllus* Sieb. ex Spreng.

Family: Convolvulaceae

Occurs in the plains of Northern India

Local names: *Pun*: Porprang, Dodak.

Uses: The plant extract is exhibited marked hypoglycemic effect.

**Coptis teeta** Wall.

Family: Ranunculaceae

A perennial herb, root stock horizontal, woody, bitter. Leaves ternately dissected, leaflets ovate–lanceolate, incised. Flowers on leafless scapes, white. Fruit of 6–8 follicles.

Usually in peaty soil in shaded places in Arunachal Pradesh, Sikkim and Darjeeling.

Fl. & Fr.: July–September.

Local names: *Ben*: Tita; *Guj*: Haladio vachnag; *Hin*: Mamila; *Mishmi*: Tita.

Trade name: Coptis, Gold thread.

Uses: Rhizome useful for the treatment of diabetes.

**Corallocarpus epigaeus** Clarke

Syn: *Bryonia epigaea* Rottl. & Willd.

Family: Cucurbitaceae.

Thick stemmed climber, root stock large, tuberous, branches glabrous. Leaves broadly suborbicular, angled or deeply 3–5-lobed, densely villose. Flowers unisexual. Male flowers in crowded racemes on long axillary peduncles, female flowers usually solitary on short peduncles from the same axis. Fruit ellipsoid berry, glabrous, apex beaked, 6–9-seeded.

Common in many parts of India.

Fl. & Fr.: September–March.

Sanskrit: Pathalagaruda.

Local names: *Hin*: Akash gaddah; Rakash gaddah; *Kan*: Akashagarudagadde; *Mal*: Kollanhova-kizhauna; *Mar*: Akash Garudand; *Tam*: Akasha Garudan; *Tel*: Nagadonda, Murudonda.

Uses: Plant useful for the treatment of diabetes.

**Corchorus olitorius** L.

Family: Tiliaceae

Annual erect herb, up to 75cm tall. Leaves oblong, lanceolate or elliptic, two lower serratures prolonged into long sharp points. Flowers yellow, solitary or 2–3 fascicled, axillary or extra-axillary. Fruit capsule, cylindric.
Fl. & Fr.: September–January.

Uses: Leaves useful in the treatment of diabetes.

**Cordia dichotoma** Forst. f.

Syn: *Cordia obliqua* Willd.
*Cordia myxa* Forst. f.

Family: Boraginaceae

Deciduous tree, up to 10m tall. Leaves broadly ovate. Flowers white to cream-coloured, in lax axillary and terminal cymes. Fruit ovoid drupe, cream coloured, mucilaginous, seed solitary.
Occasional in forests and hedges of fields.
Fl. & Fr.: December–January.
Sanskrit: Shleshmanthaka, Bahuvaraka.
Local names: *Ben*: Bahubara; *Guj*: Bargund; *Hin*: Lasora, Chota lasora; *Kan*: Chikkachalle; *Mal*: Viri, Cheruviri; *Mar*: Shelvant; *Tam*: Naruvili; *Tel*: Chinna nakkeru, Bankiriki.

Uses: Aerial parts useful in the treatment of diabetes.

**Coriandrum sativum** L.

Family: Apiaceae (Umbellifereae).

Annual erect herb, 30–45 cm tall. Leaves dimorphic, decompound, lower leaflets orbicular, deeply lobed, upper leaflets nearly sessile, bi or tripinnate with linear segments. Flowers white in terminal and leaf-opposed umbels, polygamous. Fruit globose or ellipsoid schizocarp.
Cultivated for seeds and foliage.
Fl. & Fr.: November–December.
Sanskrit: Dhanyaka.
Local names: *Ben*: Dhane; *Guj*: Konphir; *Hin*: Dhania, Dhanya; *Kan*: Kothambari; *Mal*: Kothum palari; *Mar*: Dhanna kothimber; *Tam*: Kottamalli; *Tel*: Dhaniyalu, Kothimeera.
Trade name: Coriander.
Propagation: By seeds.

Uses: Seeds useful in the treatment of diabetes.

**Corydalis govaniana** Wall.

Family: Fumariaceae

Gregarious, fleshy, perennial herb with coiled root-stocks. Flowers bright yellow.

Sanskrit: Bhutakisi

Local names: *Ben & Hin*: Bhutkis.

Propagation: From seed or by division.

Uses: Likely to be threatened medicinal plant

**Crescentia cujete** L.

Family: Bignoniaceae

Trees. Fruit ovoid or rounded.

Introduced and commonly found in gardens.

Uses: Plant used to treat diabetes mellitus.

**Crinum defixum** Ker–Gawl.

Family: Amaryllidaceae

A stout herb with bulbous stock, bulb ovoid. Leaves canaliculate, gradually tapering. Flowers white, in terminal umbels, fragrant at night. Fruit capsule.

Common in Deccan and West Bengal.

Sanskrit: Vishamandala.

Local names: *Ben*: Sukdarsan; *Guj*: Nagrikand; *Tel*: Kesar chettu.

Uses: Whole plant useful in diabetes.

**Crotalaria medicaginea** Lam.

Family: Fabaceae (Papilionaceae)

Diffuse herb. Leaves 3-foliolate, leaflets narrow-oblanceolate. Flowers in terminal racemes. Fruit pod, sub-globose.

Throughout India.

Fl. & Fr.: July–December.

Local names: *Hin*: Gulabi; *Mar*: Zenzue, Jenjarn.

Fl. & Fr.: July–December.

Uses: Whole plant used to treat diabetes.

**Crotalaria retusa** L.

Family: Fabaceae (Papilionaceae)

Undershrubs, up to 1.5m tall, branchlets terete, pubescent. Leaves simple, oblanceolate. Flowers yellow in terminal racemes. Fruit pod, oblong, turgid 10–15-seeded.

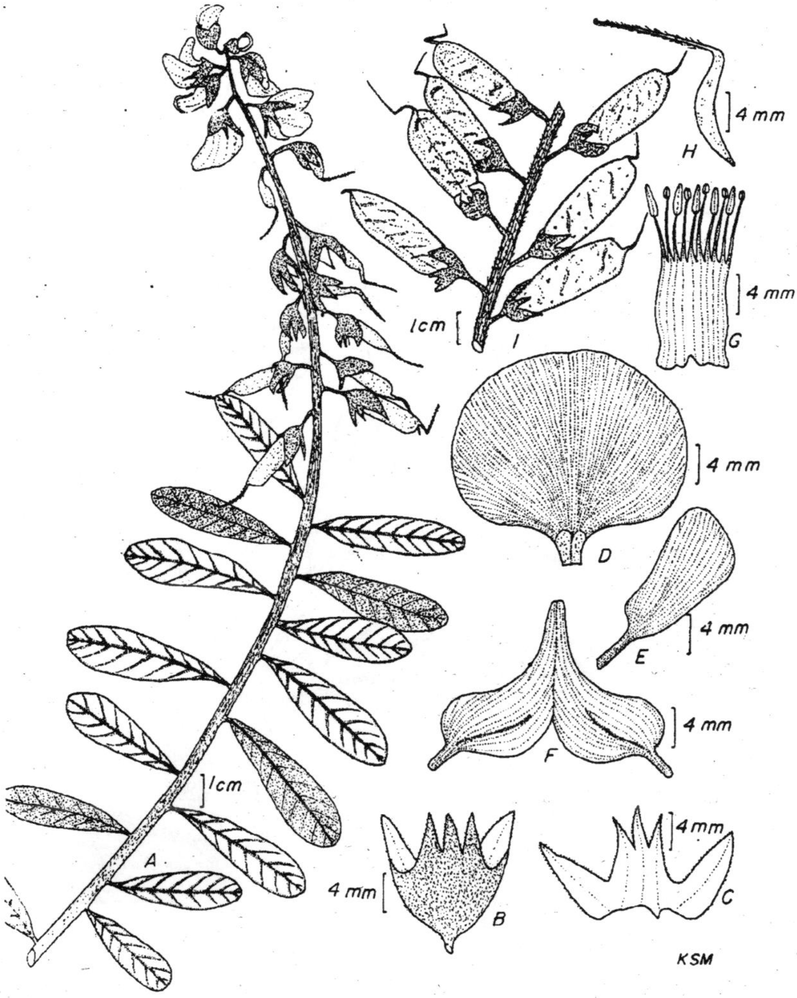


Fig. 37: *Crotalaria retusa* L.
A. Twig; B. Calyx; C. Calyx split open; D. Standard petal; E. Wing petal; F. Keel petals; G. Staminal column; H. Pistil; I. Fruiting twig.

Common weed in cultivated fields and waste lands.

Fl. & Fr.: August–December.

Sanskrit: Sanapuspi, Sanaghantika.

Local names: *Ben*: Bil jhunjun; *Hin*: Ghunghuniyan; *Mar*: Ghagri; *Tam*: Kilu kiluppai; *Tel*: Potti giligicha.

Trade name: Green yellow Sweet Pea.

Propagation: By seeds

Uses: Aerial parts useful for the treatment of diabetes.

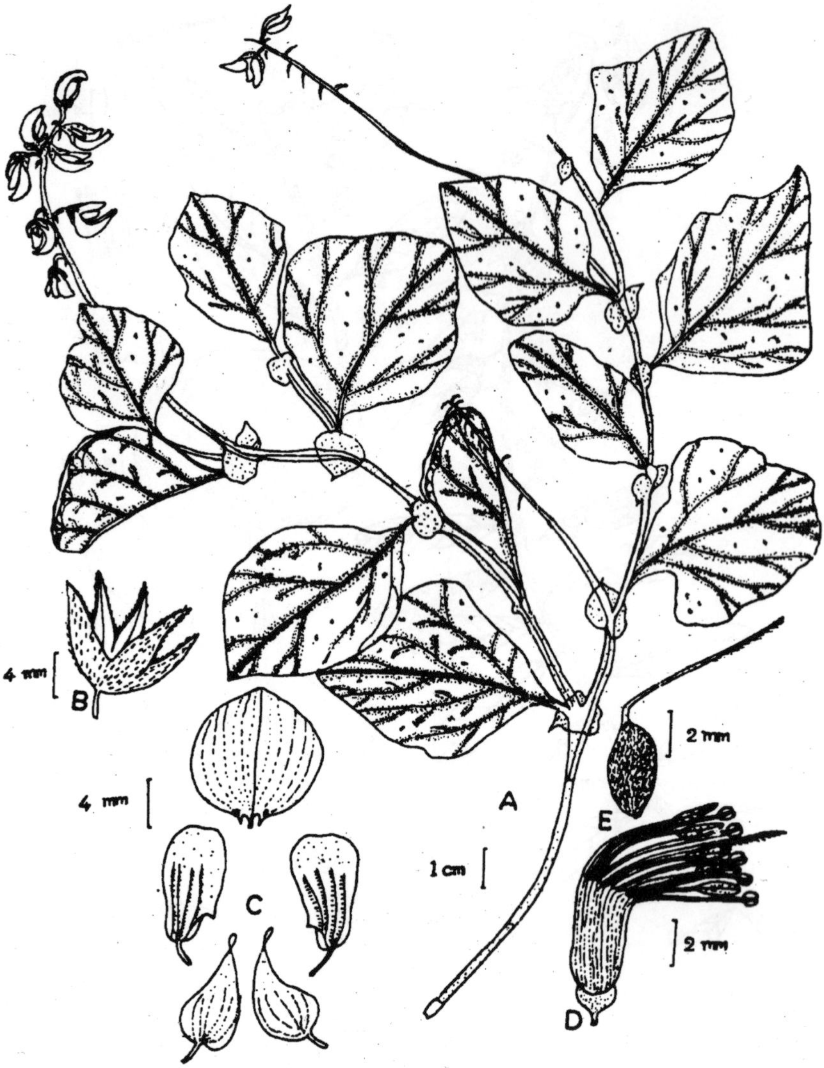


Fig. 38: *Crotalaria verrucosa* L.
A. Twig; B. Calyx; C. Corolla; D. Staminal column with Pistil; E. Pistil.

## Crotalaria verrucosa L.

Family: Fabaceae (Papilonaceae).

Erect subshrubs, up to 1m tall, branchlets 4-angled, appressed pubescent. Leaves simple, ovate or broadly rhomboid. Flowers bluish white in terminal racemes. Fruit pod, oblong, cylindric, turgid.

Common in open waste lands.
Fl. & Fr.: December–February.
Local names: *Tel*: Giligicha.
Propagation: by seeds.

Uses: Whole plant useful for the treatment of diabetes.

**Crypstostegia grandiflora** Wight

Family: Asclepiadaceae

Woody climbing shrub with plenty of latex. Leaves elliptic-oblong. Flowers large, pale purple or rose-coloured in axillary dichotomous cymes. Fruit paired follicles.
Found throughout India.
Fl. & Fr.: August–December.

Uses: Aerial parts useful for the treatment of diabetes.

**Cucumis melo** L.

Family: Cucurbitaceae

Annual climbing or creeping herb, stem angular, scabrous. Leaves orbicular-reniform, 5-angled or 5-lobed, scabrous on both surfaces. Flowers unisexual, yellow. Fruit slender and elongate up to 90cm long, pale or dark green in colour, smooth or ridged.
Cultivated throughout India.
Propagation: By seeds
Sanskrit: Karkati, Ervaruh.
Local names: *Hin*: Kakkri, Tar-Kakkri, *Mal*: Kakkarikka; *Tam*: Kakkarikkay, Vellarikkay; *Tel*: Kharbuja.
Trade name: Snake cucumber.

Uses: Whole plant useful for the treatment of diabetes.

**Cucumis sativus** L.

Family: Cucurbitaceae.

Annual monoecious herbs, trailing or climbing, stems hirsute. Leaves broadly cordate-ovate, palmately 3–5-lobed, densely hairy. Flowers yellow, solitary, axillary. Fruits of various shapes, narrowly or broadly oblong, pale to dark-green or pale yellow, glabrous, many—seeded.
Cultivated for fruit vegetable.
Fl. & Fr.: Through out the year.
Sanskrit: Sukasa.
Local names: *Ben, Hin & Mar*: Khira; *Tel*: Dosakaya.

Trade name: Common cucumber.
Propagation: By seeds.

Uses: Whole plant useful for the treatment of diabetes.

**Cucurbita maxima** Duchesne ex Lam.

Family: Cucurbitaceae

Trailing tendrillar annual herb with some what prickly or hairy stem. Leaves orbicular to reniform in out line. Flowers large, yellow, unisexual, solitary, axillary. Fruit rounded or oval, bluntly ribbed pepo, seeds many, compressed.

Cultivated throughout India

Sanskrit: Pitakusmandah

Local names: *Hin*: Lalkumra, Kaddu; *Kan*: Kumbalakai; *Mal*: Mathan; *Tam*: Pusanikkay; *Tel*: Gummadi.

Trade name: Squash, Red gourd, Pumpkin.

Propagation: By seeds.

Uses: Plant useful for the treatment of diabetes.

**Cucurbita moschata** Duchesne ex Poir.

Family: Cucurbitaceae

Annual trailing herb. Leaves velvety. Fruit variable in shape and colour. Seeds flattened, greyish white.

Cultivated for its fruits.

Uses: Seeds used in the treatment of diabetes.

**Cucurbita pepo** L.

Family: Cucurbitaceae

Annual hispid herb. Leaves orbicular, shallowly lobed. Fruit pepo. Cultivated.

Local names: *Hin*: Kumra, Safed kaddu; *Tam*: Suraikayi

Trade name: Vegetable marrow, Field pumpkin.

Uses: Plant used in the treatment of diabetes

**Curculigo orchioides** Gaertn.

Family: Hypoxidaceae.

Perennial acaulescent herbs, root stock stout, to 30 cm. Leaves lanceolate, prominently nerved, base sheathing. Flowers bright yellow in racemes

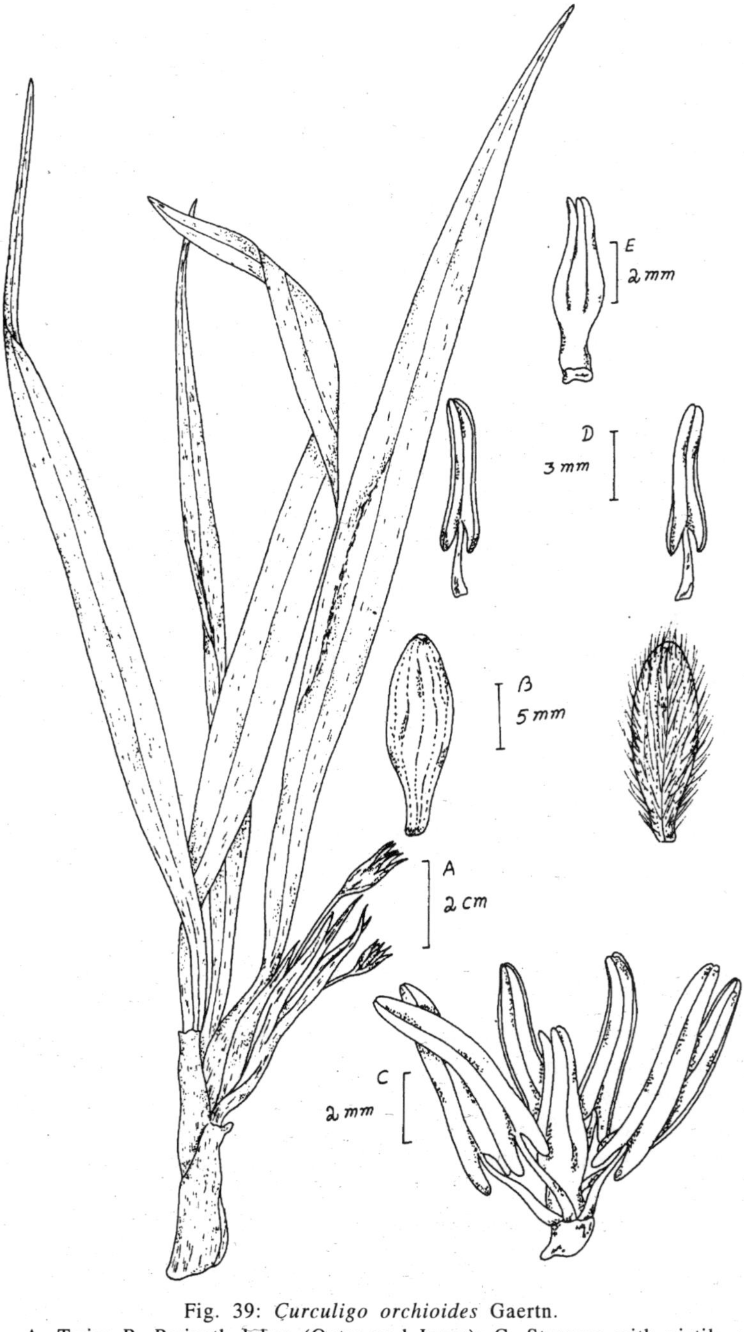


Fig. 39: *Curculigo orchioides* Gaertn.
A. Twig; B. Perianth lobes (Outer and Inner); C. Stamens with pistil; D. Stamens; E. Pistil.

or subcapitate clusters, lower ones bisexual, upper ones often male. Fruit oblong, succulent, 1–4-seeded.

Occasional in forest undergrowth in Subtropical Himalayas from Kumaon Eastwards, Western Ghats and Andhra Pradesh.

Sanskrit: Talmulika, Mushali.

Local names: *Ben*: Tala muli; *Hin*: Kali musli; *Kan*: Nela tati-gadde; *Tel*: Nelathatigedda.

Trade name: Black Musli.

Uses: Whole plant useful for the treatment of diabetes.

**Curcuma longa** L.

Syn: *Curcuma domestica* Valeton

Family: Zingiberaceae

Perennial herb with thick underground rhizome. Leaves born in a tuft, broadly lanceolate. Flowers borne on a separate peduncle arising directly from the rhizome. Fruit capsule, seeds arillate.

Cultivated for its rhizome.

Sanskrit: Haridra.

Local names: *Ben*: Haldi, Pitras; *Guj*: Halada; *Hin*: Haldi; *Kan*: Arashina, Acishina; *Mal*: Mannal, Marinalu; *Mar*: Halede; *Pun*: HaldarHlja; *Tam*: Manjal; *Tel*: Pasupu. *Urdu*: Haladi.

Trade name: Turmeric.

Propagation: Rhizomes.

Uses: Rhizome used for the treatment of diabetes.

**Cyamopsis tetragonaloba** (L.) Taub.

Syn: *Cyamopsis psoralioides* DC.

Family: Fabaceae (Papilionaceae).

Aannual erect herb, with appressed hairs. Leaves tripinnate, leaflets broad-elliptic, pubescent. Flowers small, purplish in axillary racemes. Fruit legume, 3–5cm long.

Cultivated for its fruit vegetable and seeds.

Sanskrit: Bakuchi, Dridhabija, Goraksha-phalini, Gorani.

Local names: *Hin*: Gowar; Gowar; *Guj*: Guwar; *Kan*: Gorikayi; *Mar*: Bavachi, Gowar; *Ori*: Guar; *Pun*: Kulti, Guar, Kuwara; *Tam*: Kothavarai; *Tel*: Matikkayalu, Chowlekayalu, Goruchikkudu.

Trade name: Guar Gum, cluster bean.

Uses: Fruit, gum and seeds are useful for the treatment of diabetes.

**Cydonia oblonga** Mill.

Syn: *Cydonia vulgaris* Pers.

Family: Rosaceae

Shrub or small tree. Fruits are pear or apple-shaped.
Cultivated in Punjab, Kashmir and Nilgiris.
Sanskrit: Amritphala
Local names: *Hin*: Bihi; *Tam*: Simaimathala; *Tel*: Simadanimma.

Uses: Plant useful in treating diabetes

**Cymbopogon citratus** (DC.) Stapf

Syn: *Andropogon citratus* DC.

Family: Poaceae (Gramineae)

Tall, tufted perennial grass with a short rhizome. Leaf blades linear, sheath terete. Flowers in spikelets in loose panicles.
Cultivated throughout India
Sanskrit: Bhustrnah
Local names: *Hin*: Gandhtrnin, *Kan*: Majjigahullu; *Mal*: Cennampullu, Vasanapullu; *Tam*: Vasanapillu; *Tel*: Nimmagaddi.
Trade name: West Indian Lemon grass
Propagation: By slips

Uses: Root useful for the treatment of diabetes.

**Cymbopogan flexuosus** (Nees ex Steud.) Watson

Syn: *Andropogon flexuosus* Nees ex Steud.

Family: Poaceae (Gramineae).

A perennial tufted grass, up to 3 m tall. Leaf sheaths 6–15 cm long glabrous, blade lanceolate. Spikelets in lax panicles.
Common among hill tops and open forests.
Fl. & Fr.: July–December
Local names: *Mal*: Kodi-pulla; *Tel*: Nimma gaddi.
Trade name: Lemon grass.
Propagation: By slips.

Uses: Whole plant useful for the treatment of diabetes.

**Cymbopogon martinii** (Roxb.) Watson

Syn: *Andropogon martinii* Roxb.

Family: Poaceae (Gramineae)

A perennial tufted, sweet scented grass up to 2m tall. Leafsheaths 7–15 cm long,

Blades linear-lanceolate. Spikelets in panicles.

Occasional in forests.

Fl. & Fr.: July–December.

Sanskrit: Rohisah, Dhyama Kah.

Local names: *Guj*: Rauns; *Hin*: Gandh bel; *Mal*: Sambharappullu; *Mar*: Roshegavat; *Tam*: Kavatham pillu; *Tel*: Kamakshi Kasuvu.

Trade name: Palma Rosa, Rosha grass.

Propagation: By slips.

Uses: Whole plant useful for the treatment of diabetes.

**Cynara scolymus** L.

Family: Asteraceae (Compositae)

Perennial herb, up to 1.5m tall. Flowers in heads.

Cultivated occasionally.

Local names: *Ben & Hin*: Hatichak, Hathichoke.

Trade name: Globe Artichoke

Propagation: By seeds and by suckers.

Uses: Flowers useful for the treatment of diabetes.

**Cynodon dactylon** (L.) Pers.

Syn: *Panicum dactylon* L.

Family: Poaceae (Gramineae)

Perennial, stoloniferous grass. Leafsheaths glabrous, ligule ciliate, blade linear. Flowers in terminal spikes. Fruit caryopsis, oblong.

Common in plains throughout India.

Fl. & Fr.: August–October.

Sanskrit: Durva, Niladurva.

Local names: *Ben*: Durba, Dubh; *Hin*: Dub, Durba; *Kan*: Kudigarkai; *Mal*: Karuka, Karikapullu; *Mar*: Haryali, Karala; *Tam*: Arukampillu, Muyalpul; *Tel*: Garikagaddi, Garike.

Trade name: Dhub grass, Bahama grass, conch grass.

Propagation: By cuttings and rootings

Uses: Plant useful for the treatment of diabetes.

**Cyperus iria** L.

Syn: *Cyperus parviflorus* Nees

Family: Cyperaceae

Annual, erect, tufted, marshy herb, up to 50cm tall. Leaves flat, channelled, 30×0.6cm. Flowers in decompound umbel. Fruit nut.
Throughout India.
Fl. & Fr.: July–December.

Uses: Whole plant useful in the treatment of diabetes.

**Cyperus pangorei** Rottb.

Syn: *Cyperus tegetum* Roxb.

Family: Cyperaceae

Perennial, erect, rhizomatous, marshy herb, up to 1.3m tall. Leaves flat, 25×1cm. Flowers in compound umbels. Fruit nut.
Throughout India.
Fl. & Fr.: September–December.

Uses: Plant useful in the treatment of diabetes.

**Dahlia pinnata** Cav.

Family: Asteraceae

Found in northern India.

Uses: Aerial parts are used in treatment of diabetes mellitus.

**Dalbergia spinosa** Roxb.

Family: Fabaceae (Papilionaceae)

Spiny shrub.
Found in the coastal parts of peninsula and West Bengal.

Uses: Aerial parts used in the treatment of diabetes.

**Datisca cannabina** L.

Family: Datiscaceae

Bushy, glabrous, dioecious herb, up to 2m tall.
Found in subtropical Himalayas from Kashmir to Nepal.
Local names: *Hin*: Akalbir, *Pun*: Bhangjala, Bujrabanga.

Uses: Whole plant used in the treatment of diabetes.

**Daucus carota** L. var. **sativa** DC.

Family: Apiaceae (Umbelliferae)

Biennial herb with thick orange fleshy tap root. Leaves pinnately divided, upper leaves linear-lanceolate. Flowers white in terminal much branched umbels. Fruit oblong with bristly hairs along ribs.

Cultivated throughout India.

Sanskrit: Garjarah

Local names: *Ben, Hin, Pun & Guj*: Gajar; *Kan*: Gajjari; *Mal*: Karattu, Mannamullanki; *Mar*: Gazara; *Tam*: Gajjarakilangu, Mancalmullanki; *Tel*: Gajjaragadda.

Propagation: From seeds.

Uses: Root powder, one teaspoonful twice a day with hot water for 20 days lowers the glucose level.

**Decalepis hamiltonii** Wight & Arn.

Family: Asclepiadaceae.

Large glabrous climbing shrub, branches jointed, branchlets terete. Leaves obovate-orbicular, glabrous. Flowers white, small in axillary peduncled, trichotomous cymes.

Fruit follicle, oblong-lanceolate.

Endemic to Eastern Ghats and Western Ghats, in Andhra Pradesh, Tamil Nadu, Karnataka and Kerala.

Fl.: April–September. Fr.: September–February.

Sanskrit: Sariba, Sweta Sariva.

Local names: *Kan*: Maakali beru, Magali beru; *Mal*: Nannari, Naruninti; *Tam*: Makalikkilanku, Mavillinga; *Tel*: Nannari, Maredu kommulu.

Propagation: By seeds.

Uses: Roots useful for the treatment of diabetes.

**Decaschistia crotonifolia** Wight & Arn.

Family: Malvaceae

Erect undershrub, up to 1.5m tall, branchlets appressed stellate tomentose. Leaves ovate-lanceolate or elliptic. Flowers yellow with a deep purple eye in the centre, axillary, solitary or in terminal racemose clusters. Fruit capsule.

Occasional in Kerala, Tamil Nadu, Andhra Pradesh, Karnataka and Maharashtra.

Uses: Whole plant used in the treatment of diabetes.

**Derris scandens** (Roxb.) Benth.

Syn: *Dalbergia scandens* Roxb.

Family: Fabaceae (Papilionaceae)

Large straggler. Leaves odd-pinnate, leaflets to 6 pairs, obovate. Flowers cream coloured in terminal or axillary panicles. Fruit pod, thin.

Throughout India.

Local names: *Ori*: Kentia; *Tam*: Thekil; *Tel*: Nallatiga.

Uses: Aerial parts used in the treatment of diabetes.

**Descurainia sophia** (L.) Webb. ex Prantl

Syn: *Sisymbrium sophia* L.

Family: Brassicaceae (Cruciferae).

Annual or biennial herb, up to 50cm tall. Flowers pale yellow. Seeds compressed, ellipsoid, light brown.

Temperate Himalayas from Kashmir to Kumaon.

Trade name: Flax weed, Flix weed.

Uses: Whole plant is used to treat diabetes mellitus.

**Desmostachys bipinnata** (L.) Stapf

Syn: *Briza bipinnata* L.
*Eragrostis cynosuroides* (Retz.) Beauv.
*Poa cynosuroides* Retz.

Family: Poaceae (Gramineae)

Perennial, stoloniferous grass, stolons very stout, covered with shining sheaths. Leaf sheaths glabrous, lingule hairy, blades linear. Panicle narrowly pyramidal, spikelets sessile, crowded, 30-flowered. Fruit caryopsis.

Throughout India.

Sanskrit: Darbhah, Kusah

Local names: *Hin*: Dab, Davoli; *Kan*: Darbha; *Mal*: Darbha, Darbhappullu; *Tam*: Darbhaipul; *Tel*: Dharbha, Kusa dharbha.

Uses: Plant useful for the treatment of diabetes.

**Dichanthium pertusum** (L.) Clayton

Syn: *Bothriochloa pertusa* (L.) Camus
*Holcus pertusus* L.
*Andropogon pertusus* (L.) Willd.

Family: Poaceae

Perennial stoloniferous grass, up to 50cm tall. Leaves linear. Spikelets in digitate racemes.

Common in plains of India.

Uses: Whole plant useful in the treatment of diabetes.

**Dicliptera roxburghiana** Nees

Family: Acanthaceae

Medium sized tufted herb.
Found in plains of Punjab and Assam.

Uses: Whole plant is used to treat Diabetes mellitus.

**Dioscorea alata** L.

Syn: *Dioscorea atropurpurea* Roxb.
*Dioscorea globosa* Roxb.
*Dioscorea pupurea* Roxb.

Family: Dioscoreaceae.

A large climber, up to 15m long, with stems twining to the right. Leaves opposite or rarely alternate, usually 5-nerved. Bulbils globose, ovoid. Tubers brown to black in colour, non poisonous, edible.
Cultivated in all states of India.
Fl. & Fr.: September–December.
Sanskrit: Pindalu.
Local names: *Ass*: Katalu, Racta guranialu; *Ben & Hin*: Chupri alu, Khamalu; *Kan*: Onthalargasu, Tung-genasu; *Mal*: Kachchilkilangu, Kaavathu; *Tam*: Perumvalli, Kizhanga; *Tel*: Pendalamu.
Trade name: Greater yam, Asiatic yam.

Uses: Rhizome useful for the treatment of diabetes.

**Dioscorea bulbifera** L.

Syn: *Dioscorea sativa* Thunb. non L.

Family: Dioscoreaceae.

A vine. Stems twining to the left, bulbiferous. Roots tuberous, globose. Leaves broadly ovate-sub-orbicular. Flowers unisexual, male flowers green or purplish, female flowers in axillary spikes. Fruit capsule, recurved.
Common in dry deciduous forests.
Fl. & Fr.: September–December.
Local names: *Ben*: Banalu, Kukuralu, Gaichaalu; *Hin*: Ratalu; Suaralu, Pitaalu: *Kan*: Heggenasu; *Mal*: Kattu kachil; *Mar*: Mana-kund; *Tam*: Kodikilangu, Punnukilangu; *Tel*: Adavi dumpa.
Trade name: Potato yam.

Uses: Aerial parts useful for the treatment of diabetes.

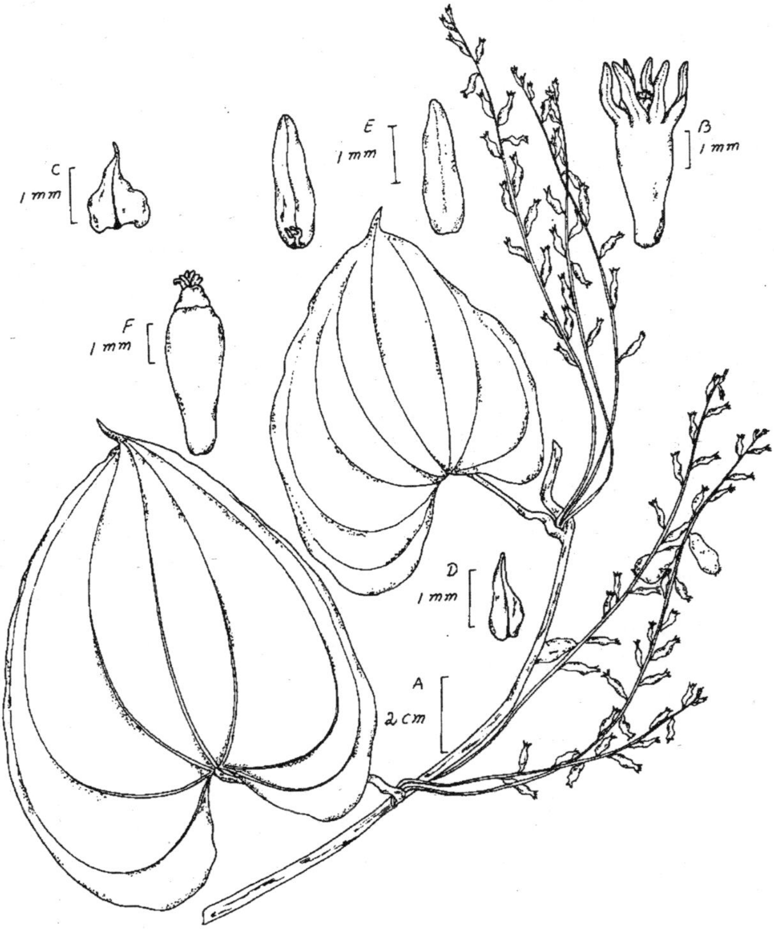


Fig. 40: *Dioscorea bulbifera* L.-Female.
A. Twig; B. Female flower; C. Bract; D. Bracteole;
E. Perianth lobe (Dorsal and Ventral); F. Pistil.

**Dioscorea hispida** Dennst.

Syn: *Dioscorea daemona* Roxb.
*Dioscorea hirsuta* Dennst.
*Dioscorea triphylla* L.

Family: Dioscoreaceae

Climber with prickly stem, twining to the left. Leaves alternate, 3-foliolate, leaflets broadly obovate. Flowers unisexual, in spikes. Fruit capsule.

Throughout India

Fl. & Fr.: October–December.

Local names: *Hin*: Karukandu; *Mal*: Podavakilangi; *Tam*: Periperandal; *Tel*: Tellaginigeddalu, Puli–dumpa.

Uses: Plant useful in the treatment of diabetes.

**Dioscorea oppositifolia** L.

Family: Dioscoreaceae

Climber, stem twining to the right. Leaves oblong or ovate-suborbicular. Flowers unisexual, flowers in pedunculate spikes.
Fruit capsule.
Throughout Deccan.
Local names: *Tam*: Kavalakodi, Vemilaivalli; *Tel*: Yellagadda, Adavidumpa.

Uses: Aerial parts useful in the treatment of diabetes.

**Dipteracanthus prostratus**

Syn: *Ruellia prostrata* Poir.

Family: Acanthaceae

Diffuse undershrub. Leaves ovate or elliptic. Flowers solitary, axillary, blue to violet. Fruit capsule.
Fl. & Fr.: July–December.
Local names: *Tel*: Nela neelambarmu.

Uses: Plant useful for the treatment of diabetes.

**Diospyros insignis** Thw.

Family: Ebenaceae

Large tree, about 20m tall.
Distributed in Kerala and Tamil nadu.
Local name: *Tam*: Pottuttuvarai

Uses: Aerial parts used in the treatment of diabetes.

**Diospyros peregrina** (Gaertn.) Guercke

Syn: *Diospyros embryopteris* Pers.
*Diospyros malabarica* Desr.

Family: Ebenaceae

Medium sized evergreen tree, up to 15m tall. Leaves oblong, thick coriaceous. Flowers dioecious, yellowish in colour, male few in axillary cymes, female solitary. Fruit berry, globose.

Throughout India.
Sanskrit: Tinduka, Krishmasara.
Local names: *Ben*: Gab, Tendu; *Hin*: Gab, Kalatendu; *Kan*: Holetupale, *Mal*: Panachi, Vananji, *Mar*: Timburi, Temburni; *Tam*: Kattatti, Kavi-Kattai, Tumbi; *Tel*: Tinduki; Gabu.

Uses: Aerial parts used to cure diabetes.

**Dipterocarpus indicus** Bedd.

Syn: *Dipterocarpus turbinatus* Gaertn.

Family: Dipterocarpaceae

Tall evergreen tree, bark yellowish brown with grey and white patches. Flowers white and pink shaded in axillary racemes. Fruit winged nut.
Endemic to Western Ghats in Karnataka, Tamil Nadu and Kerala.
Local names: *Hin*: Gujun; *Kan*: Ennamara, Vanasapige; *Mal*: Kalpayin, Karanjili; *Tam*: Enneimaram.
Trade name: Wood oil tree of Malabar.
Propagation: From seeds.

Uses: Aerial parts useful for the treatment of diabetes.

**Dodonaea viscosa** (L.) Jacq.

Family: Sapindaceae

Gregarious evergreen shrubs. Leaves simple, elliptic-oblanceolate. Flowers greenish-yellow, polygamous in lateral or terminal branched racemes. Fruit 2–3-winged capsule, seeds black.
Common in scrub jungles through out India.
Fl. & Fr.: August–January.
Sanskrit: Aliar, sanatta.
Local names: *Hin*: Sinatha, Aliyar; *Kan*: Bandara; *Mal*: Unnataruvi; *Ori*: Mohra Mahada; *Pun*: Benmenu; *Tam*: Velari; *Tel*: Bandaru.
Trade name: Jamaica Switch Sorrel.

Uses: Whole plant useful for the treatment of diabetes.

**Drimia indica** (Roxb.) Jessop.

Syn: *Urginea indica* (Roxb) Kunth.
*Urginea coromandeliana* (Roxb.) Hook.f.
*Urginea wightiana* Hook.
*Scilla coromandeliana* Roxb.

Family: Liliaceae.

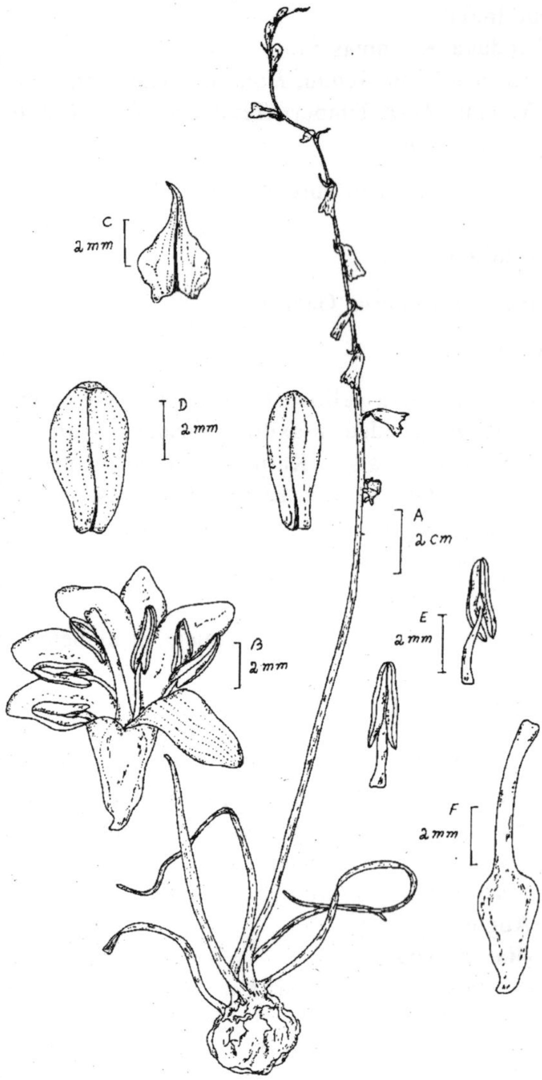


Fig. 41: *Drimia indica* (Roxb.) Jessop.
A. Habit; B. Flower; C. Bract; D. Perianth lobe; E. Stamens; F. Pistil.

A herb with tunicate bulb, bulb the size of an apple, pale, ovoid, thick. Leaves appearing after the flowers, nearly flat, linear. Flowers dingy brown in slender lax flowered racemes. Fruit ellipsoid capsule, the cells 6–9-seeded, seeds elliptic, black.

Found throughout the plains of India and in the dry hills of the lower Himalayas up to an altitude of 1500m in shady localities of forest; also cultivated in Deccan peninsula.

Fl. & Fr.: March–April.
Sanskrit: Kola kanda, Vanpandan.
Local names: *Guj*: Jangli kanda, Rankanda; *Hin*: Jangli piyaz, Han piyaz; *Kan*: Adairirulli; *Mal*: Kattulli; *Mar*: Ranacha kanda, Rankanda; *Pun*: Kachwassal; *Tam*: Nari-vangayam; *Tel*: Nakkavulligadda, Adavi Tellagadda.
Trade name: Indian squill.
Propagation: By bulbs.

Uses: Bulbs useful for the treatment of diabetes.

**Drypetes roxburghii** (Wall.) Hurusawa

Syn: *Putranjiva roxburghii* Wall.

Family: Euphorbiaceae.

Tree, to 20m tall. Leaves elliptic–oblong or lanceolate. Flowers unisexual, male flowers in axillary clusters. Fruit ellipsoid drupe, pubescent, seed crustaceous.
Occasional in forests.
Fl. & Fr.: July–December.
Local names: *Ben*: Putranjiva, Jiaputa; *Hin*: Putranjivika, Putijia, Jiaputa, Juti; *Kan*: Amani, Putranjiva; *Mal*: Pongalam, *Mar*: Jewanputra, Putajan; *Ori*: Pointundia; *Tam*: Irukolli, Karupalai; *Tel*: Putrajivika.
Trade name: Putrajivika.

Uses: Plant useful for the treatment of diabetes.

**Dysoxylum binectarfernim** Hook.f.

Family: Meliaceae

Evergreen tree.
Found in Sikkim, Assam, Bengal and Western Ghats.
Local names: *Ben*: Lassuni, *Kan*: Agilu, Kadugandha; *Tam*: Agunivagil.

Uses: Fruit used in the treatment of diabetes.

**Elaegnus conferta** Roxb.

Syn: *Elaegnus latifolia* auct non L.

Family: Elaegnaceae

Unarmed scandent shrubs, young shoots scaly. Leaves elliptic or oblong. Flowers in many-flowered axillary fascicles. Nut enclosed by fleshy pericarp, red, nut 4-angled.
Himalayas and Hills of Southern India in semievergreen forests.

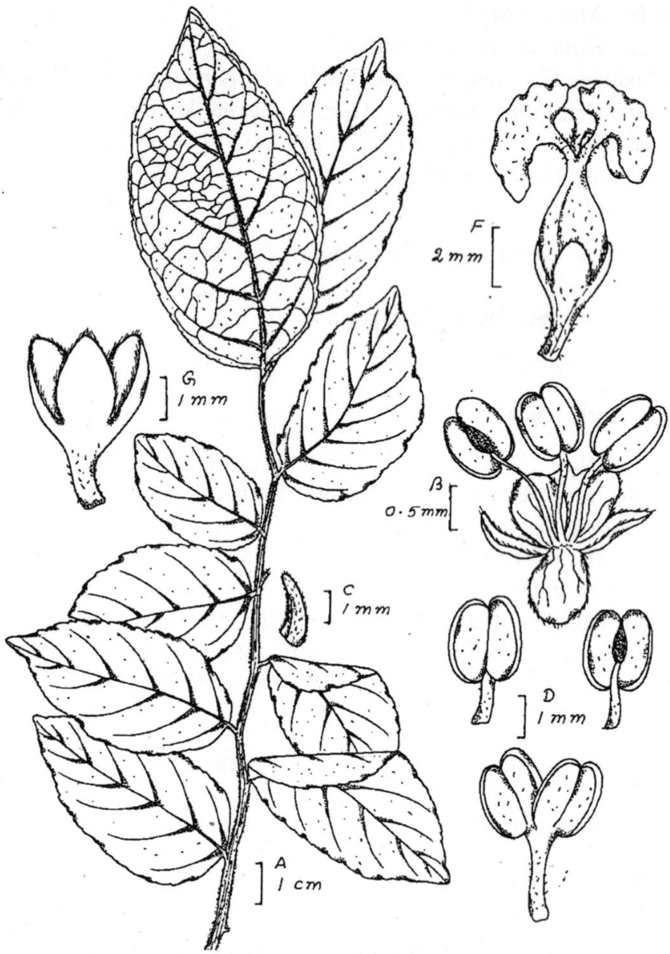


Fig. 42: *Drypetes roxburghii* (Wall.) Hurusawa
A. Female flower; B. Bract; C. Stamens; D. Anthers male; E. Twig; F. & G. Tepals.

Local names: *Hin*: Ghiwain; *Kan*: Kerahuli, Hulige; *Mal*: Kayalampuvalli; *Mar*: Nurgi; *Tam*: Kulangi, Kulari.

Propagation: From seeds and through cuttings.

Uses: Aerial parts used for the treatment of diabetes.

**Elaeocarpus ganitrus** Roxb.

Syn: *Elaeocarpus sphaericus* (Gaertn.) K.Schum.

Family: Elaeocarpaceae

Medium sized tree. Leaves oblong-lanceolate. Flowers white in dense racemes arising mostly from old leaf axils. Fruit drupe, globose or ovoid, bluish purple enclosing hard, tubercled stone.

Occur in Bihar, West Bengal, Assam, Madhya Pradesh and Maharashtra.

Sanskrit: Rudraksha

Local names: *Ben*: Rudrakhya; *Hin*: Rudraki; *Ori*: Rudrakhyo. *Kan, Mal, Tam & Tel*: Rudraksha.

Uses: Stem bark is used to treat diabetes.

**Elaeocarpus serratus** L.

Family: Elaeocarpaceae

Moderate sized tree. Leaves ovate or obovate. Flowers white, in axillary racemes. Drupe ovoid, greenish containing a much tubercled 1-seeded stone.

Found in Eastern Himalayas, forests of North Kanara and Western Coast down to Travancore.

Local names: *Ben*: Jalpai; *Kan*: Perinkara; *Mal*: Avil, Nallakara, Valiyakara, Karamava; *Tam*: Ulang karei.

Trade name: Ceylon olive.

Uses: Aerial parts useful for the treatment of diabetes.

**Elaeocarpus sphaericus** (Gaertn.) K. Schum.

Syn: *Elaeocarpus ganitrus* Roxb.

Family: Elaeocarpaceae

Medium sized evergreen tree. Leaves oblong-lanceolate. Flowers white in dense racemes. Fruit globose, drupe, purple, stone tubercled, longitudinally grooved.

Maharashtra, Bihar, West Bengal, Madhya Pradesh and Assam.

Sanskrit: Rudraksah.

Local names: *Hin*: Rudraki, Rudraks. *Kan*: Rudraksa; *Mal*: Rudraksam; *Tam*: Ruttiratcam; *Tel*: Rudraksi.

Trade name: Utrasam, Bead tree.

Uses: Stem bark useful for the treatment of diabetes.

**Enicostemma axillare** (Lam.) Roynal

Syn: *Enicostemma hyssopifolium* (Willd.) Verdc.
*Enicostemma littorale* auct.
*Exacum hyssopifolium* Willd.

Family: Gentianaceae.

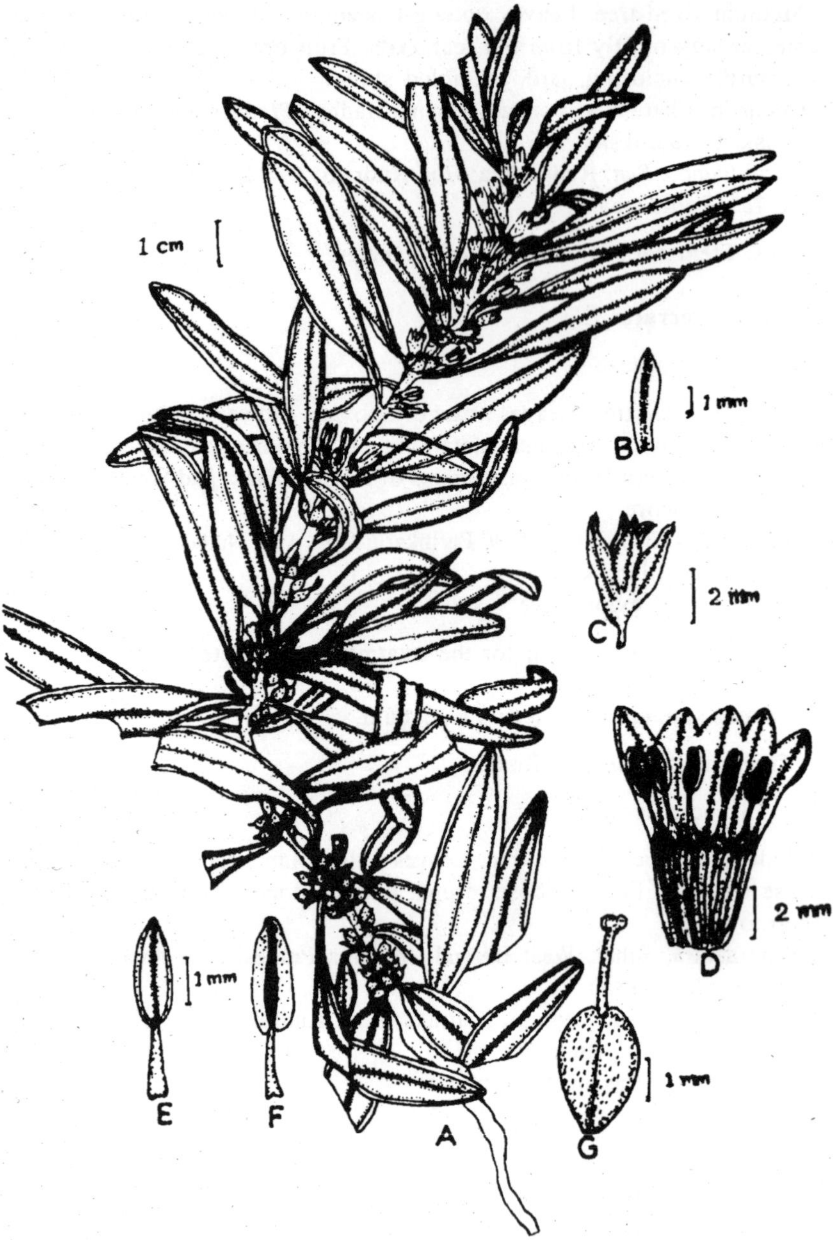


Fig. 43: *Enicostema axillare* (Lam.) Roynal.
A. Twig; B. Bract; C. Calyx; D. Corolla split open; E–F. Stamens; G. Pistil.

Perennial, erect, glabrous herb, up to 40m tall, stem 4-angular. Leaves decussate, lanceolate-oblong. Flowers white, sessile, in dense, axillary, clusters. Fruit septicidal capsule, 2-valved.

Occasional in moist places.

Fl. & Fr.: June–January.

Sanskrit: Nagaguha.

Local names: Chota chirayata; *Mar*: Kadavinayi, *Guj*: Mamijeva; *Kan*: Karibandita, Sogade; *Mal & Tam*: Vellaragu, Vallari; *Tel*: Nelagolimidi, Nelagurugudi.

Trade name: Indian Gentian.

Propagation: By seeds.

Uses: Whole plant useful for the treatment of diabetes.

**Entada pursaetha** DC.

Syn: *Entada scandens* auct non Benth.
*Mimosa entada* L.

Family: Mimosaceae.

Unarmed lianas, up to 30m long. Leaves alternate, bipinnate, pinnae 2 pairs, leaflets about 4 pairs, ovate-obovate, main rachis generally ending in a bifid tendril. Flowers pale green, in panicled spikes. Pods elongate, flat, up to 1m long, woody, falcate, indented between seeds, seeds orbicular, shining.

Hill forests throughout India.

Fl. & Fr.: March–July.

Local names: *Ben & Hin*: Gila; *Kan*: Doddakampi, Hallekayi balli; *Mal*: Kakkavalli, Malamanchadi; *Mar*: Garambi, Garbe; *Ori*: Geredi; *Tam*: Vattavalli, Chillu; *Tel*: Gilatiga.

Trade name: Elephant creeper, Mackay bean, Garbee bean.

Uses: Aerial parts useful for the treatment of diabetes

**Epilobium hirsutum** L.

Family: Onagraceae

Robust pubescent herb, up to 1.5m tall. Leaves oblong-lanceolate. Flowers pink purple.

Distributed in Western Himalayas

Trade name: Hairy willow weed.

Uses: Plant useful in the treatment of diabetes.

**Eragrostis pilosa** Beauv.

Family: Poaceae

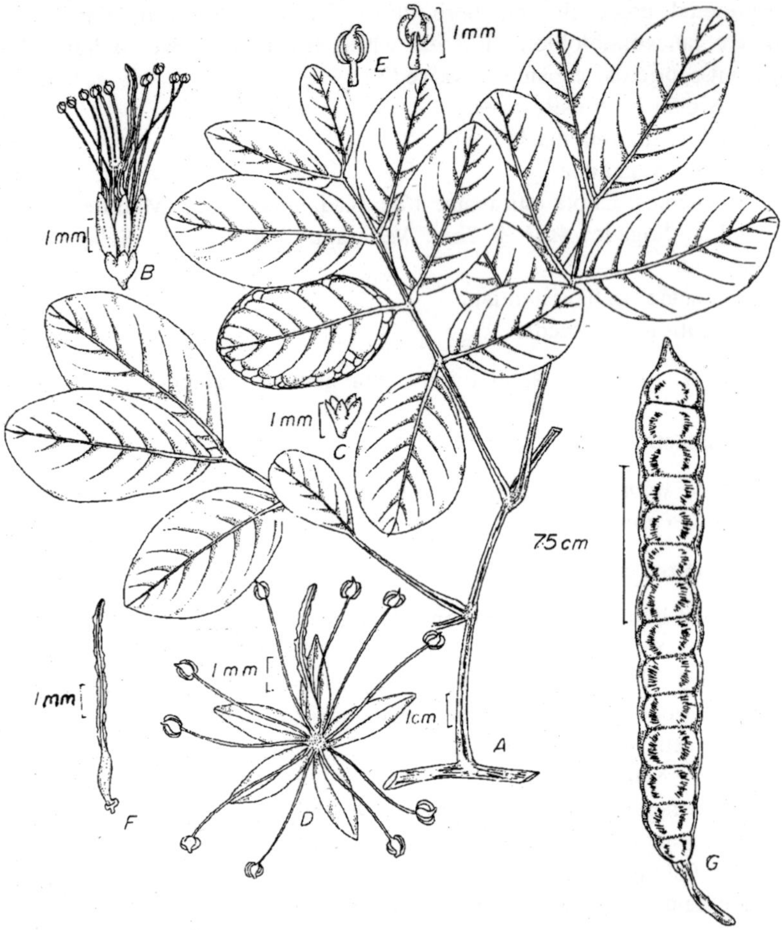


Fig. 44: *Entada pursaetha* DC.
A. Twig; B. Flower; C. Calyx entire; D. Upper view of the flower entire and with stamens; E. Anthers; F. Pistil; G. Pod.

Tufted annual, erect grass, up to 90cm tall. Leaves linear. Spikelets in terminal panicle.

Found throughout India.

Local names: *Kan*: Kadusannasamai hullu; *Tam*: Kuthiral val pul.

Uses: Plant useful in the treatment of diabetes.

**Erigeron canadensis** L.

Syn: *Conyza canadensis* (L.) Cronquist

Family: Asteraceae

Erect, much branched annual herb, up to 1m tall. Leaves linear-lanceolate. Flowers pale rose or purplish.
Found in Punjab, upper Gangetic plain, Western Ghats and Nilgiris.
Sanskrit: Jarayupriya, Makshikavisha.
Trade name: Canada fleabane.

Uses: Leaves and stem used to treat diabetes mellitus.

**Eriobotrya japonica** Lindl.

Family: Rosaceae

Medium sized evergreen tree, up to 8m tall. Flowers white, fragrant. Fruit oval.
Cultivated for its fruit in U.P., Punjab and Nilgiris.
Local names: *Hin*: Lokat; *Kan*: Lakkote; *Tam*: Ilakotta, Nakkotta.
Trade names: Loquat, Japanese mellar.

Uses: Aerial parts useful in the treatment of diabetes.

**Eryngium foetidum** L.

Family: Apiaceae (Umbelliferae)

Much branched aromatic herb. Leaves spathulate, spinous. Flowers white. Fruits ellipsoid, seeds semiterete.
Occurs in Assam up to 1500m.
Local names: *Ass*: Mandhania.

Uses: Plant useful for the treatment of diabetes.

**Erythrina suberosa** Roxb.

Family: Fabaceae (Papilionaceae)

Deciduous prickly trees, up to 10m tall. Leaves 3-foliolate, leaflets broadly ovate, glabrous above, tomentose below. Flowers red in 8 cm long racemes. Pod stipitate, torulose, 2–5-seeded.
Occasional in deciduous forests.
Fl. & Fr.: February–May.
Sanskrit: Mandala.
Local names: *Ass*: Mandal; *Guj*: Jagri vokharo, Janghario; *Hin*: Dauldhak, Madara, Panpranasat, Kanti palas, Rungra; *Kan*: Kaduparivala, Mulluharivara; *Mal*: Murukku; *Mar*: Pangra; *Ori*: Piri; *Tam*: Mullumurukku; *Tel*: Mulumoduga, Munimoduga.
Trade name: Corky coral tree.

Uses: Stem bark useful for the treatment of diabetes.

**Erythrina variegata** L.

Syn: *Erythrina indica* Lam.

Family: Fabaceae (Papilionaceae).

Large unarmed tree, up to 18m tall. Leaves 3-foliolate, leaflets rhomboid-ovate. Flowers red in racemes. Fruit pod, curved.

Throughout India.

Fl. & Fr.: March–July

Sanskrit: Mandar

Local names: *Ben*: Palita; *Guj*: Bangaro, Panarvbeo; *Hin*: Dadap; Mandar; *Kan*: Varjipe; *Ori*: Paladhua; *Tam*: Kalyanamurungai;. *Tel*: Badise, Badita.

Uses: Plant used in the treatment of diabetes.

**Eucalyptus citriodora** Hook.

Family: Myrtaceae

Tall tree, bark smooth, grey, decorticating in small flakes. Leaves lanceolate, often falcate, strongly lemon scented. Flowers cream, in 3–5-flowered umbels. Fruit ovoid-urceolate.

Planted in Malabar, Nilgiris and Coorg.

Fl. & Fr.: May–July.

Trade name: Lemon—scented Eucalypt.

Uses: Leaves useful in the treatment of diabetes.

**Eucalyptus globulus** Labill.

Family: Myrtaceae.

Large trees, bark smooth, sheds in long strips or sheet. Leaves elliptic-ovate, lanceolate or falcate. Flowers whitish, solitary or rarely three, axillary. Fruit globular, sessile.

Planted on roadsides, wastelands and degraded forest by Forest Department.

Local names: *Hin*: Yukeliptus; *Mal & Tam*: Yukkalimaram; *Tel*: Neelagiri thailamu chettu, Eucalyptus.

Trade name: Blue gum, Eucalyptus.

Uses: Leaves useful in the treatment of diabetes.

**Euonymus echinatus** Wall.

Family: Celastraceae

Found in Temperate Himlayas from Garhwal to Sikkim.

Uses: Aerial parts used in the treatment of diabetes.

**Euonymus glaber** Roxb.

Family: Celastraceae

Found in Himalayas, Assam, Bengal and Bihar.

Uses: Aerial parts used in the treatment of diabetes.

**Euphorbia chamaesyce** L.

Syn: *Euphorbia prostrata* Ait.

Family: Euphorbiaceae

Spreading herb. Leaves elliptic-obovate. Flowers in axillary cyathea, unisexual. Fruit capsule.

Fl. & Fr.: July–February.

Local names: *Tel*: Pala alumu.

Uses: Aerial parts useful for the treatment of diabetes.

**Euphorbia hirta** L.

Syn: *E. pilulifera* sensu Hook.f. non L.

Family: Euphorbiaceae.

Annual ascending hispid herb, to 60cm tall. Leaves elliptic-lanceolate, opposite, base obliquely acute. Flowers in cyathia, male florets 4–6, female floret laterally pendulous. Fruit capsule, pubescent, seeds 4-angled.

Common weed along road sides, wastelands and cultivated fields.

Fl.& Fr.: Through out the year.

Sanskrit: Pusitoa.

Local names: *Ben*: Baro–kheruie; *Guj*: Dudeli; *Mar*: Dudhi, Mothi dudhi, Didhli; *Hin*: Dudhi; *Tam*: Amam patchaiarisi; *Mal*: Nea-palai; *Tel*: Reddivarinanubalu.

Trade name: Snake weed.

Uses: Whole plant useful for the treatment of diabetes.

**Euphorbia tirucalli** L.

Family: Euphorbiaceae

Succulent shrub or small tree, up to 5m tall. Leaves small, linear, caducous. Flowers in terminal cyathia. Fruit globose capsule.

Fl. & Fr.: January–April.

Uses: Plant useful in the treatment of diabetes.

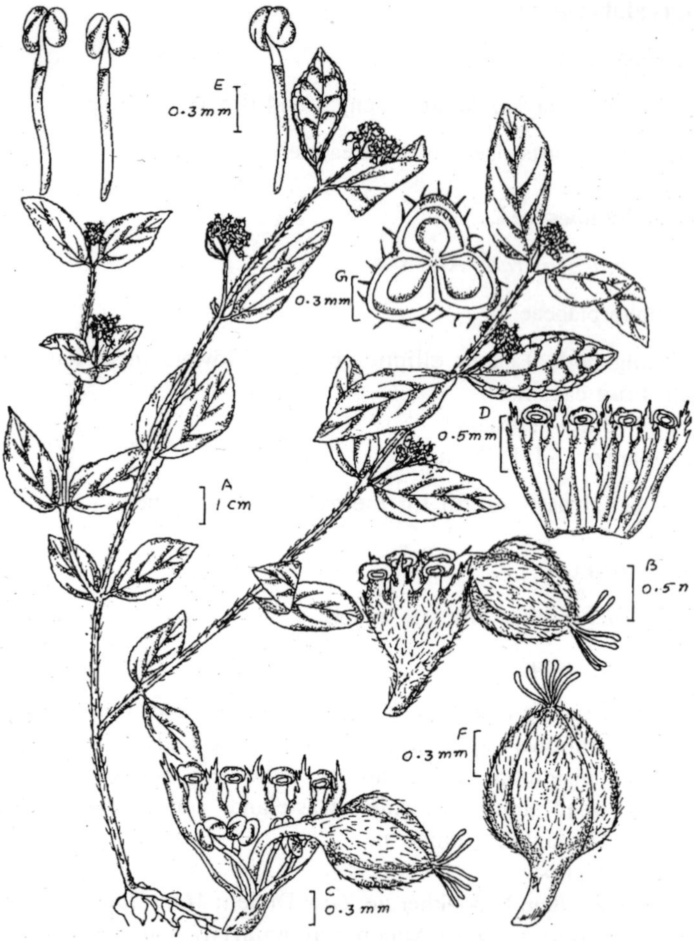


Fig. 45: *Euphorbia hirta* L.
A. Twig; B. Cyathium; C. Cyathium split open; D. Involucre split open; E. Stamens; F. Pistil; G. Ovary T.S.

**Exacum bicolor** Roxb.

Family: Gentianaceae.

Annual erect herb, stem quadrangular. Leaves ovate–lanceolate or elliptic. Flowers in terminal cymes. Fruit capsule.

Found in the Deccan Peninsula.

Local names: *Hin*: Barachirayita,

Uses: Aerial parts used in the treatment of diabetes.

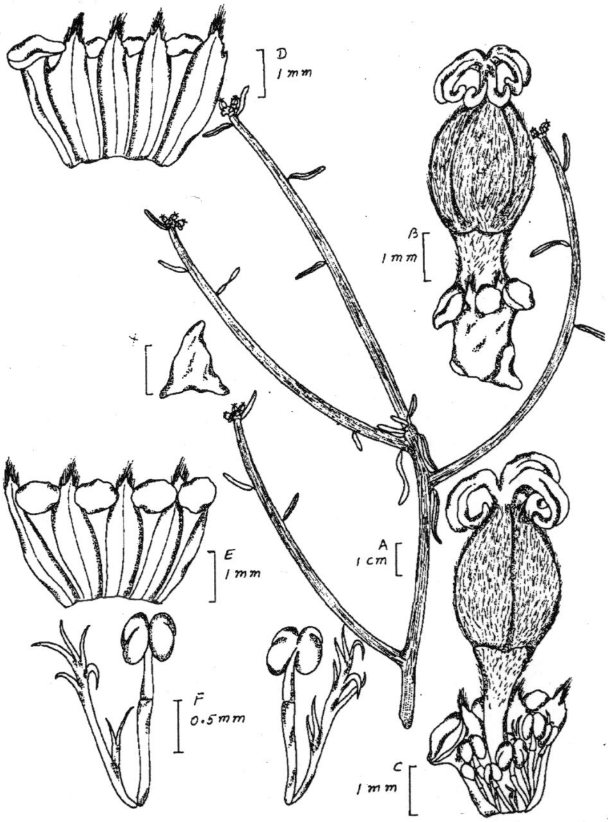


Fig. 46: *Euphorbia tirucalli* L.
A. Twig; B. Cyathium; C. Cyathium split open; D. & E. Involucre split open; F. Stamens with bracteoles.

**Fagopyrum cymosum** Meissn.

Family: Polygonaceae

Tall, branched annual with perennial roots. Leaves ovate, long petioled. Found in temperate Himalayas from Kashmir to Sikkim and Khasi hills.

Uses: Whole plant useful in the treatment of diabetes.

**Fagopyrum esculentum** Moench

Family: Polygonaceae

Annual herb, up to 1.5m tall. Leaves alternate, hastate. Flowers pinkish white in axillary or terminal cymes, fragrant. Fruit achene.

Grown for its grains in the higher altitudes of Himalayas from Kashmir to Sikkim, Khasi hills, Manipur and in Nilgiris.

Local names: *Hin*: Kotu, Phaphra.
Trade name: Common buckwheat.

Uses: Seeds useful in treating diabetes.

**Ferula asafoetida** L.

Family: Apiaceae (Umbelliferae).

A tall perennial, having carrot-shaped rhizome. Leaves upper one much divided into numerous parts. Flowers yellow in umbels. Fruit ovate, flat, thin, flaky.

Wild in Punjab and Kashmir.

Sanskrit: Hingu

Local names: *Hin*: Himg; *Kan*: Hingu; *Mal*: Kayam, Karikayam, Perunkayam; *Tam*: Perunkayam, Kayam; *Tel*: Inguva.

Trade name: Asafoetida

Propagation: by seeds

Uses: Gum useful for the treatment of diabetes.

**Ficus benghalensis** L.

Syn: *Ficus indica* L.

Family: Moraceae.

Very large trees, sending down many aerial roots from the main trunk and large branches which descend to the soil. Leaves elliptic-ovate, alternate, coriaceous, glabrous above, puberulous below. Flowers in figs, axillary, sessile, in pairs, globose, puberulous, red when ripe.

Common all over India.

Fl. & Fr.: December–May.

Sanskrit: Vata, Bahupada.

Local names: *Ben*: Bar, Bot; *Guj*: Vad, Vadlo, War; *Hin*: Bar, Bargad, Bhor; *Kan*: Ala, Alada, Batam; *Mal*: Ala, Vatam; *Mar*: Vada, Vadio, Vor; *Ori*: Baro; *Tam*: Al, Alam; *Tel*: Marri.

Trade name: Banyan tree.

Uses: Stem bark and sap useful for the treatment of diabetes.

**Ficus benjamina** L.

Family: Moraceae.

Large trees with numerous small aerial roots, all parts are glabrous. Leaves elliptic-ovate, alternate, subcoriaceous. Flowers in axillary figs, figs sessile, paired, globose, yellowish when ripe.

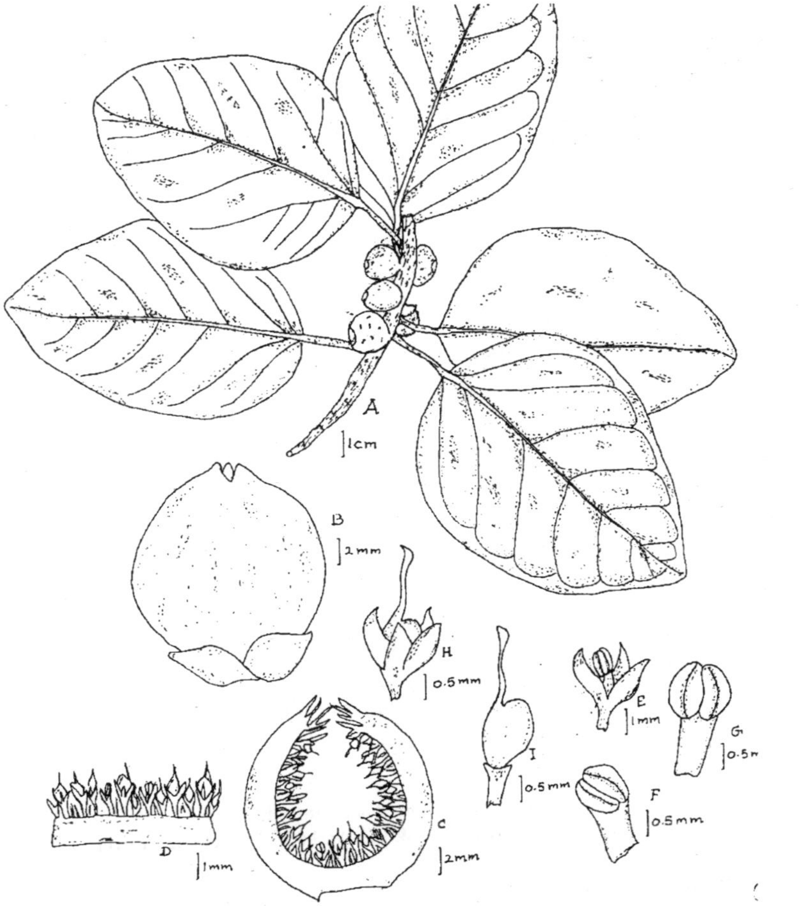


Fig. 47: *Ficus benghalensis* L.
A. Twig; B. Fruit; C. & D. Receptacle L.S and part enlarged; E. Male flower; F. & G. Anthers; H. Female flower; I. Pistil.

Occasional.
Fl. & Fr.: January–April
Local names: *Tel*: Konda golugu, Konda juvvi, Putra Juvvi.
Trade name: Benjamin fig, Java fig.

Uses: Aerial parts useful for the treatment of diabetes.

**Ficus carica** L.

Family: Moraceae

Small or modertate sized deciduous trees. Leaves ovate or nearly orbicular, more or less deeply 3–5-lobed, rough above and pubescent below. Fruit axillary, usually pear-shaped, variable in size and colour.

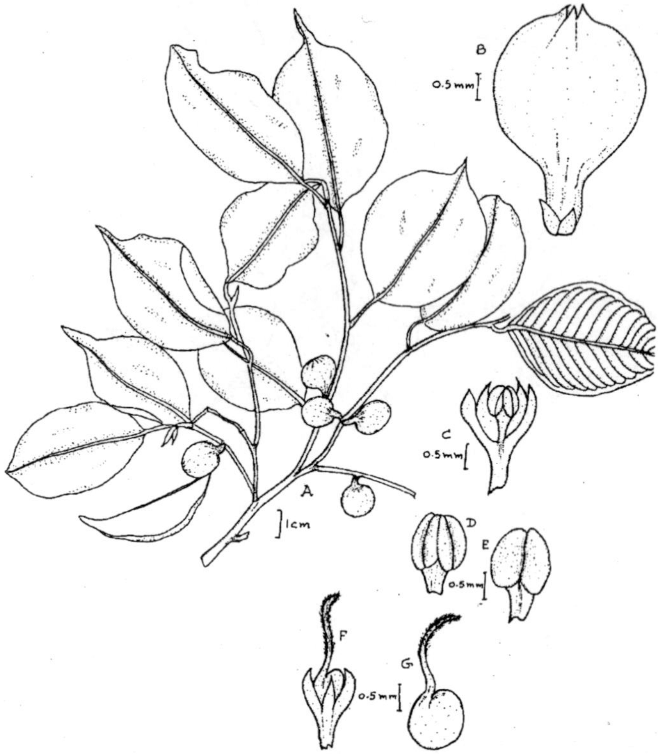


Fig. 48: *Ficus benjamina* L.
A. Twig; B. Fruit; C. Male flower; D. & E. Anthers; F. Female flower; G. Pistil.

Cultivated occasionally.

Sanskrit: Ansira.

Local names: *Ben, Guj, Hin & Mar*: Anjir; *Kan*: Anjura; *Mal*: Simayatti; *Tam*: Simayatti, Tenatti; *Tel*: Anjooramu.

Trade name: Common fig.

Propagation: By stem cuttings.

Uses: Decoction of leaves as supplement to breakfast in IDDM could be of help to control postprandial glycemia.

**Ficus hispida** L.f.

Family: Moraceae.

Shrub or small trees, generally with hollow internodes, without aerial roots, bark grey, rough, all parts very hispid. Leaves sub-obovate or ovate-oblong, opposite, at times alternate. Figs on special shoots and branchlets at the base, densely hispid, yellow when ripe.

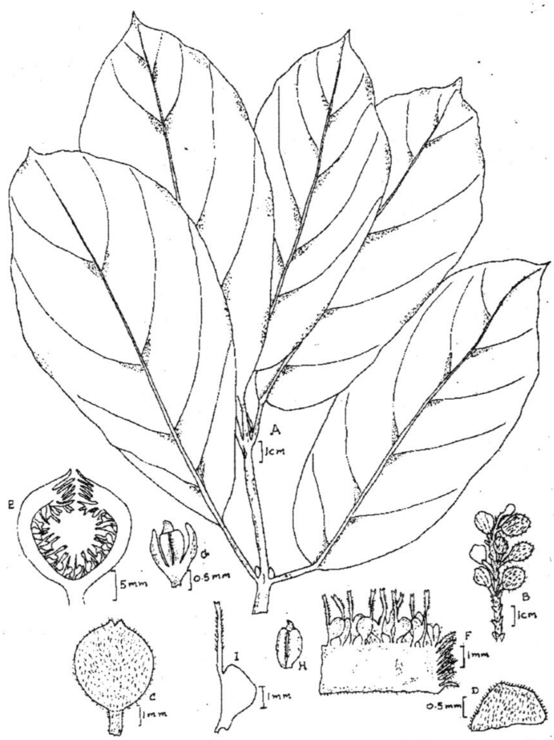

Fig. 49: *Ficus hispida* L.f.
A. Twig; B. Fruiting twig; C. Fruit; D. Bract; E. & F. Receptacle L.S. and part enlarged; G. Male flower; H. Stamen; I. Female flower.

Common in forests in damp localities in Central and South India.

Fl. & Fr.: December–March.

Sanskrit: Kakodumbarika, Bhadradumbarka.

Local names: *Ben*: Dumoor, Kakodumar; *Guj*: Dhedaumaro, Jangliangir; *Hin*: Daduri, Dagarin, Gobla, Kagsha, Katgularia; *Kan*: Adavi atti, Kadatti; *Mal*: Erumanakku, Peyatti; *Mar*: Bhokada, Bokria, Kalaumber, Kharoti; *Tam*: Peyatti, Sonatti; *Tel*: Adaviathi, Kakimedi.

Trade name: Wild fig, Devil fig, Crow fig.

Propagation: By seeds and stem cuttings.

Uses:Aerial parts useful in the treatment of diabetes.

**Ficus racemosa** L.

Syn: *Ficus glomerata* Roxb.

Family: Moraceae.

Large deciduous tree, with a few or no aerial roots, bark smooth, greyish white, branchlets white-pilose. Leaves elliptic-lanceolate, alternate. Figs monoecious, cauliflorous, globose, white pilose, ripening red.

Common in forests.

Fl. & Fr.: Through out the year.

Sanskrit: Udumbhara, Sadaphala.

Local names: *Ben*: Dumur, Jagyadumur, Yagnadumur; *Guj*: Umar, Umaro, Umbar, Umbro; *Hin*: Dimere, Gular, Lelka, Parao, Umar, Umrai, Tue; *Kan*: Athi, Atti, Rumadi; *Mal*: Atti, Audumbaram, Jantuphalam, Udumbgaram; *Mar*: Atti, Gular, Raumadi, Umar, Umbar, Umbra, Umbara; *Ori*: Dimiri, Jaagnondumboro, Dumuro; *Pun*: Batbar, Rumbal, Dadburi, Kakammal, Palak; *Tam*: Atti Adam, Adavam, Adaru, Anai, Anjiram, Asamarudam, Asuvattam, Tumbaram, Tuniangam, Udumbaram; *Tel*: Atti, Medi; *Urdu*: Gular.

Trade name: Gular fig, cluster fig.

Propagation: by seeds and stem cuttings.

Uses: Stem bark and fruit useful for the treatment of diabetes.

**Ficus religiosa** L.

Family: Moraceae.

Large glabrous tree, bark greenish. Leaves broadly ovate, alternate. Figs monoecious, axillary, sessile, paired, obovoid or depressed globose, ripening dark purple or black.

Commonly planted on village sites and as an avenue tree.

Fl. & Fr.: May–August.

Sanskrit: Ashwatha, Pippala.

Local names: *Ben*: Aswatha, Aswat, Asud, Asvatha; *Guj*: Pipul; *Hin*: Asvattha, Pipal; *Kan*: Arali, Aswattha, Rangi, Basri, Arole, Haspath, Ragi, Asvatt; *Mal*: Arasu, Arayal; *Mar*: Asvath, Pipal; *Ori*: Zari; *Pun*: Pipal; *Tam*: Arasa, Atti, Aswartham; *Tel*: Raavi, Ashwathamu, Bodi.

Trade name: Peepal tree, Sacred Fig.

Propagation: by seeds.

Uses: Root bark and root used for the treatment of diabetes.

**Ficus talboti** King

Family: Moraceae.

Large evergreen tree without aerial roots, all parts glabrous, milky juice abundant, yellowish. Leaves broadly ovate-elliptic or ovate, alternate. Figs monoecious, axillary, in pairs, sessile, yellowish when ripe.

Occasional in forests in Peninsular India.

Fl. & Fr.: December–February.

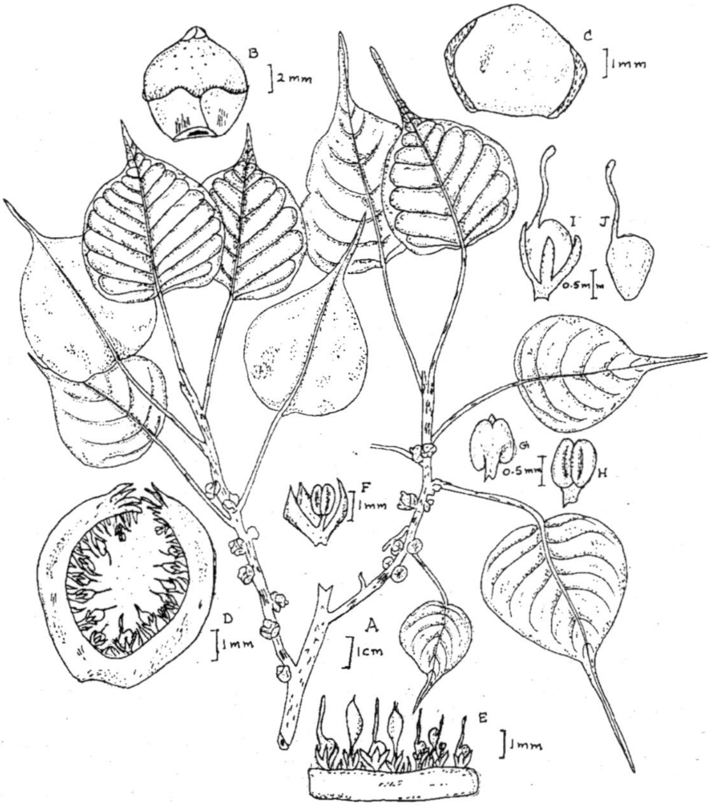


Fig. 50: *Ficus religiosa* L.
A. Twig; B. Fruit; C. Bract; D. & E. Receptacle L.S and part enlarged; F. Male flower; G. & H. Anthers; I. Female flower; J. Pistil.

Sanskrit: Plaksah.

Uses: Aerial parts used for the treatment of diabetes.

**Flacourtia montana** Grah.

Family: Flacourtiaceae

Medium–sized or large tree. Fruit red or purple, edible.
Found in Evergreen forests of Western Ghats and Orissa.
Local names: *Kan*: Han sampige, Gudda; *Mar*: Attak, Champari

Uses: Aerial parts used in the treatment of diabetes.

**Fragaria vesca** L.

Family: Rosaceae

Erect, perennial herb. Leaves serrate-dentate. Flowers white in clusters. Fruit ovoid, red when ripe.

Found at higher altitudes in Kashmir and Sikkim.

Trade name: Perpetual strawberry.

Uses: Leaves used in the treatment of diabetes.

**Garcinia indica** (Dupetit-Thours) Choisy

Syn: *Brindonia indica* Dupetit-Thours

Family: Clusiaceae (Guttiferae)

Moderate sized tree with drooping branches, bark dark brown, smooth, thin. Leaves opposite, lanceolate or obovate-oblong, shiny, dark brown. Flowers white, solitary, terminal. Fruit globose berry, orange-pink when ripe with persistintent calyx lobes.

Found in tropical evergreen forests of Maharashtra, Goa, Karnataka, Tamil Nadu and Kerala.

Sanskrit:Vrksamla, Amlavetasa.

Local names: *Guj*: Kokan; *Hin*: Kokam, Vishambil; *Kan*: Murginahuli-mara, Devana huli; *Mal*: Punampuli; *Mar*: Amsol, Bhirand, Katambi, Kokam, Ratamba; *Tam*: Murgal, Murgal-mara; *Tel*: Ratamba, Kokam.

Trade name: Wild mangosteen, Indian gamboge.

Propagation: By seeds, through cuttings and grafts.

Uses: Aerial parts used for the treatment of diabetes.

**Garcinia pedunculata** Roxb.

Family: Clusiaceae

Tall tree, up to 15m tall. Leaves obovate or oblanceolate. Seeds enclosed in a pulpy aril.

Found in upper Assam and Manipur.

Local names: *Ben*: Tikul; Tikur.

Uses: Aerial parts used in the treatment of diabetes.

**Geranium nepalense** Sweet

Family: Gentianaceae

Slender, much branched diffuse, perennial herb. Leaves palmately 3–5-lobed. Flowers pink or purple.

Found throughout Himalayas and in Khasi, Nilgiri and Pulney hills.

Local names: *Hin*: Bhanda.

Trade name: Nepal Geranium.

Uses: Whole plant used in the treatment of diabetes.

**Glinus lotoides** L.

Family: Aizoaceae

Spreading herb. Leaves obovate, suborbicular or spathulate. Flowers greenish-white in axillary fascicles. Fruit ovoid capsule, enclosed in persistent calyx.

Found throughout the plains of India.

Fl. & Fr.: March–July.

Uses: Whole plant useful for the treatment of diabetes.

**Glochidion hohenackeri** Bedd.

Syn: *Glochidion lanceolarium* Dalz.

Family: Euphorbiaceae

Small or medium sized evergreen tree.

Konkan and North Kanara.

Uses: Aerial parts used to treat diabetes.

**Gloriosa superba** L.

Family: Liliaceae.

Climbing herbs, root stock with cylindric tubers, branchlets terete. Leaves alternate, opposite or whorled, oblong-lanceolate, sessile, glabrous, base cordate, margin entire. Flowers large, axillary, solitary at the ends of branches, greenish at first, then yellow, passing through orange and scarlet to crimson. Fruit oblong-ellipsoid capsule, seeds numerous, globose, warty.

Common throughout tropical parts of India, climbing on bushes and hedges.

Fl. & Fr.: August–September.

Sanskrit: Langali, Agnisikha.

Local names: *Ben*: Bishalanguli, Ulatchandal; *Guj*: Dudhiovachnag, Varhvardi; *Hin*: Languli, Karihari, Karadikanninagadde, Nangulika; *Kan*: Kolikuttuma; *Mal*: Ventoni, Mentonni; *Mar*: Karianag, Nagakaria; *Ori*: Ognisikha, Garbhoghhatono, Panjangulia, Meheriaphulo; *Pun*: Kariari, Mulim; *Tam*: Kantal, Kalappaikkilanku; *Tel*: Adavi nabhi, Kalappa gadda, Vanka vajramu.

Trade name: Glory lily.

Propagation: Through seeds collected during october and through tubers.

Uses: Whole plant useful for the treatment of diabetes.

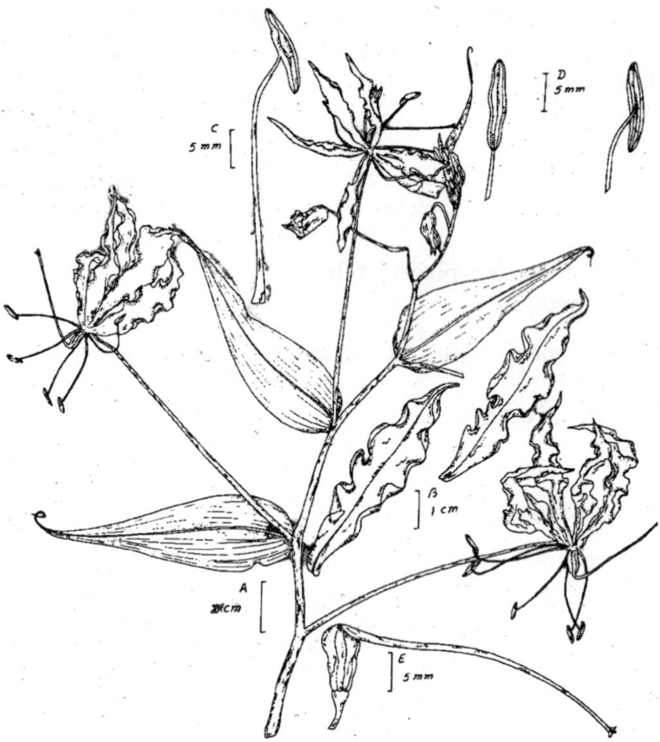


Fig. 51: *Gloriosa superba* L.
A. Twig; B. Perianth lobe (Dorsal and Ventral); C. Stamen; D. Anthers; E. Pistil.

**Glycine max** Merr.

Syn: *Glycine soja* Sieb. & Zucc.

Family: Fabaceae (Papilionaceae)

Annual erect or climbing herb, densely pubescent. Leaves trifoliolate, leaflets ovate-lanceolate. Flowers small, white or purple in axillary racemes. Fruit pod, 2–4-seeded. Cultivated for its seeds.

Local names: *Ben*: Garjkalai; *Hin*: Bhat Bhatwar, Bhetmas

Trade name: Soyabean, Soya.

Uses: Aerial parts used in the treatment of diabetes.

**Glycyrrhiza glabra** L.

Family: Fabaceae (Papilionaceae)

Erect perennial herb, 1–2m tall. Leaves alternate, odd pinnate, leaflets 3–8 pairs. Flowers lilac or light violet, in slender axillary spikes. Fruit pod, flat, sutures thick, glabrous, 3–5-seeded.

Cultivated.

Sanskrit: Madhuyashti

Local names: *Ben*: Jashtimadhu; *Hin*: Mulethi, Mulathi; *Kan*: Yashtimadhukam; *Mal*: Irati-madhuram; *Tam*: Atimadhuram; *Tel*: Yashtimadhukam

Trade name: Liquorice

Propagation: By seeds.

Uses: Root used for the treatment of diabetes.

**Gmelina arborea** Roxb.

Family: Verbenaceae.

Unarmed medium sized trees, up to 10m tall, branches terete. Leaves broadly ovate. Flowers yellow or yellowish brown in threes in panicles. Fruit ovoid or pyriform drupe, orange yellow when ripe.

Occasional in the deciduous forests.

Fl. & Fr.: March–May.

Sanskrit: Gambhari, Kasmari, Gandhari, Shriparni, Bhadraparni.

Local names: *Ben*: Gumbhar; *Hin*: Gumbhar, Kumbhar; *Kan*: Kumizhu, Kumil; *Mal*: Kumilu, Kumpil, Kumil; *Mar*: Shewan, Gamar; *Ori*: Gambari, Bhodropornni; *Tam*: Kumil, Gumadi; *Tel*: Gummadi teku.

Trade name: Coomb Teak, White Teak.

Uses: Stem useful for the treatment of diabetes.

**Gomphrena globosa** L.

Family: Amaranthaceae

Erect herb, up to 40cm tall. Leaves elliptic to obovate, oblong. Flowers in globose heads. Seeds black.

Cultivated all over India as ornamental.

Fl. & Fr.: Throughout the Year.

Local names: *Tel*: Rudraksha poolu.

Uses: Plant useful for the treatment of diabetes.

**Gomphrena serrata** L.

Syn: *Gomphrena decumbens* Jacq.

Family: Amaranthaceae

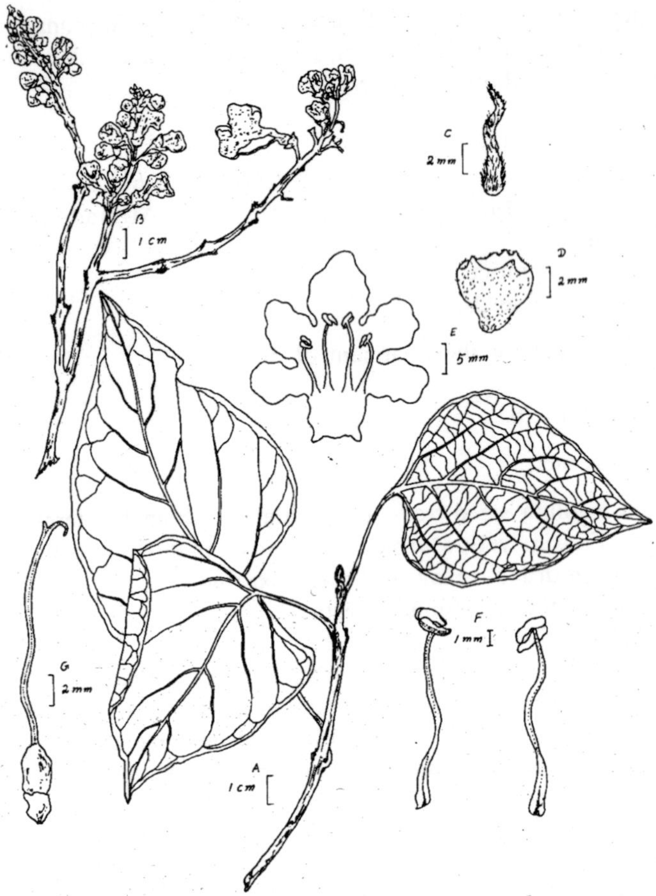


Fig. 52: *Gmelina arborea* Roxb.
A. Branch; B. Inflorescence; C. Bract; D. Calyx; E. Corolla open;
F. Stamens; G. Pistil.

Erect herb, up to 40cm tall. Leaves opposite-decussate, lanceolate. Flowers white in subglobose spike. Seeds brown.

Fl. & Fr.: Throughout the year.

Local names: *Tel*: Tella pogada banthi.

Uses: Plant useful in the treatment of diabetes.

**Gordonia obtusa** Wall.

Family: Theaceae; Ternstroemiaceae

Tall evergreen tree. Leaves elliptic-lanceolate. Flowers large, white or creamy. Fruit capsule, woody.

Found in Western Ghats.

Local names: *Kan*: Nagette; *Mal*: Kattukarana; Atangi, ola; *Tam*: Miyilai, Atangi, Ola, Nagatte, Thorilla.

Uses: Aerial parts used in the treatment of diabetes.

**Gossypium herbaceum** L.

Family: Malvaceae

Small shrub, up to 2.5m tall, twigs and young leaves are sparsely hairy. Leaves cleft into 3–7 lobes, lobes ovate. Flowers yellow with purple centre, axillary, solitary. Fruit rounded capsule, beaked, seeds with two coats of hairs.

Cultivated throughout India.

Sanskrit: Karpasah

Local names: *Hin*: Kapas; *Kan*: Janivaro, Hitti-Mara; *Mal*: Parutti, Nulparutti, Kuruparutti, Pannipparutti; *Tam*: Karpasam, Panju; *Tel*: Pathi.

Propagation: By seeds

Uses: Leaves useful in the treatment of diabetes.

**Grewia hirsuta** Vahl

Family: Tiliaceae

Erect shrubs, softly rufous-pubescent. Leaves oblong or lanceolate, stellate pubescent above, woody below. Flowers polygamous (male + bisexual), pale to bright yellow, in axillary, extra-axillary, umbellate cymes. Fruit globose drupe.

Fl. & Fr.: May–October.

Uses: Aerial parts useful for the treatment of diabetes.

**Grewia serrulata** DC.

Syn: *G. disperma* Rottl

Family: Tiliaceae

Shrub or small tree.

Found in North East India and Western Ghats.

Uses: Aerial parts useful in the treatment of diabetes.

**Grewia tiliaefolia** Vahl

Family: Tiliaceae

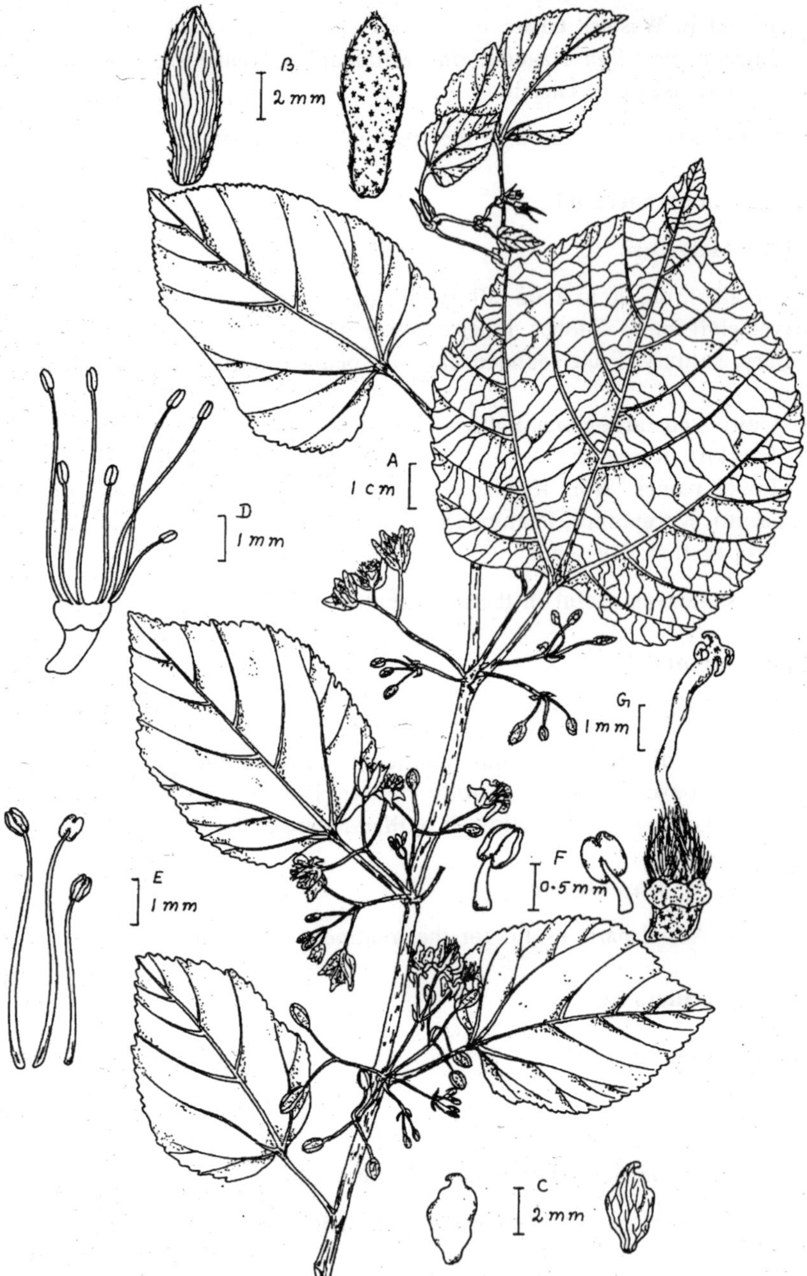


Fig. 53: *Grewia tiliaefolia* Vahl
A. Twig; B. Sepals; C. Pistil; D. Androecium; E. Stamens; F. Anther; G. Gynoecium.

Moderate sized tree, up to 10m tall, bark grey to blackish brown. Leaves broadly ovate or oblong, hoary-tomentose beneath. Flowers yellow in axillary or extra-axillary cymes. Fruit globose drupe, 2–4-lobed, black when ripe.

Common in deciduous and semievergreen forests throughout India.

Fl. & Fr.: July–December.

Sanskrit: Dhanvangah, Dhanurvrksah.

Local names: *Ben & Hin*: Dhamni, Dhaman; *Guj*: Dalmon, Dhamana; *Kan*: Dadasalu; *Mal*: Catacci, Dhanvanavrksah; *Mar*: Damem, Damani; *Tam*: Catacci, Unnu; *Tel*: Pedda Tena.

Trade name: Dhaman.

Uses: Aerial parts and stem bark useful for the treatment of diabetes.

**Gymnema sylvestre** (Retz.) R. Br.ex Schult.

Syn: *Periploca sylvestris* Retz.

Family: Asclepiadaceae.

Large, woody much branched climber running over the tops of high trees, young stems and branches pubescent. Leaves ovate-elliptic or ovate-lanceolate. Flowers minute, greenish-yellow or tinged pink in axillary pedunculate cymes. Fruit follicles, beaked at apex, glabrous. Seeds with thin broad marginal wing.

Occasional in forests in Central and Peninsular India.

Fl. & Fr.: September–December.

Sanskrit: Madhunosini, Mesharingi.

Local names: *Ben*: Mera singi; *Guj*: Dhuleti, Mardasingi; *Hin*: Meshasingi, Gudmar; *Kan*: Madhunaasha, Sanna garase; *Mal*: Chakkarakkolli, Madhunasini; *Mar*: Kavali, Vakundi; *Tam*: Ciru kurincan, Ayagam; *Tel*: Podapatri.

Trade name: Periploca of the woods, sugar killer.

Propagation: By stem cuttings and by seeds.

Uses: Leaves used for treating diabetes.

**Hamiltonia suaveolens** Roxb.

Family: Rubiaceae

Shrub, up to 3m tall. Leaves large, elliptic–lanceolate. Flowers blue or white, fragrant, in terminal branched panicles. Fruit capsule, ellipsoid.

Throughout India.

Local names: *Ori*: Janamirgiri, Pitondi; *Pun*: Kanera, Muskei, Kantalu, Tulenni; *Tel*: Kondauritidi.

Uses: Root is reported to be used in the treatment of diabetes.

**Hedychium spicatum**

Family: Zingiberaceae

Perennial rhizomatous herb, up to 90cm tall. Flowers white in terminal dense spikes.

In Western and Central Himalayas.

Sanskrit: Karpurakachali, Gandhashati.

Local names: *Ben, Guj, Hin & Mar*: Kapurakachari; *Kan*: Gandhashati. *Tam*: Shimai-kich-chilik-kishangu,

Uses: Rhizome useful in the treatment of diabetes.

**Hedyotis biflora** (L.) Wight & Arn.

Syn: *Oldenlandia biflora* L.

Family: Rubiaceae

Erect or diffuse annual herb. Leaves elliptic. Flowers white in terminal or axillary few-flowered cymes. Fruit capsule.

Found in North-east India and Carnatic coast.

Local names: *Ben*: Khet-Papra; *Hin*: Daman–Papra.

Uses: Whole plant used in the treatment of diabetes.

**Helianthus annuus** L.

Family: Asteraceae (Compositae).

Annual, erect herb, up to 4m tall. Leaves alternate, broadly ovate to cordate, pubescent. Flowers in terminal heads, bright yellow. Fruit compressed cypsela, pappus falling early.

Cultivated throughout India.

Sanskrit: Adityabhakta, Suryamukhi.

Local names: *Ben & Hin*: Surajmukhi; *Kan*: Adityabhakti; *Mal*: Suryakanti, Suryappu; *Mar*: Suraja-mukha, Suryaphul; *Tam*: Suryakanti; *Tel*: Suryakanthi, Poddutirugudu chettu.

Trade name: Sunflower.

Propagation: By seeds.

Uses: Plant useful in the treatment of diabetes.

**Helianthus tuberosus** L.

Family: Asteraceae (Compositae).

Erect, tuberous, perennial herb. Leaves ovate. Flowers in heads, yellow. Fruit achene.

Cultivated occasionally.

Local names: *Ben*: Brahmokha; *Hin*: Hatichuk; *Pun*: Hathipich.

Trade name: Jerusalem artichoke; Girasole.

Uses: Root tuber used to treat Diabetes mellitus.

**Helicteres isora** L.

Family: Sterculiaceae.

Shrubs or trees, up to 5m tall, branchlets apically stellate-tomentose. Leaves obovate or elliptic-oblong, scabrous above, pubescent beneath. Flowers crimson in axillary cymes. Fruit of 5 spirally twisted follicles, seeds minutely tuberculate.

Common in forests from Jhelum eastwards to Nepal, Bihar, West Bengal, Central, Western and Southern India.

Fl. & Fr.: July–December.

Sanskrit: Mrigashringa, Murva, Avarttani.

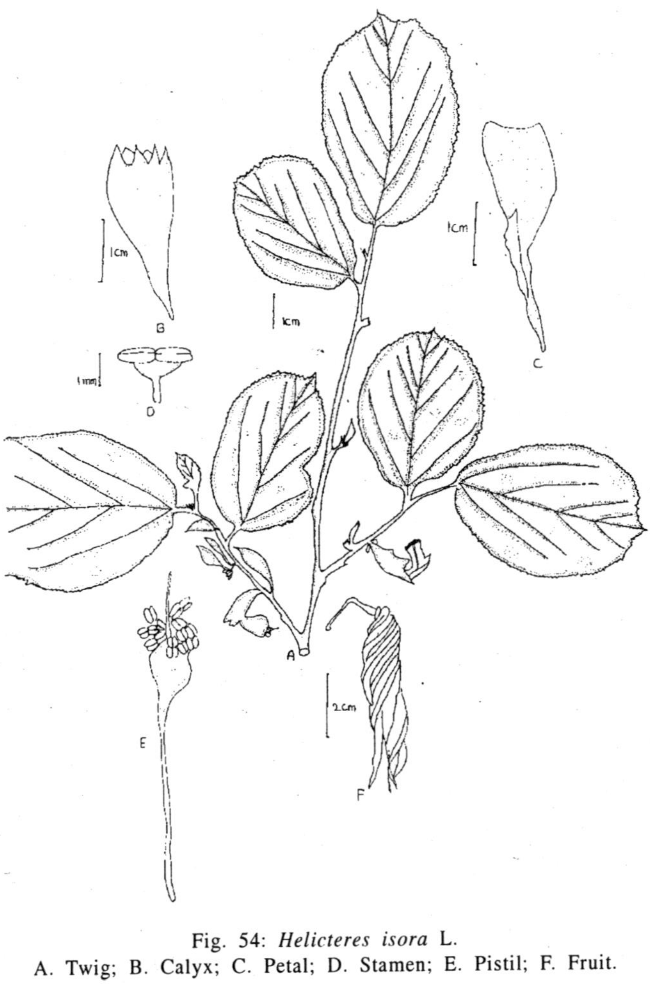


Fig. 54: *Helicteres isora* L.
A. Twig; B. Calyx; C. Petal; D. Stamen; E. Pistil; F. Fruit.

Local names: *Ben*: Atmora; *Guj*: Murdasing; *Hin*: Marosi, Maraphali; *Kan*: Kavagi, Yedamuri; *Mal*: Valampiri, Kayyuna; *Mar*: Muradasinge, Kewan; *Ori*: Murmuria; Murimuri; *Pun*: Marorphali; *Tam*: Tirukupalai, Valampuri; *Tel*: Godratada, Valumbari, Peddashamala.

Trade name: East Indian Screw Tree.

Propagation: Both by seeds and vegetative means.

Uses: Seeds, stem and root bark useful in the treatment of diabetes.

**Heliotropium subulatum** Hochst.

Syn: *Heliotropium zeylanicum* C.B.Clarke

Family: Boraginaceae

Erect, scabrous, hispid, annual herb.

Found in North-Western India and Deccan Peninsula.

Local names: *Guj*: Pilo Hathisundho.

Uses: Ethanolic extract of the plant showed hypoglycemic activity in albino rats.

**Helleborus niger** L.

Family: Ranunculaceae

Small perennial herb, about 30cm tall, rhizome black, jointed. Leaves pale green, ovate. Flowers white or pink.

In Kashmir.

Sanskrit: Katurchini, Katuroum.

Local names: *Ben*: Kalakutki; *Hin*: Khorasani; *Mal & Tam*: Kadagaruganie; *Tel*: Katkaro-gani.

Trade name: Setter wort, The black Hellebore.

Uses: An unani drug 'QS' containing *Helleborus niger* and *Anacyclus pyrethrum* (3:1) reduced the cholesterol levels in patients of diabetus mellitus. Use of the drug in patients with insulin dependent diabetes reduced the dose of insulin.

**Heritiera minor** Lam.

Syn: *Heritiera formes*

Family: Sterculiaceae

Small to moderate-sized evergreen tree. Leaves oblong-lanceolate. Flowers small, orange-coloured, unisexual, in tomentose panicles.

Found in the deltaic regions of the Ganges, Brahmaputra and Mahanadi.

Local names: *Ben & Ori*: Sundri
Trade name: Sudri

Uses: Aerial parts used in the treatment of diabetes.

**Hibiscus syriacus** L.

Family: Malvaceae

Deciduous, much branched shrub, up to 3m tall. Leaves sub-rhomboid, 3-lobed. Flowers solitary, axillary, bell-shaped. Fruit capsule, oblong, seeds pilose.
Native of China, cultivated in gardens throughout India.
Local names: *Ben*: Swet Jaba; *Ori*: Gurhul; *Pun*: Gurhul.
Trade name: Rose of Sharon, Shrubby Althaea.

Uses: Leaves useful in the treatment of diabetes.

**Hibiscus tiliaceus** L.

Family: Malvaceae

Much branched tree, up to 10m tall. Leaves orbicular. Flowers solitary or in racemes, yellow with crimson centre. Fruit capsule, globose, seeds punctate, black.
East and West coast near back waters and mangroves.
Fl. & Fr.: January–November.
Local names: *Ben & Hin*: Bola, Chelwa; *Mal & Tam*: Nirparathi; *Mar*: Belapata;
*Tel*: Etagogu.

Uses: Aerial parts useful in the treatment of diabetes.

**Holarrhena pubescens** (Buch.-Ham.) Wall. ex G. Don

Syn: *Holarrhena antidysenterica* Wall. ex DC.
*Echites pubescens* Buch.-Ham.

Family: Apocynaceae

Small tree, up to 6m tall, with milky latex, elliptic, glabrous, very large, nerves on the leaves conspicuous. Flowers white in axillary and terminal cymes, fragrant. Fruit paired follicles. Seeds with a tuft of brown hairs.
Common in forests throughout India.
Fl.& Fr.: April–October.
Sanskrit: Kutaja, Indra.
Local names: *Hin*: Khurchi; *Ori*: Kherwa, Patrukurwa, Indrojabafair; *Tel*: Pala kodisa.

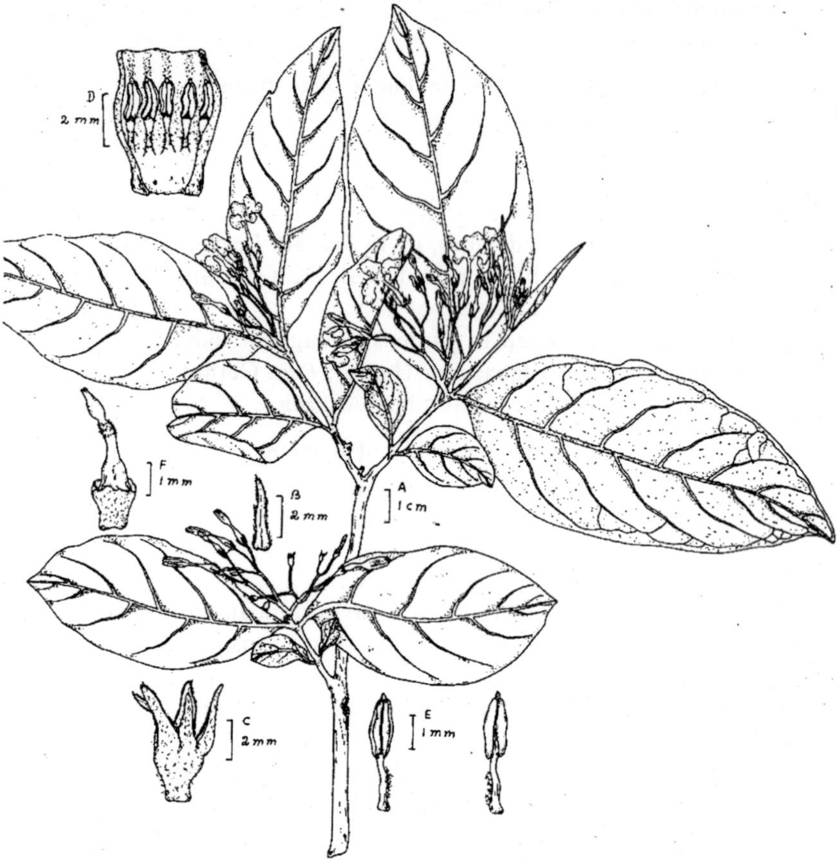


Fig. 55: *Holarrhena pubescens* (Buch-Ham.) G.Don
A. Twig; B. Bract; C. Calyx; D. Corolla split open with stamens; E. Stamens; F. Pistil.

Trade name: Kurchi, Tellicherry Bark.
Propagation: By seeds.

Uses: Fruits useful in the treatment of diabetes.

**Holigarna grahamii** Hook.f.

Family: Anacardiaceae

Medium–sized to large tree. Leaves oblanceolate, coriaceous. Flowers small, unisexual in terminal panicles. Fruit drupe, oblong–ovoid.

Found in Western Ghats and parts of Deccan.

Uses: Apical parts are used to treat Diabetes mellitus.

**Holigarna nigra** Bourd.

Family: Anacardiaceae

Tree.
Found in Evergreen forests of Kerala.

Uses: Aerial parts are used to treat Diabetes Mellitus.

**Holmskioldia sanguinea** Retz.

Family: Verbenaceae

Large climbing or scrambling shrub with drooping branches. Leaves ovate–elliptic. Flowers scarlet in axillary or terminal cymes.
In Himalayas, Bihar and Assam.
Local names: *Hin*: Kapni
Trade name: Chinese hat plant, parasol flower

Uses: Aerial parts are used to treat diabetes.

**Holostemma ada-kodien** Schult.

Syn: *Holostemma annulare* (Roxb.) K. Schum.
*Asclepias annularis* Roxb.

Family: Asclepiadaceae.

Extensive perennial twining shrub with milky latex. Leaves ovate, cordate at base, glabrous. Flowers pinkish red, fleshy, in axillary few-flowered lax cymes. Fruit paired follicles, seeds many, ovoid with silky coma.
Common in forests of Peninsular India and tropical Himalayas.
Fl. & Fr.: April–October.
Sanskrit: Jivanti, Shitala.
Local names: *Guj*: Kharner, Khiravel, Khordodi, *Hin*: Chhirvel; *Kan*: Jeeva haale balli, Muraligana kasa; *Mal*: Ada-kodien, Atakkoti; *Mar*: Shidodi, Tulatule; *Tel*: Palagurugu, Dudidapalatiga, Bandiguruvinda teega.
Trade name: Ring-coronel, Swallow-wort.
Propagation: By seeds and by vegetative methods.

Uses: Plant useful in the treatment of diabetes.

**Hordeum vulgare** L.

Family: Poaceae (Gramineae).

Annual, erect, tufted herb, up to 1m tall. Leaves linear, upper ones close to the spike, sheath smooth. Spike terminal, linear oblong, compressed. Fruit caryopsis, grooved on the inner face, elliptic.

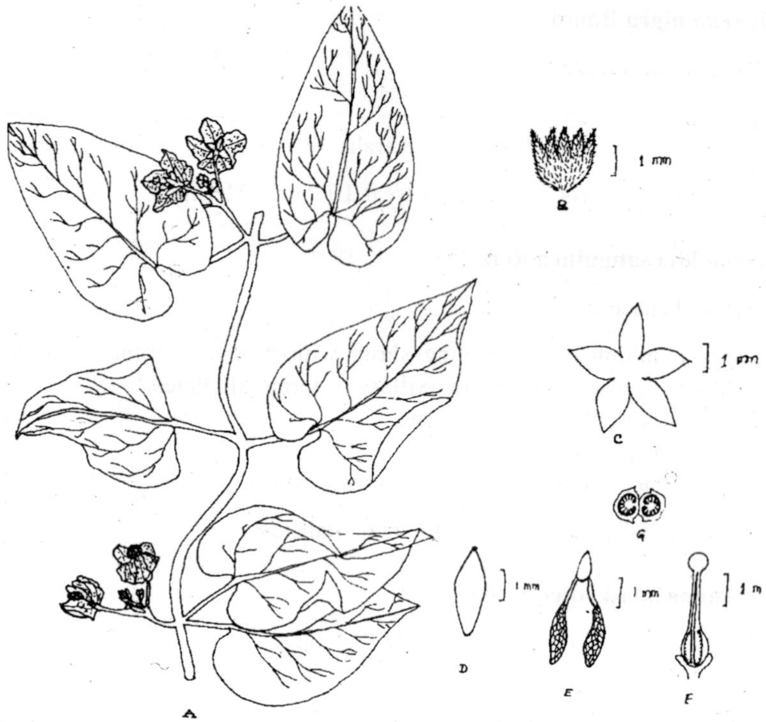


Fig. 56: *Holostemma ada-kodien* Schult.
A. Twig; B. Calyx split open; C. Corolla split open; D. Corona; E. Pollinia; F. Pistil.

Cultivated in hill stations.

Sanskrit: Yavah.

Local names: *Ben*: Jab, Jau; *Guj*: Jau, Jav; *Hin*: Jav, Jau; *Kan*: Yava, Jave-godhi; *Mal*: Yavam, Barli; *Mar*: Java; *Tam*: Barliarisi; *Tel*: Barli, Yava.

Trade name: Barley.

Propagation: By seeds.

Uses: Seeds useful in the treatment of diabetes. Chapati prepared with the flour of barley and chana, taken hot is very useful for treating diabetes. One/two chapatis are to be taken daily for several days.

**Hugonia mystax** L.

Family: Linaceae

Rambling or climbing shrubs, branchlets tomentose. Leaves elliptic, obovate or obovate-oblong, glabrous. Flowers large, yellow in terminal and /or axillary cymes, lower peduncles spirally hooked. Fruit globose, drupe, red when ripe.

Occasional in forests.
Fl. & Fr.: Through out the year.
Sanskrit: Kamsamarah.
Local names: *Kan & Mar*: Modirakkani; *Mal*: Karttotti, Motirakkanni; *Ori*: Chulijinka; *Tam*: Agori, Motirakkanni; *Tel*: Kakibira.
Trade name: Climbing Flax.
Propagation: By seeds.

Uses: Aerial parts useful in the treatment of diabetes.

**Humboldtia brunonis** Wall.

Family: Fabaceae

Small tree.
Found in Southern Western Ghats.

Uses: Aerial parts used in the treatment of diabetes.

**Hydnocarpus alpina** Wight

Family: Flacourtiaceae

Dioecious tree, 20–30m tall. Leaves alternate, elliptic-oblong to lanceolate, deep green, brilliant red when young. Flowers few, in axillary racemes. Fruit ovoid berry.
Forests of Western Ghats from South Kanara to Kerala.
Local names: *Kan*: Tirathi, Sanuasolti; *Mal*: Malamaravetti; *Mar*: Kastel; *Tam*: Attuchankalai.

Uses: Aerial parts useful for the treatment of diabetes:

**Hydrangea anomala** D. Don

Syn: *Hydrangea altissima* Wall.

Family: Saxifragaceae

Large deciduous shrub. Leaves ovate-lanceolate. Flowers whitish, greenish or bluish, in terminal clusters.
Found in Himalayas from Ravi eastwards to Assam.

Uses: Aerial parts useful in the treatment of Diabetes.

**Hydrolea zeylanica** Vahl

Family: Hydrophyllaceae

Erect or diffuse often succulent herb. Leaves lanceolate. Flowers blue on short lateral branches. Fruit ovoid capsule enclosed in enlarged persistent calyx.

Found in moist and swampy places throughout India.

Sanskrit: Langali

Local names: *Ben*: Isha–langula, Kasschra; *Mal*: Cheruvallel.

Uses: Whole plant used in the treatment of diabetes.

**Hygrophila auriculata** (Schum.) Heine

Syn: *Asteracantha longifolia* (L.) Nees
*Barleria auriculata* Schum.
*Barleria longifolia* L.

Family: Acanthaceae

A stout, erect, armed unbranched strigose-hispid herb, up to 75 cm tall. Leaves whorled, subsessile, 6 at a node, each having a sharp, yellow spine in its axil. Flowers bluish purple to pink, in axillary whorls. Fruit linear capsule, seeds orbicular.

Common in wet places, marshes and margins of tanks throughout India.

Fl. & Fr.: October–April.

Sanskrit: Kokilaksha.

Local names: *Ben*: Kulia khara; *Hin & Mar*: Talimkhana; *Tam*: Nirmulli; *Tel*: Nirugubbi, Gobbichettu.

Trade name: Talamakhana.

Fl. & Fr.: October–April.

Uses: Whole plant useful for the treatment of diabetes.

**Hyoscyamus niger** L.

Family: Solanaceae

Erect, biennial herb, up to 1.5m tall, densely covered with glandular hairs. The root is fusiform and turnip-like at the top. The leaves are oblong, basal leaves are petiolate and cauline leaves are stem clasping. Flowers yellowish pale in one-sided, leafy and revolute spikes. Fruit pyxidium, globose, seeds numerous, grey-brown, pitted.

Cultivated in Nilgiri Hills, Kashmir, Uttar Pradesh, Madhya Pradesh, Maharastra and Punjab.

Trade name: Henbane.

Propagation: The plant can be propagated from seeds. The seeds are first raised in nursery during october. 5Kg of seeds are sufficient for one hectare. Seeds germinate with in a week after sowing in nursery beds and can be transplanted after about a month. When the seedlings attain 4 to 5

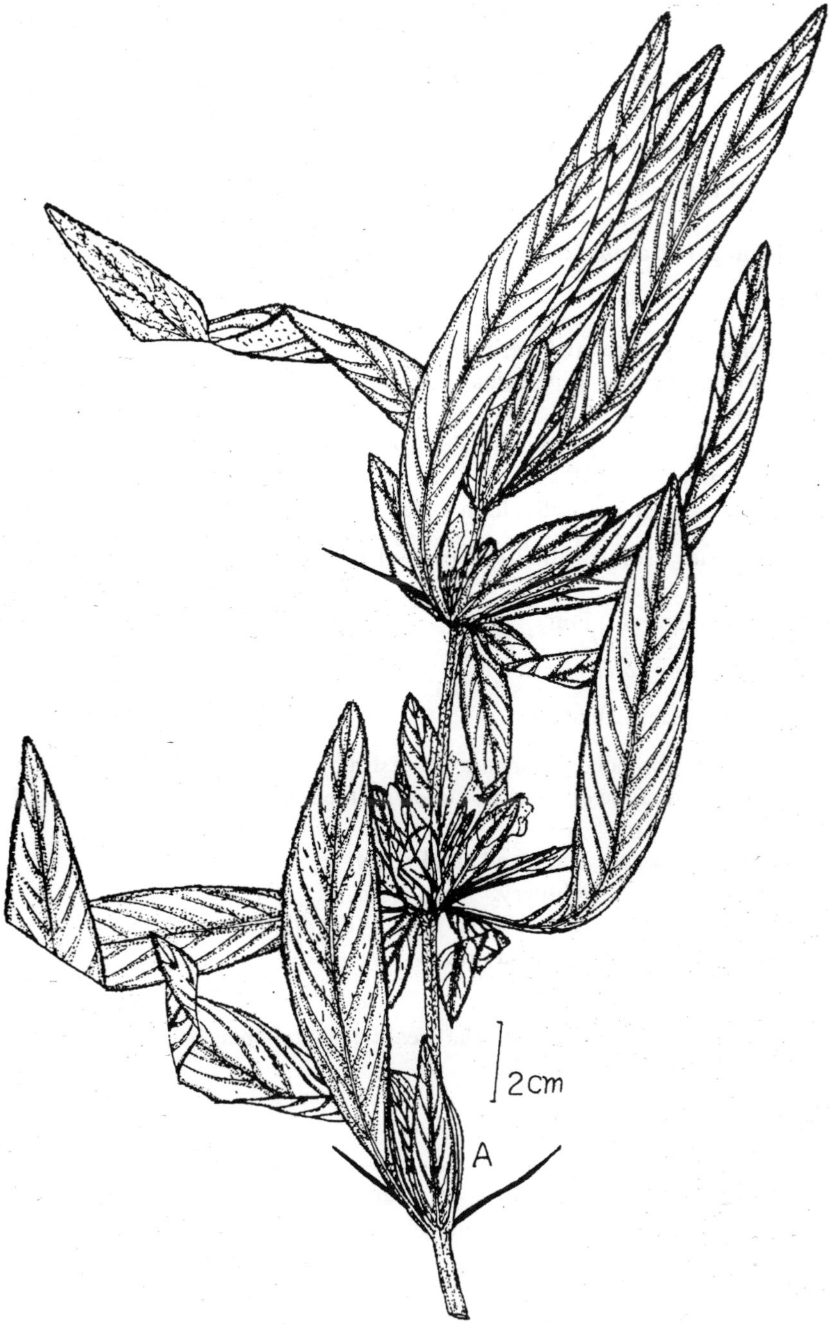


Fig. 57: *Hygrophila auriculata* (Schum.) Heine
A. Twig.

leaves, seedlings are planted with spacing of 30 × 45cm. The crop requires 3–4 irrigations. When plants reach flowering stage, they are cut at the ground level. The entire herbage is spread in the shade and dried. From one hectare the yield of leaves is about 15 quintals while stalks, pedicels and leaves is about 30q/ha.

Uses: Plant useful in the treatment of diabetes.

**Hypericum perforatum** L.

Family: Hypericaceae

Rhizomatous perennial herb, up to 1m tall. Leaves oblong, ovate or linear. Flowers yellow, in terminal corymbose cymes. Fruit ovoid capsule, seeds many.

In Western Himalayas at altitudes 1000 to 3000m.

Local names: *Hin*: Bassant, Balsana, Dendhu.

Trade name: Common St. John's wort, Kalmath weed.

Uses: Plant useful in the treatment of diabetes.

**Hyptis suaveolens** (L.) Poit.

Syn: *Ballota suaveolens* L.

Family: Lamiaceae (Labiatae).

Erect, much branched aromatic undershrub, up to 2m tall, stem tetragonal. Leaves ovate. Flowers blue or violet, scented, in axillary cymes. Fruit of nutlets.

Common in waste lands and road sides.

Fl. & Fr.: August–February.

Local names: *Ben*: Bilati tulsi; *Hin*: Wilayati tulsi; *Ori*: Ganga tulsi, Purodo; *Tel*: Sima Tulasi, Mahavira.

Propagation: By seeds.

Uses: Aerial parts useful in the treatment of diabetes.

**Impatiens balsamina** L.

Family: Balsaminaceae

Erect herb, up to 1m tall. Leaves ovate–lanceolate. Flowers pale pink, solitary or in clusters. Fruit capsule, oblong.

Fl. & Fr.: September–March

Uses: Plant useful for curing diabetes.

**Imperata cylindrica** (l.) Raeusch.

Syn: *Imperata arundinacea* Cyr.
*Lagurus cylindricus* L

Family: Poaceae

Perennial tufted grass, up to 2.8m tall. Spikelets in terminal dense panicle, silky. Fruit caryopsis, brown.

Throughout hotter parts.

Sanskrit: Darbha

Local names: *Ben*: Ooloo, Ulu; *Hin*: Dabh, Srni, *Kan*: Sanna dabbai hullu; *Mal*: Vidulam; *Tam*: Dharbhai pul, Inankapillu; *Tel*: Darbhagaddi.

Uses: Roots useful in the treatment of diabetes.

**Indigofera arrecta** Hochst

Family: Fabaceae (Papilionaceae)

Erect undershrub, up to 2m tall. Leaves imparipinnately compound, leaflets 7–8 pairs, with one odd terminal leaflets. Flowers pinkish red, in axillary racemes. Fruit pod, straight.

Cultivated in Bihar.

Trade name: Natal Indigo, Bengal Indigo.

Uses: Use of root powder three times a day helps in reducing glucose levels in diabetics.

**Indigofera glandulosa** Willd.

Family: Fabaceae (Papilionaceae)

Annual herb, Leaves trifoliolate. Flowers red in racemes. Fruit pod, brown, seeds 1–2, reddish.

Common in dry and sandy soils of Deccan and Gujarat.

Local names: *Guj*: Vekhariyo; *Mar*: Bargadan; *Tel*: Baragadam, Barapatalu, Barapatam.

Uses: Whole plant used in the treatment of diabetes.

**Indigofera tinctoria** L.

Syn: *Indigofera sumatrana* Gaertn.

Family: Fabaceae (Papilionaceae)

Woody, stiff undershrubs, up to 2m tall, branches terete. Leaves compound, 9-foliolate, leaflets bluish-green, appressedly pubescent, ovate-oblong. Flowers pink in axillary racemes. Fruit cylindric pod, slightly falcate towards tip, seeds 10–12, globose.

Common in waste lands all over India.

Fl.& Fr.: August–November.

Sanskrit: Nilini, Nilika.

Local names: *Hin*: Gauchi, Nil; *Kan & Tan*: Nili; *Mar*: Guli; *Tel*: Nili.

Trade name: Common Indigo.

Propagation: By seeds.

Uses: Aerial parts useful for the treatment of diabetes.

**Inula racemosa** Hook.f.

Family: Asteraceae (Compositae).

Erect herb, up to 1.8m tall, young parts densely hairy. Leaves elliptic-lanceolate or obovate, amplexicaul. Flowers in heads, yellow. Fruit achene.

Along bunds of cultivated fields in Jammu & Kashmir.

Fl. & Fr.: July–September.

Sanskrit: Pauskaram, Puskaram

Local names: *Hin*: Pohakarmul, Puskarmul; *Kan*: Rasnabheda; *Mal*: Puskkaramulam; *Tam*: Puskkaramulam; *Tel*: Puskaramu.

Uses: Roots useful in the treatment of diabetes.

**Ipomoea aquatica** Forssk.

Syn: *Ipomoea reptans* Poir.

Family: Convolvulaceae

A twiner or prostrate herb, rooting at nodes. Leaves variable in shape, ovate, ovate–oblong or linear. Flowers purple, solitary or in cymes. Fruit capsule, ovoid.

In moist localities or in ponds.

Fl. & Fr.: Round the year.

Uses: Plant useful for the treatment of diabetes.

**Ipomoea batatas** (L.) Lam.

Family: Convolvulaceae

Slender, prostrate perennial herbaceous vine with tuberous roots. Leaves alternate, ovate-cordate, entire, angular or deeply lobed. Flowers purple, solitary or in cymose clusters. Fruit capsule, globose or ovoid, seeds 2–4, black.

Cultivated throughout India.

Sanskrit: Pindalah, Raktaluh.

Local names: *Ben*: Lal alu, Ranga alu; *Guj*: Kanangi, Sakaria; *Hin*: Mithaalu, Sakkara kand; *Kan*: Sehigenasu; *Mar*: Ratalu; *Ori*: Kanda; *Tam*:

Sakkaravallikilangu; *Tel*: Genusugadda, Chilagadadumpa.

Trade name: Sweet potato.

Propagation: By seeds

Uses: The tuberous roots are useful in treating diabetes.

**Ipomoea nil** (L.) Roth

Syn: *Ipomoea hederacea* auct.
*Convolvulus nil* L.

Family: Convolvulaceae.

Slender, twining climbers with retrorsely villous stem. Leaves ovate-cordate, irregularly 3-lobed. Flowers bluish pink, in axillary umbellate cymes. Fruit capsule, subglobose.

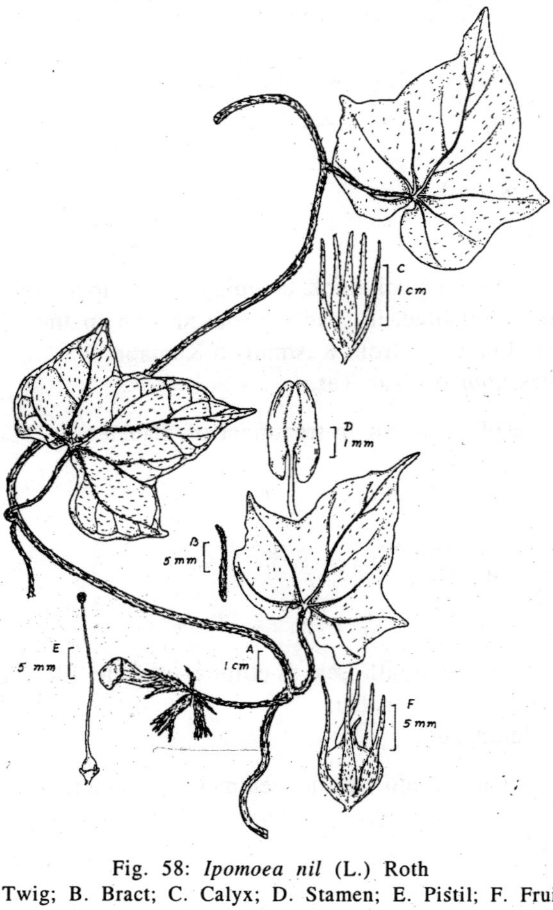


Fig. 58: *Ipomoea nil* (L.) Roth
A. Twig; B. Bract; C. Calyx; D. Stamen; E. Pistil; F. Fruit.

Common in jungles through out India.
Fl. & Fr.: Most part of the year.
Sanskrit: Krisnabijah.
Local names: *Ben*: Kaladanah, Nikalmi; *Guj*: Kaladana, Kalkumpan; *Hin*: Kaldana, Mirchai; *Kan*: Garibija; *Mal*: Talitari; *Mar*: Nilpushpi, Nilyel; *Ori*: Khanikhondo; *Tam*: Kakkattan, Sirikki; *Tel*: Kolli-vittulu.
Trade name: Morning Glory, Pharbitis seeds.
Propagation: By seeds.

Uses: Plant useful in the treatment of diabetes.

**Ipomoea purpurea** (L.) Roth

Family: Convolvulaceae

Twining, annual herb. Leaves broadly ovate–cordate. Flowers large, funnel–shaped, varying in colour from white to dark purple in axillary cymes. Fruit capsule, globular.
Throughout India, also grown in gardens.

Uses: Whole plant used in the treatment of diabetes.

**Iris kumaonensis** Wall.

Family: Iridaceae

Perennial herb, root stock thick, creeping, stems up to 30cm tall. Leaves linear. Flowers bright lilac, in spadix enclosed by a spathe. Fruit capsule.
In Western Himalayas from Kashmir to Kumaon.
Local names: *Pun*: Karkar, Tezma.

Uses: Whole plant useful in treatment of diabetes.

**Ixora arborea** Roxb. ex Smith

Syn: *Ixora pavetta* Andrews
*Ixora parviflora* Vahl

Family: Rubiaceae

Small tree, up to 2.5m tall. Leaves elliptic–obovate. Flowers in terminal branched cymes, white. Fruit berry.
Fl. & Fr.: March–June.

Uses: Aerial parts useful in the treatment of diabetes.

**Ixora coccinea** L.

Family: Rubiaceae.

Shrub. Leaves elliptic-obovate to oblanceolate. Flowers red or yellowish in terminal corymbose panicles. Fruit subglobose, fleshy, red in colour, crowned with persistent calyx.

Cultivated as an ornamental.

Fl. & Fr.: Round the year.

Sanskrit: Bandhuka, Paranti.

Local names: *Ben*: Rangan, Rookmini, Rajana; *Hin*: Rangan, Ranjana; *Kan*: Kepala, Kissargida; *Mal*: Thechi, Cetti; *Mar*: Pentgul; Pankul;*Ori*: Bonhuko, Romoniphulo; *Tam*: Vetci, Sedaram; *Tel*: Bandhukamu, Manmadhabanam.

Trade name: Jungle Flame Ixora, Flame flower.

Propagation: By seeds as well as through stem cuttings.

Uses: Aerial parts useful in the treatment of diabetes.

**Jasminum rigidum** Zenker non Thw.

Family: Oleaceae

Flowers white

Found in Deccan & Carnatic, Plains and hills and Western Ghats.

Fl. & Fr.: March–April.

Uses: Aerial parts used in the treatment of diabetes.

**Jatropha curcas** L.

Family: Euphorbiaceae.

Shrub or small tree, up to 5m tall. Leaves cordiform, shallowly 3–5-lobed. Flowers unisexual, monoecious, yellowish green in loose panicle of cymes. Fruit ovoid capsule.

Common hedge plant, along roadsides and outskirts of villages.

Fl. & Fr.: August–March.

Sankrit: Dravanthi, Hanaleronda.

Local names: *Ass*: Bongalibhotora; *Ben*: Bagharinda, Eranda Guchhi; *Guj*: Jamalgota, Ratanjota; *Hin*: Bagberanda, Bheranda; *Kan*: Adaluharerlu, Battadaharallu, Doddaharalu, Kadi, mario, Ucharel, Marayavudala, Kinnocchi; *Mal*: Kattavankku, Kadalavankka; *Mar*: Mogalierenda, Ramayerandi; *Ori*; Jahajin, Bamprijada, Dhuma jara; *Tam*: Tiravaadi, Kat-amanak, Kurubaravuni, Njaligaddi; *Tel*: Nepalamu, Adavi amudamu.

Trade name: Purging nut, physic nut.

Propagation: By cuttings and seeds.

Uses: Aerial parts useful in the treatment of diabetes.

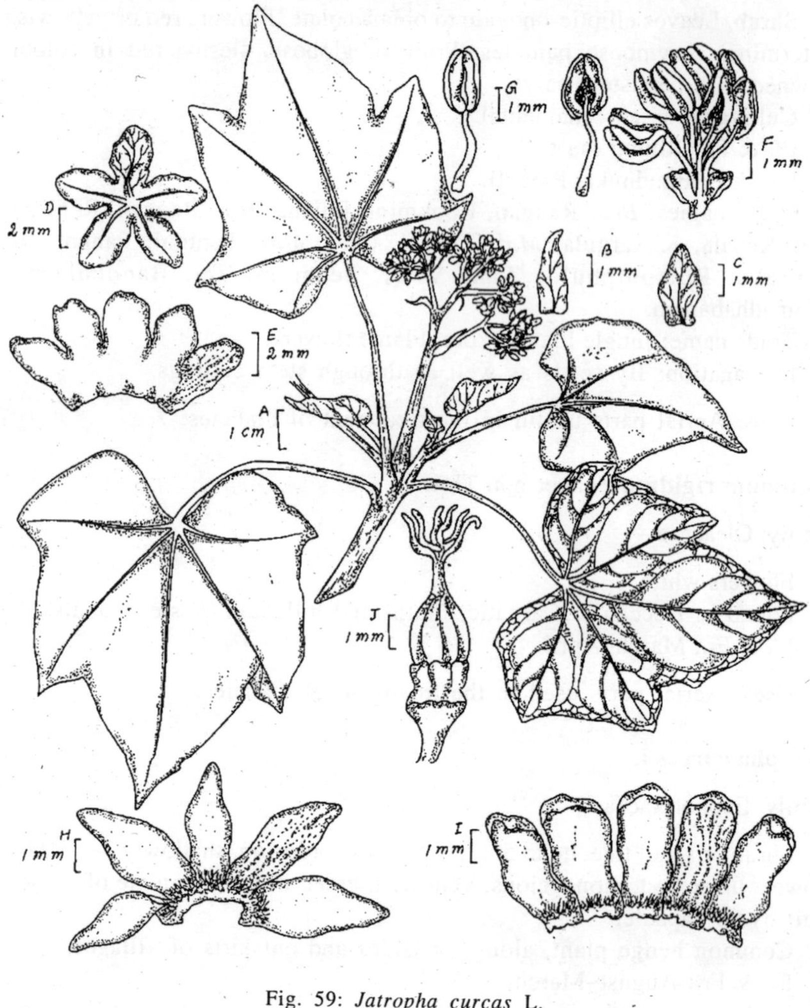


Fig. 59: *Jatropha curcas* L.
A. Twig; Male: B. Bract; C. Bracteole; D. Outer tepals; E. Inner tepals split open; F. Androecium; G. Stamens: Female: H. Outer tepals split open; I. Inner tepals split open; J. Pistil.

**Jatropha gossypifolia** L.

Family: Euphorbiaceae.

Shrubs, to 3m tall, monoecious, branchlets dark purple, glandular hairy. Leaves glaucous, cordiform, deeply 3–5-lobed, lobes obovate. Flowers in axillary cymes. Fruit capsule, subglobose, seeds oblong.

Common in waste lands and roadsides.

Fl. & Fr.: Through out the year.

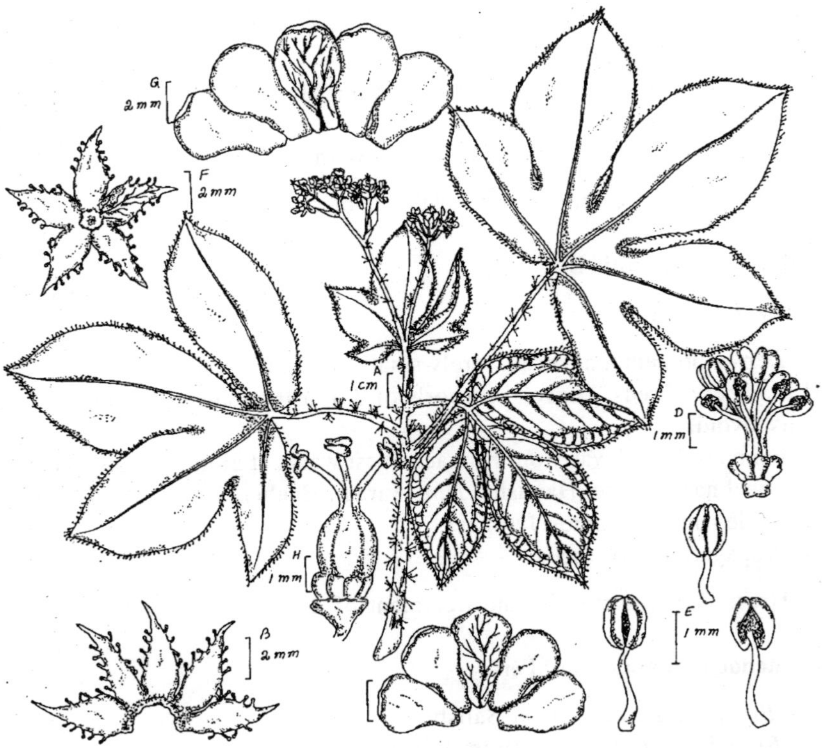


Fig. 60: *Jatropha gossypifolia* L.
A. Twig; Male: B. Outer tepals split open; C. Inner tepals split open; D. Androecium; E. Stamens: Female: F. Outer tepals; G. Inner tepals split open; H. Pistil.

Sanskrit: Nikumba.

Local names: *Ben*: Lalbherenda; *Hin*: Bherenda, Verenda; *Tam*: Atalai; *Tel*: Seema Nepalamu, Nela Amudamu.

Trade name: Bellyache Bush.

Propagation: By seeds.

Uses: Plant useful in the treatment of diabetes.

## **Juglans regia** L.

Family: Juglandaceae

Large, deciduous, monoecious tree. Leaves alternate, imparipinnate, leaflets 5–13, elliptic to oblong. Flowers yellowish green, male in catkins, female in terminal catkins. Fruit drupe with leathery exocarp and wrinkled, hard endocarp, seed edible.

Throughout Himalayas and Khasi hills of Assam.
Sanskrit: Aksotah
Local names: *Hin*: Akhor, Akhrot; *Kan*: Akrodu; *Mal & Tam*: Akrottu; *Tel*: Akrotu.
Trade name: Common walnut, persian walnut, Europaean walnut, Akhrot.

Uses: Leaves useful in the treatment of diabetes.

**Juniperus communis** L.

Family: Pinaceae

Dense, procumbent shrub, rarely small tree, bark reddish brown, peeling off in papery shreds. Leaves in whorls of 3, linear-subulate. Cones axillary. Seeds ovoid.
Found in Himalayas from Kumaon West wards at altitudes 1500–4000m.
Local names: *Ben*: Havusha; *Hin*: Aaraar, Haubera, Abhal; *Mar*: Hosha.
Trade name: Common Juniper.
Propagation: By seeds.

Uses: Cones useful for the treatment of diabetes

**Kalanchoe pinnata** (Lam.) Pers.

Syn: *Bryophyllum calycinum* Salisb.
*Bryophyllum pinnatum* (Lam.) Oken.
*Cotyledon pinnata* Lam.

Family: Crassulaceae

Succulent herb, up to 1m tall. Leaves opposite decussate, crowded in young shoots, distant in adult ones, often 3–5-foliolate, oblong or ovate-elliptic. Flowers reddish purple, pendulous in paniculate cymes. Fruit follicle, seeds numerous.
Throughout India, also grown as ornamental.
Fl. & Fr.: January–March.
Sanskrit: Parnabijah.
Local names: *Hin*: Jakh me hayat; *Kan*: Gandu Kalinga; *Mal*: Ilamulacchi, Ilayinmeltai; *Tam*: Malaikkalli; Runakkalli; *Tel*: Simajamudu.

Uses: Plant useful for the treatment of diabetes.

**Kandelia candel** (L.) Druce

Syn: *Rhizophora candel* L.
*Kandelia rheedii* Wight & Arn.

Family: Rhizophoraceae

Shrub. Leaves decussate, elliptic-oblong. Flowers white, few, in axillary cymes. Fruit ovoid.

Found in the coastal forests of India.

Fl. & Fr.: March–June.

Local names: *Ben*: Coria; *Kan*: Kandale; *Mal*: Cerukandal; *Ori*: Rasunia; *Tam*: Thuvar kandan; *Tel*: Kandigala.

Uses: Stem bark useful in the treatment of diabetes.

**Kickxia ramosissima** (Wall.) Janchen

Syn: *Linaria ramosissima* Wall.

Family: Scrophulariaceae

Prostrate, perennial herb, up to 40cm long. Leaves lower opposite, upper alternate, lower leaves 3–5-lobed or triangular. Flowers solitary, axillary, yellow. Fruit capsule, many–seeded.

Throughout India

Fl. & Fr.: August–October.

Local names: *Guj*: Bhintgalodi, Kanodi.

Uses: Whole plant useful for the treatment of diabetes.

**Kyllinga bulbosa** Beauv.

Syn: *Kyllinga triceps* Rottb.
*Cyperus triceps* (Rottb.) Endl.

Family: Cyperaceae

Perennial, rhizomatous herb, up to 15cm tall. Leaves linear. Flowers in head. Fruit achene.

Found from upper Gangetic plains to Deccan peninsula and up to West Bengal.

Uses: Plant useful in the treatment of diabetes.

**Kyllinga nemoralis** (Forst. & Forst.f.) Dandy ex Hutchins. & Dalz.

Syn: *Thryocephalon nemoralis* Forst. & Forst.f.
*Kyllinga monocephala* Rottb.
*Cyperus kyllinga* Endl.

Family: Cyperaceae

Perennial, laxly tufted, rhizomatous herb, up to 20cm tall. Leaves linear, spikelets in terminal globose head. Fruit achene.

Common throughout India.

Local names: *Ben & Hin*: Birbishi, Shwetgothubi; *Mar*: Mustu; *Mal*: Mottenga, Pimottenga.

Uses: Plant useful in treatment of diabetes.

**Lablab purpureus** L.

Syn: *Dolichos lablab* L.

Family: Fabaceae (Papilionaceae)

Annual or perennial, twining herb, up to 30cm tall. Leaves trifoliolate. Flowers white or pink in axillary racemes. Fruit legume with remains of persistent style, seeds globose, white, yellow, purple or black.

Cultivated throughout India.

Sanskrit: Nispavah.

Local names: *Ben*: Sim; *Guj*: Val; *Hin*: Sem, Bhatvas; *Kan*: Chapparada-avare; *Mal*: Amara, Avara; *Mar*: Pavata: *Tam*: Avarai; *Tel*: Chikkudu, Anapakaya.

Trade name: Indian bean, Lablab bean.

Propagation: By seeds.

Uses: Fruits and seeds useful in the treatment of diabetes.

**Lagenaria siceraria** (Molina) Standl

Syn: *Lagenaria vulgaris* Ser.
*Lagenaria leucantha* Rusby.

Family: Cucurbitaceae

Large, softly pubescent climbing or trailing herb. Leaves long-petioled, 5-lobed, cordate, pubescent. Flowers unisexual, axillary, solitary. Fruit large, bottle or dumb-bell shaped, woody when ripe, seeds many, white.

Cultivated throughout India.

Sanskrit: Kututumbi

Local names: *Ben*: Lan; *Guj*: Dudhi, Tamada; *Hin*: Titalanki, Kadvilanki; *Kan*: Kadusore, *Mal*: Peccura, Kathucura, Kaippan cura; *Tam*: Sorakkai; *Tel*: Sorakaya.

Trade name: Bottle gourd.

Propagation: By seeds.

Uses: Plant useful in the treatment of diabetes.

**Lagerstroemia parviflora** Roxb.

Family: Lythraceae

Medium sized deciduous tree. Leaves elliptic, oblong or ovate. Flowers white, in lax, axillary and terminal panicles, fragrant. Fruit capsule, ovoid or ellipsoid.

Throughout India

Local names: *Ben*: Sida; *Hin*: Dhaura; *Kan*: Channangi; *Mal*: Cimanii; *Mar*: Lend, Bondga, Bondara; *Guj*: Kankria; *Ori*: Salora; *Tam & Tel*: Chennangi.

Uses: Aerial parts used in the treatment of diabetes.

**Lagerstroemia reginae** Roxb.

Syn: *Lagerstroemia flos-reginae* Retz.
*Lagerstroemia speciosa* Pers.

Family: Lythraceae

Large deciduous tree, bark smooth, flaking off in irregular pieces. Leaves opposite, oblong-lanceolate or elliptic. Flowers purplish-lilac in large terminal panicles. Fruit capsule, broadly ovoid, pale brown.

Throughout India.

Fl. & Fr.: April–August

Local names: *Hin*: Jarul; *Ben*: Jarool; *Mar*: Tamam, Mota-bonadara; *Mal*: Manimaruthu; *Ori*: Patoli; *Tam*: Kadali, Pumaruthu; *Tel*: Varagogu.

Trade name: Jarul, Pyinma.

Uses: Decoction of the leaves and fruits contain an amorphous, slightly bitter insulin-like principle with a hypoglycemic activity.

**Lathyrus sativus** L.

Family: Fabaceae (Papilionaceae)

Much branched, annual, suberect herb. Leaves pinnately compound, leaflets modified into tendrils. Flowers reddish purple, blue or white solitary, axillary. Fruit pod.

Cultivated in northern India as a pulse crop.

Local names: *Ben*: Khesari; *Hin*: Khesari, Latri; *Guj*: Lang; *Mar*: Lakh; *Ori*: Khesra.

Trade name: Chickling vetch.

Uses: Seed used to treat diabetes.

**Launaea nudicaulis** Hook.f.

Family: Asteraceae

Decumbent herb. Leaves in a rosette at the base, lobed or runcinate. Flowers yellow in terminal heads. Fruit achene.

Throughout India.
Local names: *Pun*: Batthal, Dudhlak.

Uses: Isolate is useful in treatment of diabetes mellitus.

**Laurus nobilis** L.

Family: Lauraceae

Small evergreen tree. Leaves narrow, stiff, fragrant. Fruit berry.
Sometimes grown in Indian gardens.
Trade name: Sweet Bay, True haurd.
Propagation: By cuttings or by seed.

Uses: Leaves useful for the treatment of diabetes.

**Leea asiatica** (L.) Ridsdale

Syn: *Leea crispa* L.
*Phytolacca asiatica* L.
*Leea aspera* Edgew
*Leea edgeworthii* Sant.

Family: Leeaceae

Shrub, up to 2m tall. Leaves compound, leaflets 5–7, elliptic-ovate or oblong. Flowers pale green in terminal and axillary branched cymes. Fruit berry.
Deccan peninsula and north east India.
Local names: *Ben*: Banchalita; *Mal*: Nalugu, Nellu; *Ori*: Hatikanopotro.

Uses: Aerial parts used in the treatment of diabetes.

**Leea indica** (Burm. f.) Merr.

Syn: *Staphylea indica* Burm.f.
*Leea sambucina* (L.) Willd.
*Aquilicia sambucina* L.

Family: Leeaceae

Large shrub or small tree, up to 6m tall. Leaves 2–3-pinnate, pinnae 3-paired, leaflets oblong-lanceolate. Flowers greenish-white in lateral or leaf-opposed corymbose cymes. Fruit globose berry, black–purple when ripe.
Throughout India.
Fl. & Fr.: Throughout the year.
Sanskrit: Chatri, Kukkurajihva.
Local names: *Ben & Hin*: Kukur–Jihva; *Kan*: Gadhapatri; Andilu; *Mal*: Kutanaluku, Naluku, Nallu, Nakku, Erattayani, Maniperanti; *Tam*: Naikki, Ottanali.

Uses: Leaves useful for the treatment of diabetes.

**Lepidium ruderale** L.

Family: Brassicaceae (Cruciferae)

Annual, erect or diffuse herb.
Found in Kumaon and Kashmir.

Uses: Plant used in the treatment of diabetes.

**Leucaena latisiliqua** (L.) Gillis

Syn: *Leucaena glauca* auct non Benth.
*Leucaena leucocephala* (Lam.) de Wit.

Family: Mimosaceae

Large, unarmed deciduous trees, up to 20m tall. Leaves bipinnate, pinnae 3–8 pairs, leaflets 10–15 pairs, linear–oblong. Flowers white in dense globose heads, axillary. Fruit pod, flat.

Grown in hedges and gardens near villages.

Local names: *Guj*: Lasobaval; *Mal*: Takaranniram; *Tam*: Tagarai.

Uses: Seeds used in the treatment of diabetes.

**Limonia acidissima** L.

Syn: *Feronia limonia* (L.) Swingle
*Feronia elephatum* Correa
*Limonia elephatum* (Correa) Panigr.
*Schinus limonia* L.

Family: Rutaceae

Small armed trees, spines straight, branchlets densely tomentose. Leaves alternate, imparipinnate, leaflets 3–9, oblong or obovate, coriaceous, petiole and rachis flattened, narrowly winged. Flowers creamish in axillary and terminal panicles. Fruit globose, berry, woody, indehiscent, seeds many, embedded in pulp.

Common in dry deciduous forests.

Fl. & Fr.: March–December.

Sanskrit: Kapittha.

Local names: *Ben*: Kait, Katbel; *Hin*: Bilin, Kait kavitha; *Guj*: Kavit, Kotha kothi, Kothun; *Kan*: Bela, Byala; *Mal*: Vila vilett; *Mar*: Kavatha, Kavith, Kovith; *Tel*: Velaga.

Trade name: Wood apple.

Uses: Fruits useful for the treatment of diabetes.

**Lithospermum officinale** L.

Family: Boraginaceae

Erect, hispidly hairy perennial herb. Leaves oblong-lanceolate, rough, strigose. Flowers small, white in racemes. Fruit nutlets, small, ovoid.

Found in Kashmir and Kumaon at 1500–2700m.

Trade name: Gromwel.

Uses: Leaves and root useful for the treatment of diabetes.

**Lonicera japonica** Thunb.

Family: Caprifoliaceae.

Large climber. Leaves ovate to oblong–ovate. Flowers white or purple tinged, in axillary pedunculate pairs, often crowded at the ends of branches. Fruit berry, black.

Found in Lushai hills of Assam.

Trade name: Japanese Honey sickle

Uses: Aerial part used in the treatment of diabetes mellitus.

**Luffa acutangula** (L.) Roxb.

Syn: *Cucumis acutangula* L.
*Luffa amara* Roxb.

Family: Cucurbitaceae.

Extensive tendrillar climber. Tendrils often trifid. Leaves orbicular, palmately 5–7-angled, scabrid. Flowers pale yellow, male and female in the same axil. Fruit long, prominently 10-angled, seeds black, compressed.

Commonly cultivated for its fruits.

Sanskrit: Kosataki, Jalini.

Local names: *Ben*: Jhinga, Sataputi; *Guj*: Ghisoda; *Hin*: Torai, Jinga; *Kan*: Kahiheere balli, Heere kaayi balli; Piccinna, Peechhakam; *Mal*: Pichenga; *Mar*: Dodaki, Shirola; *Tam*: Pirkku, Pekankai; *Tel*: Beerakai.

Trade name: Ribbed gourd.

Propagation: By seeds.

Uses: Aerial parts useful for the treatment of diabetes.

**Luffa echinata** Roxb.

Family: Cucurbitaceae

Tendrillar climber, stem furrowed. Leaves orbicular, reniform, obscurely 5-angled or more or less deeply 5-lobed. Flowers unisexual, male flowers in raceme, female solitary. Fruit oblong or globose, many-seeded.

Wild in U.P Bihar, West Bengal and Gujarat.

Sanskrit: Koshaphala, Devadalika.

Local names: *Ben & Hin*: Bindal; *Guj*: Kukaravel; *Mar*: Devadali.

Trade name: Devadali

Uses: Aerial parts useful in the treatment of diabetes.

**Lycium barbatum** L.

Family: Solanaceae.

Spinous shrub, up to 3m tall. Leaves very variable, linear-oblong to spathulate. Flowers solitary or in fascicles, small, white or purplish. Fruit berry, bright red.

Found in Punjab, Rajasthan and Gujarath.

Local names: *Mar*: Gango, *Pun*: Kangu, Ganger, Chirclutta.

Uses: Fruit used in the treatment of diabetes.

**Lycium chinense** Mill.

Family: Solanaceae

Erect or rambling, armed shrub. Leaves ovate-rhomboid. Flowers axillary, solitary or fascicled. Fruit ovoid-ellipsoid, orange-brown.

Found in North–West Himalayas and West Bengal.

Uses: Fruit and root bark used in the treatment of diabetes.

**Lycopersicon esculentum** Mill.

Syn: *Lycopersicon lycopersicum* (Linn.) Karsten

Family: Solanaceae

Annual, spreading, pubescent herb. Leaves unevenly pinnate. Flowers yellow in extra axillary cymes. Fruits globose, villous when young, glabrous and shining when mature, red when ripe, seeds many.

Cultivated throughout India.

Sanskrit: Raktamachi.

Local names: *Ben & Hin*: Tamatar, Bilayati bemgan; *Kan*: Chapparabadane; *Mal*: Takkali; *Guj*: Vilayithi Vengan; *Mar*: Vel vangi; *Tam*: Takkali; *Tel*: Tamata.

Propagation: By seeds.

Uses: Plant useful for the treatment of diabetes.

**Macrotyloma uniflorum** (Lam.) Verdc.

Syn: *Dolichos uniflorum* Lam.
*Dolichos biflorus* auct non L.

Family: Fabaceae (Papilionaceae)

Climbing or twining herb, up to 1m long. Leaves 3-foliolate, leaflets ovate-lanceolate or ovate-oblong. Flowers axillary, 1–3 in a cluster, yellowish. Fruit pod, falcate.

Cultivated for its seeds.

Fl. & Fr.: September–November.

Sanskrit: Kulaththa

Local names: *Ben*: Kurtikalai; *Guj*: Kalathi, Kulit; *Hin*: Kulthi; *Kan*: Hurali; *Mal*: Muthiva, Muthera; *Tam*: Kollu; *Tel*: Ulavalu.

Trade name: Horse gram.

Uses: Seeds used in the treatment of diabetes.

**Madhuca longifolia** (Koenig) Macbr.

Syn: *Bassia longifolia.*

Family: Sapotaceae.

Deciduous trees, up to 20m tall, bark dark brown. Leaves clustered near the ends of the branches, linear-lanceolate. Flowers creamish white in terminal umbels. Fruit berry, ellipsoid, 1-seeded.

Occasional in forests.

Fl.: March. Fr.: May–June.

Sanskrit: Madhula, Gudapushpa.

Local names: *Ben*: Mahwa, Maul, Mahula; *Guj*: Mahuda; *Hin*: Mohwa, Mahua, Mauwa; *Kan*: Erappe, Hippe; *Mal*: Poonam, Ilupa; *Mar*: Mahwa, Mohwa; *Ori*: Mahula, Moha, Madgi; *Tam*: Illupei, Elupa; *Tel*: Ippa, Peddaippa.

Trade name: South Indian mahua, Butter tree.

Propagation: By seeds.

Uses: Stem bark useful for the treatment of diabetes.

**Mallotus philippensis** (Lam.) Muell-Arg.

Family: Euphorbiaceae.

Small or moderate sized tree, up to 12m tall, branchlets grey-tomentose. Leaves elliptic-ovate, tomentose with orbicular red glands below. Flowers unisexual, male flowers in axillary or terminal short spikes. Fruit capsule, red glandular, seeds subglobose, black.

Common in forests.

Fl. & Fr.: October–February.

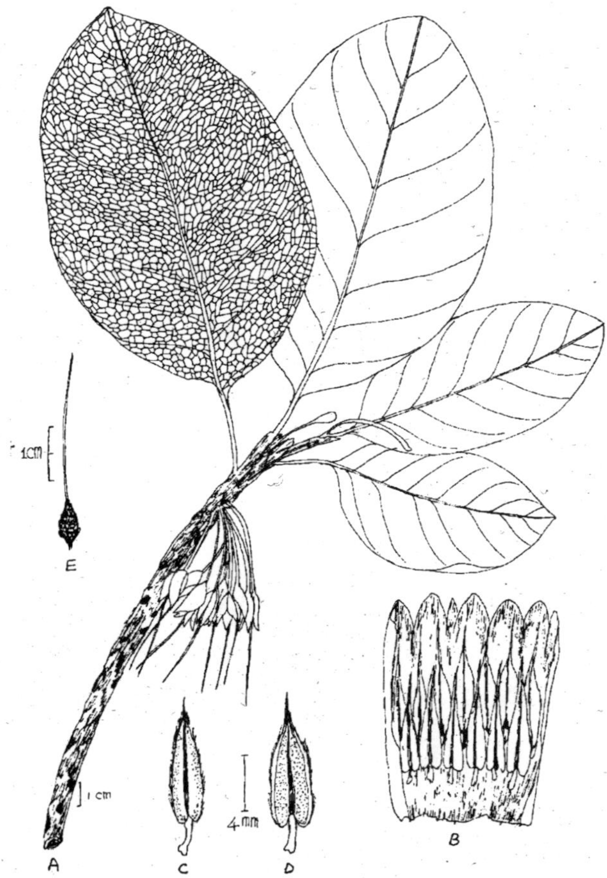


Fig. 61: *Madhuca longifolia* (Koen.) Macbr.
A. Twig; B.-E. Inner and outer calyx lobes; F. Corolla spread out with stamens; G. & H. Stamens; I. Pistil.

Sanskrit: Kampillaka, Kamela, Kapila.

Local names: *Ass*: Gangal, Jaggru, Puddum; *Ben*: Kamala, Tung, Dholasindua; *Guj*: Kapilo; *Hin*: Kamala, Kambhal, Kambila, Kamela, Kamila, Kamud, Raini, Rauni, Rohni, Roini, Roli, Rora, Ruin, Rulu; *Kan*: Chandrahittu, Honne, Honne, Ettnalige, Hullichellu, Kapila, Kesari, Kesarimava, Kunkuma, Kunkumada, Kunkume, Munnagea, Punnaga, Surapani, Suvarnakesari, Vasare; *Mal*: Chenkolli, Kapila, Kuramatukka, Manjana, Maunana, Piponnakam, Ponnakam, Punna; *Mar*: Shindri, Shindur, Kesari, Honne, Suvarnakesar, Kamala, Kapilo, Kunkum; *Ori*: Bosontogundi, Kunkumo, Kopilogudi, Punango, Sinduri, Sindurogundi; *Pun*: Kamal, Kombal, Kamela, Kumila, Reini, Reun, Rulya; *Tam*: Avam, Kabilam, Kamala, Kabilappodi, Kambosam, Kapila, Kopilapodi, Kungumam, Manjanai suvangesari; *Tel*: Sinduramu, Kunkuma

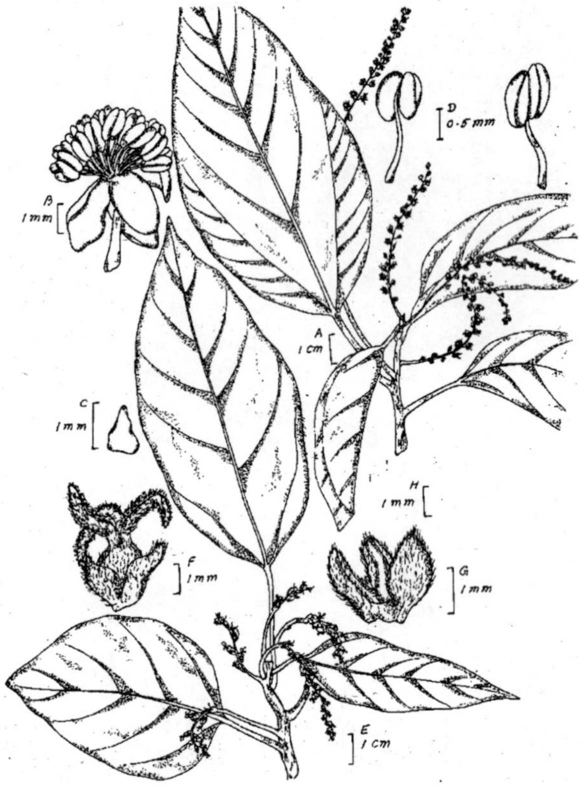


Fig. 62: *Mallotus philippensis* (Lam.) Muell.-Arg.
A. Twig; Male: B. Flower; C. Bract; D. Stamens; Female: E. Twig; F. Flower; G. Tepals; H. Pistil.

Chettu, Benduruppu; *Urdu*: Kalileh.

Trade name: Kamala Dye tree.

Propagation: By seeds.

Uses: Fruits are useful for the treatment of diabetes.

**Malva verticillata** L.

Family: Malvaceae.

Herb, up to 1.2m tall. Leaves cordate, downy pubescent. Flowers pink, crowded in clusters.

Temperate Himalayas from Punjab east-wards to Assam.

Local names: *Ben*: Lapha, napha.

Uses: Plant used in the treatment of diabetes.

**Mangifera indica** L.

Family: Anacardiaceae

Large, spreading, evergreen trees. Leaves crowded at the ends of branches, coriaceous, oblong-lanceolate, glabrous and shining. Flowers whitish in many-flowered pubescent panicles. Fruit drupe, ovoid or obliquely pyriform, 1-seeded.

In moist forests, also cultivated for its edible fruit.

Fl.: January–March; Fr.: April–July.

Sanskrit: Amrah, Chutah.

Local names: *Ass*: Am, Ghariam; *Ben*: Am; *Kan*: Amba, Ballimavu, Chandramavu, Jiregemavu, Mavina, Rasala, Simavu, Toremavu; *Hin*: Aam, Amra, Amba; *Mal*: Amram, Cutam, Tenmavu, Gommane, Manna, Mavu, Muchi, Nattumavu; *Mar*: Am, Amba; *Ori*: Ambo, Amo, Baulo; *Pun*: Am, Mawashi; *Tam*: Ambiram, Amiram, Iradam, Kachakkar, Kokku, Ma, Madi, Shudam, Tevram; *Tel*: Mamidi; *Urdu*: Amba.

Trade name: Mango tree.

Propagation: By seeds and grafting.

Uses: The tender leaves of the mango tree are considered useful in diabetes. An infusion is prepared by soaking 15 gm of fresh leaves in 250ml of water overnight, and squeezing them well in the water in the morning. This filtrate should be taken every morning to control early diabetes. As an alternative, the leaves should be dried in the shade, powdered and preserved for use when necessary. Half tea spoon of this powder should be taken twice a day.

Active Principle: Galloyl p-hydroxybenzoyl esters of maclurin-3C -glucoside (I–IV) and two galloyl esters of iriflophemone-3C-glucoside (V–VI) isolated from the leaves.

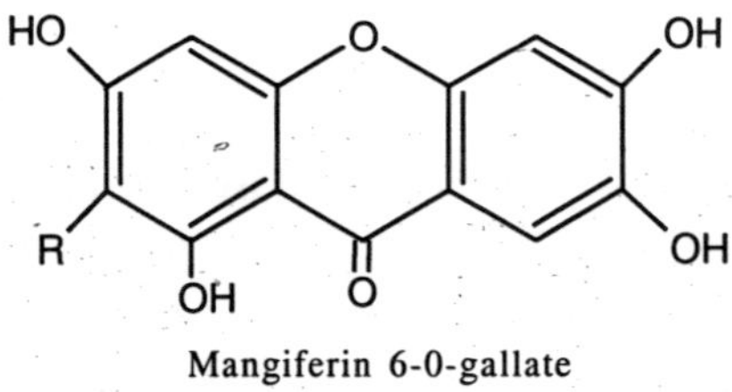


Mangiferin 6-0-gallate

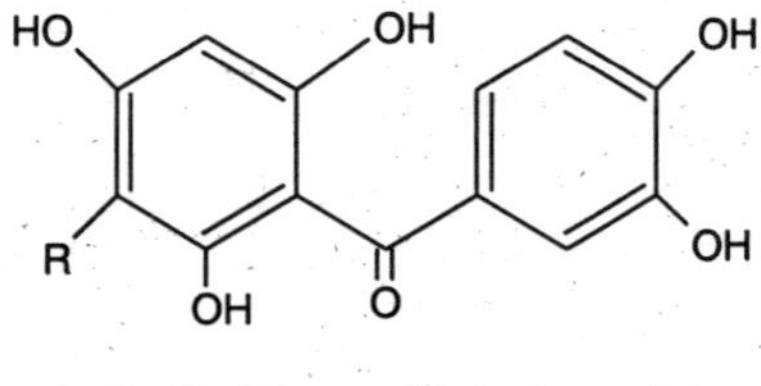


I, II, III, IV mangiferin 6-o-gallate

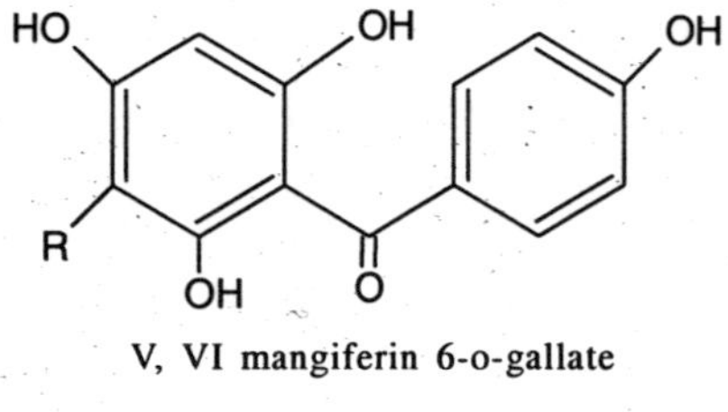


V, VI mangiferin 6-o-gallate

**Marrubium vulgare** L.

Family: Lamiaceae (Labiatae)

Tall, robust, perennial herb, up to 1m tall. Leaves orbicular or elliptic-ovate. Flowers small, white, in dense axillary whorls. Fruit nutlets.
Found in Kashmir.
Local names: *Hin*: Paharigandana.
Trade name: Horehound, Hoarhound.

Uses: Plant used in the treatment of diabetes.

**Melothria heterophylla** (Lour.) Cogn.

Syn: *Zehneria umbellata* Thw.

Family: Cucurbitaceae

Scandent herb with tuberous roots. Leaves polymorphous, ovate, sub-orbicular, oblong or narrow-lanceolate. Flowers small, yellow, male flowers in umbellate racemes, female flowers solitary. Fruit oblong, brown.
Throughout India.
Local names: *Ben*: Kudari; *Hin*: Tarali; *Pun*: Bankakra; *Tel*: Thiyyadonda.

Uses: Plant used in the treatment of diabetes.

**Memecylon umbellatum** Burm.f.

Family: Melastomataceae

Shrub or small tree, up to 4m tall. Leaves elliptic or elliptic-ovate. Flowers reddish-purple in umbellate cymes. Fruit berry, ripening black.
Occasional.

Uses: Leaves used in the treatment of diabetes.

**Mentha piperata** L.

Family: Lamiaceae

Perennial erect herb, 50–90cm tall, branches grey-tomentose. Leaves oblong-ovate, serrate. Flowers violet in false spikes. Fruits not seen.
Cultivated.
Local names: *Tel*: Pepper mint
Trade name: Pepper mint.
Propagation: By stolons.

Uses: Plant useful in the trteatment of diabetes.

**Merremia mammosa** (Lour.) Hallier. f.

Syn: *Ipomoea gomezii* C. B. Clarke

Family: Convolvulaceae

Large climber, roots tuberous.

Found in Lakimpur in Assam and Andaman and Nicobar Islands.

Uses: Tubers used locally in the treatment of diabetes.

**Michelia champaca** L.

Family: Magnoliaceae.

Medium sized evergreen tree, up to 20m tall. Leaves ovate-lanceolate, coriaceous, glabrescent. Flowers solitary, axillary, pale yellow. Fruit an aggregate of follicles.

It is distributed in the Sub-Himalayan zone of West Bengal, Assam, Bihar, and in the Western Ghats in Karnataka, Kerala and Tamil Nadu; also cultivated for its flowers.

Fl. & Fr.: March–August.

Sanskrit: Champaca.

Local names: *Ass*: Titasopa, Bolnabat, Shap; *Ben*: Champaka; *Guj*: Champo, Rae champo, Piuto-champo; *Hin*: Champa, Champe-ke-phul; *Kan*: Sampige. Kola-sampige; *Mal*: Champakam, Chembakam; *Mar*: Picala-champa, Sona-champa, Kud-champa; *Ori*: Chompa, Chompoko, Kanchana; *Tam*: Shenbuga, Chambugam; *Tel*: Sampenga, Champakamu.

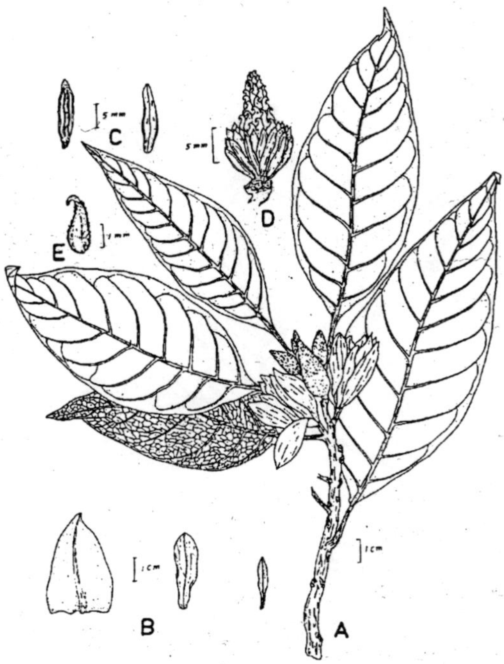


Fig. 63: *Michelia champaca* L.
A. Twig; B. Perianth lobes; C. Stamens; D. Stamens with pistil; E. Pistil.

Trade name: Champak, Golden yellow champa.
Propagation: By seeds.

Medicinal uses: Stem bark useful in the treatment of diabetes.

**Mimosa pudica** L.

Family: Mimosaceae.

Spreading herbs, branchlets glabrescent or hispid, prickles short, erect or curved. Leaves up to 4 cm long, pinnae 1–2 pairs, leaflets 15–20 pairs, elliptic-oblong, overlapping. Leaves sensitive to touch. Flowers pink in axillary heads. Fruit flat pod, slightly undulate, 2–4-jointed, bristly along margins, seeds ovoid.

Common in waste lands and road sides, especially in moist localities.

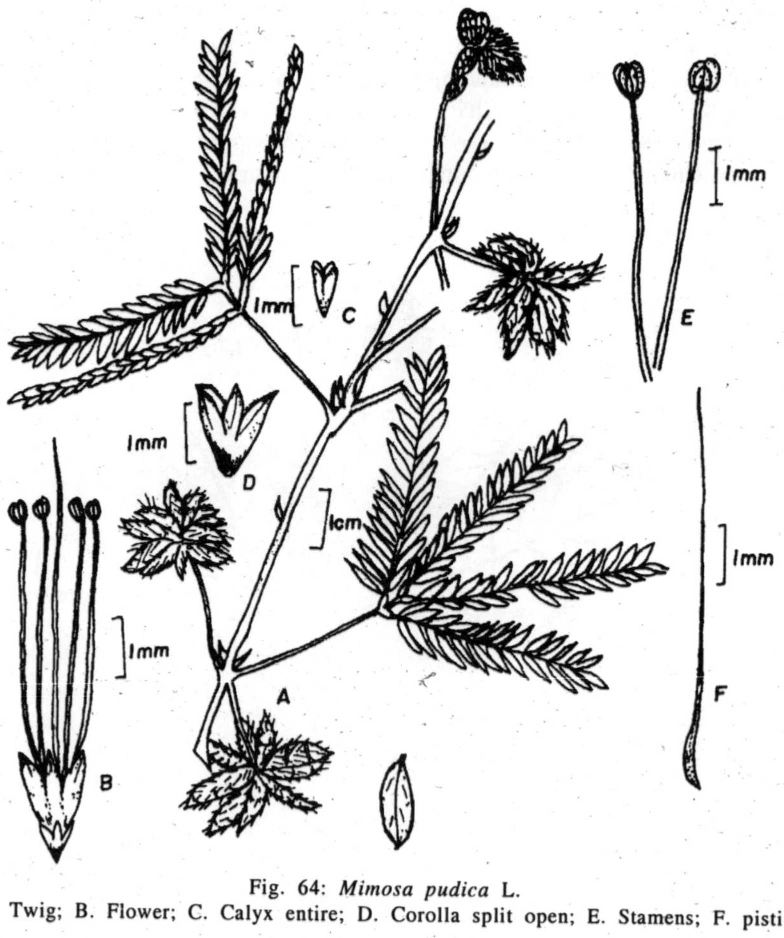


Fig. 64: *Mimosa pudica* L.
A. Twig; B. Flower; C. Calyx entire; D. Corolla split open; E. Stamens; F. pistil.

Fl. & Fr.: July–November.

Sanskrit: Lajjalu, Namaskari.

Local names: *Ben*: Lajjabati; *Hin*: Lajwanti, Chui-mui; *Kan*: Lajja, Nachike, Mudugu-davare; *Mal*: Tintarmani; *Mar*: Lajalu; *Ori*: Lajkuri; *Tam*: Tottalvadi, Tottal-chinungi; *Tel*: Attipatti, Lajja vathi.

Trade name: Sensitive plant.

Propagtion: By seeds.

Uses: Whole plant useful in the treatment of diabetes. Mixture of leaf powders of *M. pudica* and *Gymnema sylvestre* reduce blood glucose level.

**Mimusops elengi** L.

Family: Sapotaceae.

Medium sized evergreen trees, up to 10m tall, bark scaly. Leaves elliptic-oblong. Flowers solitary or few in fascicles of 2–6. Fruit ovoid berry.

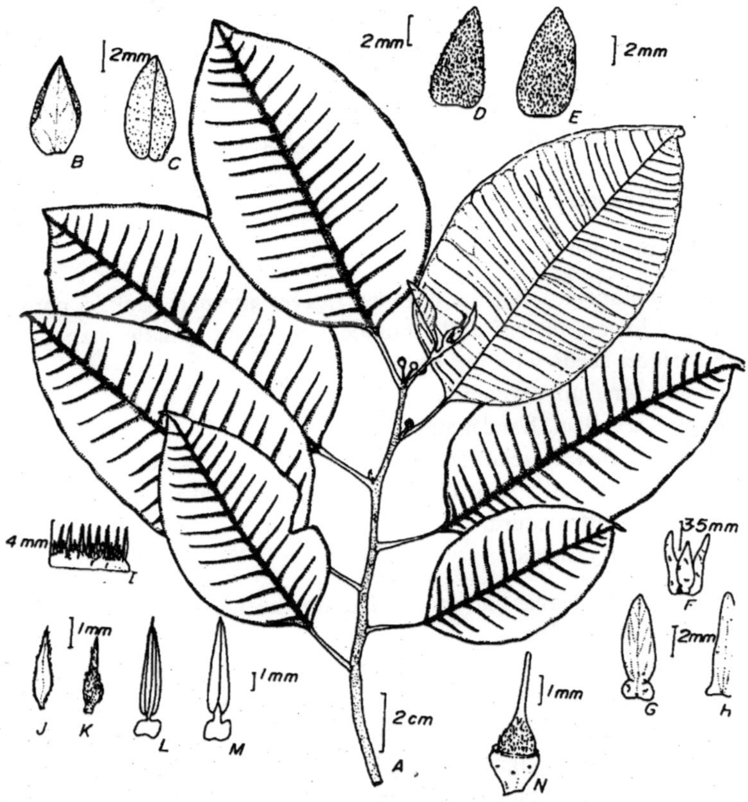


Fig. 65: *Mimusops elengi* L.
A. Twig; B.-E. Sepals; F. Part of Corolla; G. & H. Corolla lobes; I. Androecium; J. & K. Staminodes; L. & M. Stamens; N. Pistil

Deccan in ravines in the hills, also cultivated.
Fl. & Fr.: March–May.
Sanskrit: Bakula, Sinhakesara.
Local names: *Ass*: Gokul; *Ben & Ori*: Baukul; *Guj*: Barsoli, Bolsari; *Hin*: Tedu, Maulsari; *Kan*: Pokkalathu, Bakula, Pagade; *Mal*: Elangi, Elanni; *Mar*: Bakul, Ovalli; *Ori*: Bokulo baulol; *Tam*: Vagulam, Magadam, Magizham Ilangi; *Tel*: Pogada, Vekulamu, Kesara.
Propagation: By seeds.

Uses: Plant useful for the treatment of diabetes.

**Momordica balsamina** L.

Family: Cucurbitaceae

Monoecious climber. Leaves orbicular, palmately 3–5-lobed. Flowers yellow, solitary. Fruit ovoid, tuberculate, seeds ellipsoid, grey.
Found in Punjab, Western U.P., Rajasthan and Saurashtra.
Local names: *Hin*: Mokha
Trade name: Balsam apple.

Uses: Plant useful in the treatment of diabetes.

**Momordica charantia** L.

Family: Cucurbitaceae.

Annual, pubescent, tendrillar climber. Leaves alternate, simple, cordate, much lobed. Flowers in leaf axils, monoecious. Fruit spindle-shaped with wart like surface, seeds with red aril.
Cultivated for fruit vegetable.
Sanskrit: Karvellam, Kandakataka.
Local names: *Ben*: Karela; *Hin*: Karela, Kareli; *Mar*: Karele; *Kan*: Hagal; *Mal*: Kaippa, Kaippavalli; *Tam*: Pakal, Pavakka; *Tel*: Kakara.
Trade name: Bitter gourd.
Propagation: By seeds.

Uses: The fruits, leaves and roots have long been used in India as a folk remedy for diabetes mellitus.

Among the severeal herbal remedies that have proved beneficial in controlling diabetes, perhaps the most important is the use of bitter gourd. It has lately been established that bitter gourd contains a hypoglycemic or insulin-like principle, designated as plantiinsulin, which has been found valuable in lowering the blood and urine sugar levels. It should, therefore, be included liberally in the diet of the diabetics. For better results, the diabetics should take the juice of about four or five bitter gourds every morning on an empty stomach. The seeds can be added to food in a powdered form. Diabetics can also use bitter gourd in the form of decoction by boiling the pieces of fruit in water or in the form of dry powder.

Active principle: Alkaloids Momordicoside $F_1$, $F_2$, G, H, I, K,L; pure protein P-insulin and polypeptide-p isolated from fruit.

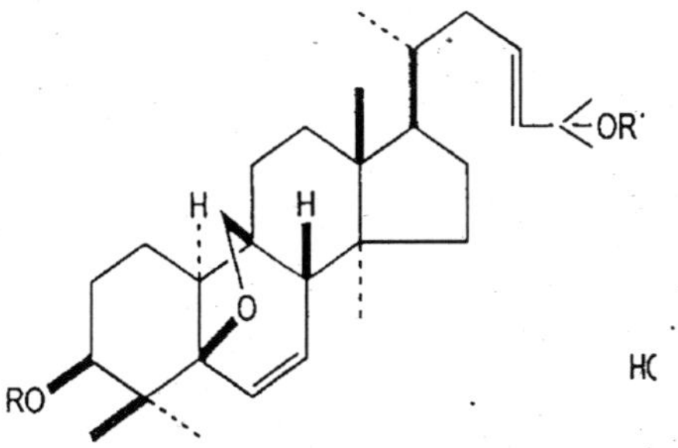


Momordicoside $F_1$
R = Glu, R′ = Me
Momocardicoside $F_2$
R = Allose, R′ = H
Momocardicoside G
R = Allose, R′ = Me
Momocard-I
R = Glu, R′ = H

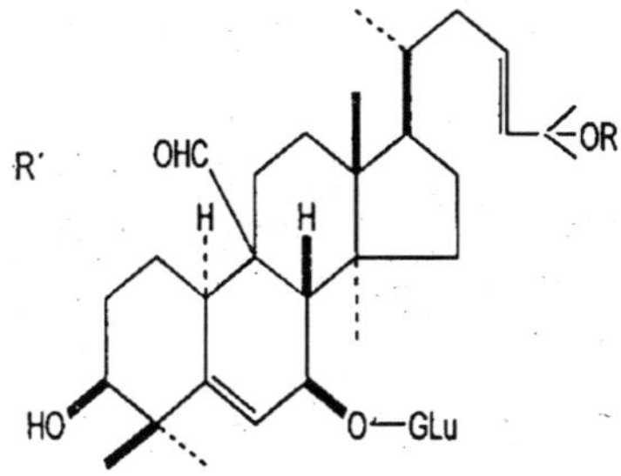


Momordicoside K
R = Me
Momordicoside L
R = H

**Momordica cochinchinensis** Spreng.

Family: Cucurbitaceae

Perennial monoecious climber with tuberous roots. Leaves suborbicular, deeply 3–5-lobed. Flowers white or pale yellow. Fruit ovoid, pointed.

Common in Assam, Bengal, South India and Andaman Islands.

Local names: *Ben*: Golkakara, Kakrol; *Hin*: Gulkakra, Gangerua; *Tel*: Adavi Kakara.

Uses: Root tubers used in the treatment of diabetes.

**Momordica cymbalaria** Fenzl. ex Naud.

Syn: *Momordica tuberosa* Cogn.
*Luffa tuberosa* Roxb.

Family Cucurbitaceae

Perennial creeping herb, roots tuberous. Tendril simple. Leaves orbicular-reniform. Flowers white, unisexual, axillary, male in fascicles, female solitary. Fruit ribbed, pyriform.

Weed in black cotton soils in Andhra Pradesh.

Local names: *Tel*: Kasara.

Uses: Fruits are useful in treating diabetes.

**Monochoria hastata** (L.) Solms-Laub.

Syn: *Pontederia hastata* L.
*Monochoria hastaefolia* Presl.

Family: Pontederiaceae.

A fresh water, floating erect herb, root creeping, rooting below, spongy. Leaves sagittate, hastate or cordate. Flowers brilliant purplish blue, crowded, racemose or subumbellate. Fruit capsule, oblong, many-seeded.

In ponds and tanks, rare.

Fl. & Fr.: August–December.

Sanskrit: Nilotpalam.

Local names: *Mal*: Karinkuvalam, Kolachempa; *Tel*: Nir-tamara.

Propagation: By seeds.

Uses: Whole plant useful in the treatment of diabetes.

**Morinda citrifolia** L.

Family: Rubiaceae.

Shrubs, up to 3m tall. Leaves coriaceous. Flowers white, in dense ovoid heads. Fruit syncarpium, white when ripe.

Throughout hotter parts of India.

Fl. & Fr.: July–October.

Sanskrit: Asyaka.

Local names: *Ben*: Ach, Achhu, Aich, Hurdi, Haldikunj; *Guj*: Al, Saroji; *Hin*: Ach, Ak, Al; *Kan*: Ainshi, Tagashe, Meddi; *Mal*: Kattapitalavam, Mannanati; *Mar*: Aal, Surangi, Al, Bartondi, Bartundi, Nagakunda; *Ori*: Achu, Gondhonagi; *Tam*: Manjatvattai, Manjanati, Nuna, Perianuna, Seyal, Tunnavu, Vellainuma; *Tel*: Togara, Togaru Mogali.

Trade name: Indian mulberry.

Propagation: By seeds.

Uses: Aerial parts useful in the treatment of diabetes.

**Moringa pterigosperma** Gaertn.

Syn: *Moringa oleifera* auct non Lam.

Family: Moringaceae.

Small trees. Leaves tripinnate, leaflets small, ovate, elliptic-obovate. Flowers white, strongly honey scented, in panicles. Fruit elongated capsule, loculicidally dehiscent, seeds rounded, winged.

Indigenous to the sub-Himalayan tracts of North-West India; Cultivated elsewhere for its fruit.

Sanskrit: Sigruh, Sobhanjanah, Madhugunjana.

Local names: *Ass*: Saijna, Sohjna; *Ben*: Sanjina; *Guj*: Midhosaragao,

Saragaro; *Hin*: Mungna; *Kan*: Nagge: *Mal*: Murinna, Sigru, Moringa; *Mar*: Shevgi, Murungamul; *Ori*: Sajina; *Pun*: Sainja; *Tam*: Murungai; *Tel*: Munaga.

Trade name: Drumstick tree.

Propagation: By seeds, cuttings

Uses: Fruits, leaves and stem useful in the treatment of diabetes.

**Morus alba** L.

Family: Moraceae

Shrub or small tree, up to 3m tall. Leaves very variable, ovate or broadly ovate. Flowers unisexual, male flowers greenish in catkins, female flowers in dense spikes. Fruit syncarp, consisting of many drupes.

Extensively cultivated for rearing Silkworm.

Local names: *Ben*: Tut; *Guj*: Shetur; *Hin*: Tut, Tutri; *Kan*; Hipnerle; *Ori*: Tuto, Tutikoli, *Mar*: Tut, Ambat; *Tam*: Musukette, Kamblichedi; *Tel*: Resham chettu.

Trade name: White mulberry.

Uses: Leaves and root bark useful in the treatment of diabetes.

Active constituents: Phytosterol, glycosides, Scopoletin, Moron, glycoprotein and Moranoline.

**Morus australis** Poir

Syn: *Morus acidosa* Griff.

Family: Moraceae

Shrub or small tree.

Found in Assam.

Uses: Plant useful in the treatment of diabetes.

**Mucuna pruriens** (L.) DC.

Syn: *Dolichos pruriens* L.
*Mucuna prurita* Hook.
*Carpopogon pruriens* L.

Family: Leguminosae (Fabaceae).

Twining herbs, branches terete, striate, downy pubescent. Leaves trifoliolate, leaflets ovate-rhomboid, appressed white-pubescent. Flowers dark purple with yellow shade on standard petal in long axillary racemes. Pods curved, prominently S-shaped, densely silky pubescent with persistent pale brown or grey irritant bristles, seeds 4–6, orbicular.

Occasional in damp places, bushes, hedges and ravines throughout India.

Fl. & Fr.: October–April.

Sanskrit: Atmagupta, Vanari.

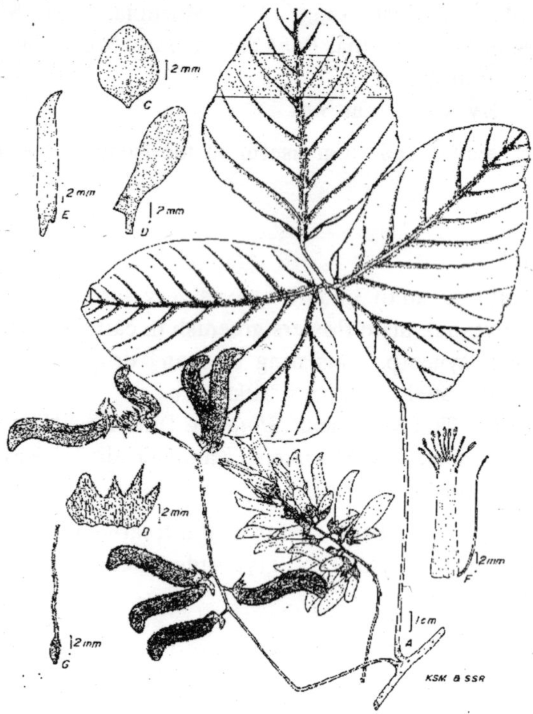


Fig. 66: *Mucuna pruriens* (L.) DC.
A. Twig; B. Calyx split open; C. Standard petal; D. Wing petal; E. Keel petal; F. Staminal column; G. Pistil.

Local names: *Ben*: Alkushi, Bichchoti; *Guj*: Kivach, Kavatch; *Hin*: Kiwach, Kivanchh; *Kan*: Turachi-gida, Nayisonangu balli; *Mal*: Naykkurana, Nayikuruma; *Mar*: Kuhili, Khag-khiri, Punaikkali, Poonaykali; *Ori*: Kaincho; *Tel*: Dulagondi.

Trade name: Common cowitch.

Propagation: It can be propagated by seeds. *Mucuna pruriens* is being cultivated all over India. The crop can be grown on a wide range of soils but it does well on sandy to clay loam type of soils, provided drainage is adequate. This species can be grown as a rainfed crop as well as irrigated crop. As a rainfed crop, sowing is done in June and final harvesting is done in December. As irrigated crop it is not season bound. The best season for planting is August and harvesting is done in January and February. A basal dose of 13–15 tonnes of Farm yard manure along with 80 kg $P_2O_5$ per hectare should be applied to the fields before ploughing. Top dressing of a mixture of 100 kg of Nitrogen and 75 kg of Potash is given in two equal split doses when the crop is 30 days old and 60 days old.

The fields are ploughed with a mould broad plough 2–3 times till a fine belt is obtained. Basal dose of manure along with phosphate should be mixed in the soil at this time. Ridges are made along the contours with a spacing of 60 cm. The seed rate is 50 kg per hectare. 60×60 cm is provided if support is given to the plants, 60×40 cm if no support is given to the plants. The crop requires 1–2 weedings in the initial stages.

Leaves may be attacked by the Cercospora leaf spot. One spray of Dithane at 1.5ml/litre at 30 days of growth are adequate as a prophylactic measure. The flowering in this crop is continuous and the pods mature periodically. The flowering starts after about 45 days growth. The dried pods should be harvested three or four times in the season. The pods are sun dried. The pods will break open on drying. These are to be winnowed and seperated from the husk.

The crop yield is about 1500–1750 kg /ha if no support is given to plants. If support is provided the yield will be 3000–3750 kg/ha.

Uses: Fruits, seeds and root useful in the treatment of diabetes.

**Murraya koenigii** (L.) Spreng.

Syn: *Bergera koenigii* L.

Family: Rutaceae.

Shrubs or small trees. Leaves pinnately compound, leaflets alternate, asymmetrical, oblong-lanceolate. Flowers white, small, in terminal corymbose panicles, fragrant. Fruit subglobose berry, purplish black when ripe, seeds 1 or 2.

Common on hill slopes in forests. Cultivated for its aromatic leaves, which are used for curry flavouring.

Fl. & Fr.: March–August.

Sanskrit: Kalasaka, Surabinimbha.

Local names: *Ben*: Barsanga, Kariaphulli; *Guj*: Goranimb, Kadhilimbdo; *Hin*: Katnim, Harri; *Kan*: Karibevu, Gandha bevu; *Mal*: Kariveppu, Kareapela; *Mar*: Karipat, Jhirang; *Ori*: Barsan, Basango, Bhursunga; *Tam*: Karuveppilai, Karuvempu; *Tel*: Karivepaku.

Trade name: Curry leaf tree.

Uses: The aqueous extract of leaves showed hypoglycemic action. Fresh leaf chatni and /or dried leaf powder are advised to be taken regularly to maintain normal glucose levels.

**Musa paradisiaca** L.

Family: Musaceae.

Perennial, rhizomatous, tall, erect herb, its robust tree like stem is composed of the sheathing spiral leaf bases. At the summit of 3–8m stem a crown of large oval deep green leaves are produced, leaves up to 3m long. Flowers in a fleshy spathe like scales which drop off as the fruit matures. Fruit fleshy, indehiscent.

Cultivated for its fruit.

Sanskrit: Kadali, Vanalakshmi.

Local names: *Ben*: Kach, Kula, Kala, Keli; *Kan*: Ble, Budibale, Chandrabale, Kaladi, Elebale, Elakkibale, Havubale, Hombale, Jenubale, Gurubale, Kandu, Karttubale, Madarangabale, Mavuju, Pachchabale, Pattubale, Rajabale, Rasabale; *Guj*: Kela; *Hin*: Kela, Amrit, Kach kula; *Mal*: Ettakkaya, Ettavala, Kandalam, Karinkadali, Kashthhila, Kunnan, Pichcha, Vanna; *Mar*: Kadali, Kel; *Ori*: Bontolo kadali, Kodoli, Konokorombha, Rombhha, Romokodoli; *Tam*: Ambanam, Angusam, Sefili; *Tel*: Aratikaya, Arati; *Urdu*: Kela.

Trade name: Banana, Plantain.

Uses: Banana flower is eaten as a vegetable and medicine for diabetes. Banana fruit is used in diabetes.

**Mussaenda glabra** Vahl

Family: Rubiaceae

Large, scandent, often climbing shrub. Leaves elliptic or oblong-lanceolate. Flowers yellow in terminal cymes. Fruit globose berry.

In Tropical Himalayas, Bihar, Bengal and Assam.

Uses: Aerial parts and fruits useful in the treatment of diabetes.

**Myrsine africana** L.

Family: Myrsinaceae.

Erect shrub or small tree, up to 1.2m tall. Leaves lanceolate or obovate. Flowers minute, white in axillary clusters. Fruit small, globose, fleshy.

Found in outer Himalayas from Kashmir to Nepal and Khasi hills.

Uses: Whole plant useful in the treatment of diabetes.

**Myrtus communis** L.

Family: Myrtaceae

Evergreen shrub, up to 3m tall. Leaves ovate to lanceolate, aromatic. Flowers white, fragrant, axillary. Fruit berry, ellipsoid, blue black when ripe.

Often grown for its attractive foliage.

Trade name: Common myrtle, clove myrtle.

Uses: Leaves and stem useful in the treatment of diabetes.

**Naravelia zeylanica** (L.) DC.

Family: Ranunculaceae.

Climbing herbs. Leaves 3-foliolate, terminal leaflet modified as a tendril, lateral leaflets ovate. Flowers greenish-yellow in axillary and terminal panicles.

Fruit achene, prolonged into a feathery style which pesrsists in fruits as twisted pilose tail.

Tropical Himalayas from East Nepal to Bengal, Assam. East and West Peninsula.

Fl.& Fr.: September–March.

Sanskrit: Dhanavalli.

Local names: *Ben*: Chagul-Bati, Murcha; *Mal*: Kuruppakodi; *Tam*: Vathomkolli, Neendavalli; *Tel*: Pulla Bachala.

Propagation: By seeds.

Uses: Aerial parts useful in the treatment of diabetes.

**Nardostachys grandiflora** DC.

Syn: *Nardostachys jatamansi* DC.
*Valeriana jatamansi* Jones

Family: Valerianaceae.

Perennial glabrous herb, up to 1m tall, stem furrowed and hollow. Leaves opposite, pinnate. Flowers white in corymbose panicle, fragrant. Fruit oblong.

In Himalayas from Kashmir to Assam at 2500m.

Trade name: Indian valerian.

Local names: *Hin*: Mushkvala.

Propagation: By seeds and through root stocks.

Uses: Plant useful in the treatment of diabetes.

**Nasturtium officinale** R. Br.

Syn: *Nasturtium fontanum* Aschers.

Family: Brassicaceae (Cruciferae).

Perennial much branched aquatic herb. Leaves pinnate, leaflets 7–11, ovate-oblong, sinuately lobed. Flowers white in short racemes. Fruit siliqua, cylindric.

Found in ditches and pools, introduced and naturalized.

Trade name: Water cress.

Uses: Plant used in the treatment of diabetes mellitus.

**Nelumbo nucifera** Gaertn.

Syn: *Nymphaea nelumbo* L.
*Nelumbium speciosum* Willd.

Family: Nelumbonaceae.

Perennial aquatic herb. Leaves peltate, rotund. Flowers rose red, white or yellow, solitary, long peduncled.

Fl. & Fr.: Throughout the year.

Uses: Rhizome, flowers and seeds useful in the treatment of diabetes. Ethanolic extract of rhizome markedly reduced the blood sugar level.

**Nepeta cataria** L.

Family: Lamiaceae (Labiatae)

Erect, hoary pubescent, perennial herb, up to 1m tall. Leaves ovate. Flowers white dotted with purple. Fruit nutlets, broadly oblong, brownish black.

Found in Western Temperate Himalayas.

Trade name: Catnip, Catmint.

Uses: Leaves and flowering tops are considered carminative, tonic, diaphoretic, refrigerant and soporific. Leaves are chewed to relieve toothache.

**Nicotiana tabacum** L.

Family: Solanaceae.

Annual erect subshrubs. Leaves cauline, broadly ovate elliptic-ovate, upper leaves narrowed, lanceolate. Flowers in terminal corymboid panicles. Fruit capsule.

Cultivated for the tobacco leaf.

Sanskrit: Tamakhu.

Local names: *Ben*: Tamak; *Guj*: Tobacu, Tamaku; *Hin*: Bujjarebhang, Tamaku, tambaka, Tambaku, Tumak; *Kan*: Higisappu; *Mal*: Pokala, Pukayila; *Mar*: Tamaku: *Tam*: Pugaiyiai; *Tel*: Pogaku.

Trade name: Tobacco.

Propagation: By seeds.

Uses: Plant useful in the treatment of diabetes.

**Nigella sativa** L.

Family: Ranunculaceae.

Small herb, up to 60cm tall. Leaves 2–3-pinnatisect, segments linear–lanceolate. Flowers pale blue, solitary, long penduncled. Seeds trigonous, black, rugulose-tubercular.

In Punjab and Bihar, often cultivated.

Sanskrit: Upakunchika, Karavi, Krishnajiraka.

Local names: *Ben*: Kalajira, Mungrela; *Guj*: Kalonji–Jiram; *Hin*: Kalajira, Kalomji; *Kan*: Karijirige; *Mal*: Karinchirigam, *Tam*: Karumjiragam; *Tel*: Nallajilakarra.

Trade name: Small fennel, Black cumin.

Uses: Seeds useful in the treatment of diabetes.

**Nymphaea nouchali** Burm.f.

Syn: *Nymphaea stellata* Willd.

Family: Nymphaeaceae.

Aquatic, rhizomatous, perennial herbs. Leaves long petioled, peltate, orbicular, pale purple below, green above. Flowers solitary, blue, white, rose or purple. Fruit berry, spongy, globose or ovoid, seeds numerous.

Common in ditches, ponds and tanks.

Sanskrit: Kumuda, Utpala.

Local names: *Ben*: Shaluk, Rakto-kambal, Nal; *Guj*: Kanval, Nilophal; *Hin*: Kanval, Kokka; *Kan*: Neela thavare, Biletavare; *Mal*: Ampal, Cit-ambel; *Mar*: Lalakamal, Raktakamal; *Ori*: Dhabalakain, Rangkain; *Tam*: Vellampal, Nilotpalam; *Tel*: Kaluva, Neetithamara, Allikada.

Trade name: Indian water lily.

Propagation: Rhizomes.

Uses: Root and other plant parts useful for the treatment of diabetes.

**Nymphaea pubescens** Willd.

Syn: *Nymphaea lotus* auct. non L.

Family: Nymphaeaceae

Large perennial herb. Leaves peltate, orbicular, sharply dentate at margin. Flowers white or red, solitary, arising from the rhizome.

Fl. & Fr.: January–November.

Uses: Root useful in the treatment of diabetes.

**Ocimum americanum** L.

Syn: *Ocimum canum* Sims.

Family: Labiatae (Lamiaceae).

Erect much branched strongly aromatic herbs, stems grooved, pubescent. Leaves elliptic-ovate. Flowers in whorls, white or creamish in terminal racemes. Fruit nutlets, oblong, black.

Common in waste lands all over India.

Sanskrit: Vanabarbarika, Aranyathulasi.

Local names: *Hin*: Kala thulsi, Mamri; *Kan* & *Tam*: Nayi tulsi; *Mal*: Kattu tulasi; *Tel*: Kukkathulasi, Kuppathulasi.

Trade name: Hoary basil.
Propagation: By seeds.

Uses: Leaves and seeds useful in the treatment of diabetes.

**Ocimum gratissimum** L.

Family: Lamiaceae (Labiatae).

A much branched aromatic subshrub, up to 2m tall. Leaves ovate, membranous. Flowers pale greenish yellow in close whorls in racemes. Fruit of 4 nutlets, subglobose, brown.

Occasional in waste lands and roadsides near villages.

Fl. & Fr.: October–March.

Sanskrit: Vriddhuthulasi.

Local names: *Ben & Hin*: Ban tulsi, Ram tulsi; *Guj*: Avachi bavachi, Ram tulsi; *Mal*: Kattu trittavu, Rama tulsi; *Mar*: Rama tulsi, Rama tulasi; *Tam*: Elumicham tulsi, Perum tulsi; *Tel*: Nimmathulasi, Lavanga thulasi.

Trade name: Shrubby Basil, Ban tulasi.

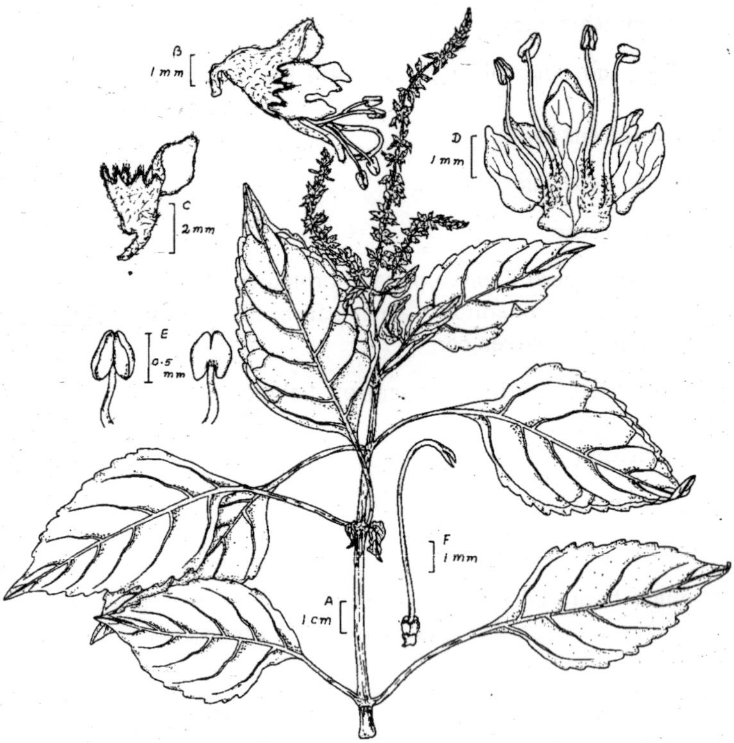


Fig. 67: *Ocimum gratissimum* L.
A. Twig; B. Flower; C. Calyx; D. Corolla split open; E. Anthers; F. Pistil.

Propagation: By seeds.

Uses: Whole plant useful in the treatment of diabetes.

**Ocimum tenuiflorum** L.

Syn: *Ocimum sanctum* L.

Family: Lamiaceae (Labiatae.)

An erect, much branched, softly pubescent aromatic subshrub. Leaves elliptic-oblong. Flowers white in terminal racemes. Fruits ellipsoid nutlets.

Cultivated in pots or on pedestals in Hindu houses, frequently run wild.

Sanskrit: Surasa, Vrinda.

Local names: *Ben*: Tulsi; *Guj*: Tulsi; *Hin*: Tulsi, Baranda, Kala tulsi; *Kan*: Vishnu tulasi, Kari tulasi, Sri tulasi; *Mal*: Trttavu; *Mar*: Tulasa, Tulasi chajadha; *Tam*: Tulasi; *Tel*: Tulasi, Krishna tulasi.

Trade name: Sacred Basil.

Propagation: By seeds.

Medicinal uses: Use of fresh leaf aqueous extract or shade dried leaf powder twice a day helps in controlling blood sugar level at initial stages of diabetes.

**Opuntia ficus–indica** (L.) Mill.

Family: Cactaceae.

Large bushy tree like cactus with oblong or elliptic joints, usually spineless. Flowers yellow. Fruit purple or red.

All over India.

Trade name: Indian Fig.

Uses: Whole plant used in the treatment of diabetes mellitus.

**Opuntia stricta** (Haw.) Haw.

Syn: *Cactus strictus* Haw.
*Opuntia dillenii* Ker-Gawl.

Family: Cactaceae.

Erect, branching, leafless xerophtic shrubs, stem jointed, joints flat, obovate, fleshy, with many areoles bearing yellowish-spines. Flowers yellow, solitary, near the margins of joints. Fruit berry, globose, fleshy.

Common in waste lands and road sides, in dry localities.

Fl. & Fr.: January–August.

Sanskrit: Vidara-Visvasraka.

Local names: *Ben*: Nagphana; *Guj*: Chorhatalo; *Hin*: Hathhathoria, Nagphana; *Kan*: Papaskalli; *Mal*: Palakkalli; *Mar*: Chapal; *Ori*: Nagophenia; *Tam*: Nagathali, Sappathikalli; *Tel*: Nagajemudu.

Trade name: Prickly pear, Snake hood Fig.
Propagation: By stem cuttings.

Uses: Fruits useful in the treatment of diabetes.

**Opuntia vulgaris** Mill.

Syn: *Opuntia monacatha* Haw.

Family: Cactaceae

Large succulent leafless shrub, up to 2.4m tall; joints bright green, areoles bearing 1–3 spines. Flowers golden yellow. Fruit reddish purple.
All over India.

Uses: Whole plant used to cure diabetes mellitus.

**Orchis latifolia** L.

Family: Orchidaceae.

Tuberous, terrestrial herb, up to 90cm tall. Leaves many, erect, oblong, linear-oblong or lanceolate. Flowers dull purple in cylindric spikes.
Himalayas from Kashmir to Nepal at altitudes of 2500–5000m in damp places.
Sanskrit: Salampamisri, Munjatakah.
Local names: *Hin*: Salampanja, Salam; *Kan*, *Mal*, *Tam* & *Tel*: Salamisri.
Trade name: Salep.

Uses: The tubers are odourless and tasteless. They are useful in diabetes.

**Orthosiphon aristatus** (Blume) Miq

Syn: *Orthosiphon spiralis* (Lour.) Merr.
*Orthosiphon stamineus* Benth.
*Orthosiphon grandiflorus* Boldingh

Family: Lamiaceae.

Erect, slender shrub, up to 1.2m tall. Leaves ovate. Flowers white or purplish in lax-flowered racemes. Fruit nutlets.
Found in Manipur, Naga and Lusai hills, Western Ghats and Nicobar Islands.
Trade name: Kidney Tea Plant, Java Tea.
Propagation: By cuttings.

Uses: Leaf extract lowers the blood sugar in diabetic patients. It stimulates glycogen formation.

**Ottelia alismoidis** (L.) Pers.

Syn: *Stratiotes alismoides* L.

Family: Hydrocharitaceae

Acaulescent submerged herb. Leaves submerged and floating, submerged leaves oblong, floating leaves obovate or cordate. Flowers white in a tubular spathe. Fruit oblong.

Found throughout India in tanks, ponds, streams and ditches.

Fl. & Fr.: May–November.

Local names: *Ben*: Parmikalla; *Kan*: Kottigenasuballi, Hasurnineerupatre; *Tel*: Nir–Veneki.

Uses: Whole plant useful in treatment of diabetes.

**Ougenia oojeinensis** (Roxb.) Hochr.

Syn: *Dalbergia oojeinensis* Roxb.
*Ougeinia dalbergioides* Benth.

Family: Fabaceae (Papilionaceae)

Moderate sized deciduous tree, bark black or dark brown. Leaves pinnately 3-foliolate, leaflets broadly ovate or suborbicular, coriaceous. Flowers white or rose-coloured, in short fascicled racemes from the nodes of old branches. Fruit 2–5-jointed pod, flat.

Occasional in Andhra Pradesh, Karnataka, Kerala, Tamil Nadu, Orissa, Bihar and Madhya Pradesh.

Fl. & Fr.: February–May.

Sanskrit: Tinisa, Syandara.

Local names: *Ben*: Tinis; *Guj*: Tanach; *Hin*: Sandan, Panjan, Tinsa, Panan; *Kan*: Kuri-mutal, Kari-honne; *Mal*: Malavema; *Mar*: Tiwas, Kalaphulas; *Ori*: Bandhona, Banjan; *Tam*: Narivengai; *Tel*: Tella moduga, Vandanam.

Trade name: Sandan.

Propagation: By seeds.

Uses: Bark has stimulant and astringent properties and is used in curing diabetes.

**Oxalis corniculata** L.

Family: Oxalidaceae.

Annual or perennial herbs, branchlets creeping, rooting at nodes. Leaves digitately 3-foliolate, leaflets obcordate. Flowers yellow, sub umbellate, axillary. Fruit capsule, oblong, beaked, seeds brown.

Common in moist localities and shade.

Fl. & Fr.: July–December.
Sanskrit: Cangeri.
Local names: *Ass*: Changeritenga; *Ben & Hin*: Amrul Sak, Chukatripati; *Kan*: Hulichikkai, Pullam Purachi; *Mal*: Puliyarel; *Mar*: Ambuti, Anjati, Bhinsarpati; *Pun*: Amlika, Khattamitha; *Tam*: Puliyarai; *Tel*: Pulichintaku, Anbotikura.
Trade name: Indian sorrel.

Uses: Leaves and stem useful in the treatment of diabetes.

**Paeonia emodi** Wall. ex Royle

Family: Ranunculaceae; Paeoniaceae.

Herbaceous or shruby perenial with a cluster of fleshy roots. Leaves divided in to distinct leaflets. Flowers white or red, usually solitary. Fruit follicles.
Distributed in Himalayas from Kashmir to Kumaon.
Local names: *Hin*: Ud-salap; *Pun*: Mamekh, Chandra.
Trade name: Himalayan paeony.

Uses: Whole plant useful in the treatment of diabetes.

**Panax ginseng** C.A. Meyer

Family: Araliaceae.

Perennial rhizomatous erect herb, with terminal whorl of 3 to 5 palmate leaves. Leaflets thin, finely serrate. Flowers greenish yellow in umbells. Fruit globular or reniform drupe, scarlet, 2-seeded.
Cultivated in Himalayan regions in India.
Trade name: Ginseng.
Propagation: By seeds, by root cuttings and grafting.

Uses: Root and leaf are used to treat diabets mellitus.
Active constituents: Ginsenosides RB–2, Panaxans a-h, q-u (A, H,ip) daucosterol, nicotinic acid (A, H po), adenosine, pyroglutamic acid.

**Pandanus fascicularis** Lam.

Syn: *Pandanus odoratissimus* L.f.
*Pandanus tectorius* auct.

Family: Pandanaceae.

A much branched shrub or tree, stem supported by prop roots. Leaves linear-ensiform, armed with prickles on margins and dorsal midrib. Flowers unisexual, male flowers white in axillary spikes, female in a solitary terminal cephalium. Fruit an oblong syncarpium.

Occasional in marshy localities.

Fl. & Fr.: July–December.

Sanskrit: Ketaki.

Local names: *Ben*: Keya, Kadki-keya, Keori; *Guj*: Kewoda; *Hin*: Keura, Kewda, Ketki, Gagandhul; *Kan*: Tale mara, Kyad-agegida; *Mal*: Kaida, Yhala; *Mar*: Keora; *Tam*: Tazhai, Thalay; *Tel*: Mogali, Ketaki.

Trade name: Fragrant screw pine.

Propagation: By offsets or suckers.

Uses: Root useful in the treatment of diabetes.

**Pandanus furcatus** Roxb.

Family: Pandanaceae.

Small gregarious tree, up to 9m tall. Leaves linear, up to 4.5m long, short stout spines on the margins and midrib. Flowers in cylindric spikes enclosed by golden yellow spathe. Fruit orange-red.

In Bengal, Assam, Konkan and North Kanara.

Uses: Aerial parts and fruits used to treat diabetes.

**Papaver somniferum** L.

Family: Papaveraceae.

Annual erect herb, 30–150 cm tall, latex milky. Leaves entire, glabrous. Flowers solitary, violet-white or red. Fruit round capsule with numerous white seeds.

Rarely cultivated. The cultivation and extraction and sale of opium is banned.

Sanskrit: Ahiphenam, Aphukam.

Local names: *Ben*: Pasto; *Guj*: Aphina, Khuskhus, Posta; *Hin*: Afim, Afyun, Kashkash, Post; *Kan*: Afim, Biligasgase, Khasakhasi; *Mal*: Afiun, Kashakhasa; *Mar*: Aphu, Khuskhus, Posta; *Tam*: Abini, Gashagasha, Kasa kasa, Postaka; *Tel*: Nallamandu (Narcotic), Gasagasalu (seeds).

Trade name: Opium poppy, white poppy.

Uses: Plant useful in the treatment of diabetes.

Active constituents: Alkaloids.

**Parthenium hysterophorus** L.

Family: Asteraceae.

Annual erect herb, up to 1.5m tall. Leaves pinnatifid, pinnules oblong-lanceolate. Flowers white in terminal heads. Fruit achene.

Abundant all over India in Wastelands and road sides.

Fl. & Fr.: Throughout the year.

Uses: Plant useful in the treatment of diabetes.

**Passiflora incarnata** L.

Family: Passifloraceae

Large climber, stems wiry. Leaves 3-lobed, serrate. Flowers pale pink. Fruit ovoid or globose.

Native of South-East USA, now grown frequently in gardens.

Trade name: Maypop.

Propagation: by seed or by layering.

Uses: Plant useful in the treatment of diabetes.

**Pentanema indicum** (L.) Ling

Syn: *Inula indica* L.
*Vicoa auriculata* Cass.
*Vicoa indica* (L.) DC.

Family: Asteraceae (Compositae).

Annual erect herb, up to 1m tall, stem reddish, terete. Leaves sessile, oblong lanceolate. Flowers yellow in terminal heterogamous heads. Fruit achene, terete.

Throughout India in drier parts.

Fl & Fr: September–December.

Local names: *Guj*: Sona Sali; *Kan*: Mugutisoppu, Hannavarikasoppu.

Uses: Whole plant useful in the treatment of diabetes.

**Perilla frutescens** (L.) Britton

Syn: *Perilla ocimoides* L.

Family: Lamiaceae (Labiatae)

Aromatic, bushy annual herb, up to 1.5m tall. Leaves broadly ovate. Flowers small, white, in axillary and terminal racemes. Fruit nutlets.

Found throughout Himalayas.

Local names: *Ben*: Ban tulsi; *Hin*: Bhanjira.

Uses: Whole plant used for treating diabetes.

**Persea americana** Mill.

Syn: *Persea gratissima* Gaertn.f.

Family: Lauraceae.

Large tree, up to 18m tall. Leaves oblong or elliptic–lanceolate. Flowers small, greenish in compact panicles. Fruit baccate.

Trade name: Avocado, Alligator pear, butter fruit.

Uses: Plant used in the treatment of diabetes.

**Petroselenium crispum** (Mill.) Airy–Shaw

Syn: *Petroselenium sativum* Hoffm.
*Petroselenium hortense* Hoffm.
*Apium crispum* Mill.

Family: Apiaceae (Umbelliferae).

Aromatic biennial herb. Leaves 2-or 3-pinnate, ultimate segments cuneate-ovate or sometimes linear–oblong, upper cauline leaves ternate. Flowers yellow or yellowish green in compound umbels. Fruit ridged.

Cultivated in high ranges.

Trade name: Parsley.

Uses: Aerial parts used to treat Diabetes mellitus.

**Peucedanum dhana** Buch.-Ham. ex C.B. Clarke

Family: Apiaceae (Umbelliferae).

Perennial herb. Flowers yellow.

Found in Maharastra, Bihar Orissa and Andhra Pradesh.

Uses: Aerial parts are used in treatment of Diabetes mellitus.

**Phaseolus coccineus** L.

Syn: *Phaseolus multiflorus* Lam.

Family: Fabaceae (Papilionaceae).

Perennial with tuberous roots. Leaves trifoliolate. Flowers large, bright red or occasionally white. Fruit pod, slightly curved.

Cultivated for its edible pods.

Trade name: Multiflora bean, scarlet runner bean.

Uses: Plant used in the treatment of diabetes

Active constituent: Glucokinin.

**Phaseolus vulgaris** L.

Syn: *Phaseolus nanus* L.

Family: Fabaceae (Papilionaceae).

Annual twining or suberect herbs. Leaves trifoliolate. Flowers white to violet-purple. Fruit pod, straight or slightly curved.

Cultivated for the fruit vegetable.

Local names: *Hin*: Bakla, Lobia, Rajmah; *Guj*: Phanasi; *Kan*: Tingalavari; *Mar*: Shravan ghevda; *Tel*: Chikkudu.

Trade name: French bean, Kidney bean.

Propagation: by seeds.

Uses: Beans are found to be more effective in reducing plasma glucose levels. It is advised to take overnight soaked fresh or cooked beans.

**Phoenix dactylifera** L.

Family: Arecaceae (Palmae).

Tall palm, up to 36m tall, trunk covered with persistent bases of petioles. Leaves pinnate, lower pinnae modified into spines. Flowers in branched spadices, unisexual, small. Fruit an oblong berry, reddish brown when ripe, seed cylindric, hard, with a longitudinal furrow.

Cultivated occasionally.

Sanskrit: Kharjurah.

Local names: *Ben*, *Guj*, *Hin* & *Mar*: Kharjur; *Kan*: Kharjura; *Mal*: Ittappazham; *Ori*: Khorjjuri; *Tam*: Perichchankay; *Tel*: Kharjuramu.

Trade name: Date palm.

Propagation: By seeds.

Uses: Plant useful in the treatment of diabetes.

**Phragmites communis** Trin.

Family: Poaceae.

Coarse reed, with thick creeping rhizome, stems erect, up to 3m tall, stout, hollow. Leaves linear-lanceolate. Inflorescence panicle, purple-brown. Fruit oblong.

Himalayas from Kashmir to Kumaon in marshes and on the banks of lakes and streams.

Trade name: Common reed.

Uses: Rhizomes and roots are used in diabetes.

**Phyllanthus amarus** Schum. & Thonn.

Syn: *Phyllanthus niruri* auct. non L.

Family: Euphorbiaceae.

Annual erect herb, up to 50 cm tall, branchlets slender. Leaves elliptic-obovate or oblong. Flowers axillary, unisexual, male flowers solitary in lower axils. Fruit capsule, depressed globose.

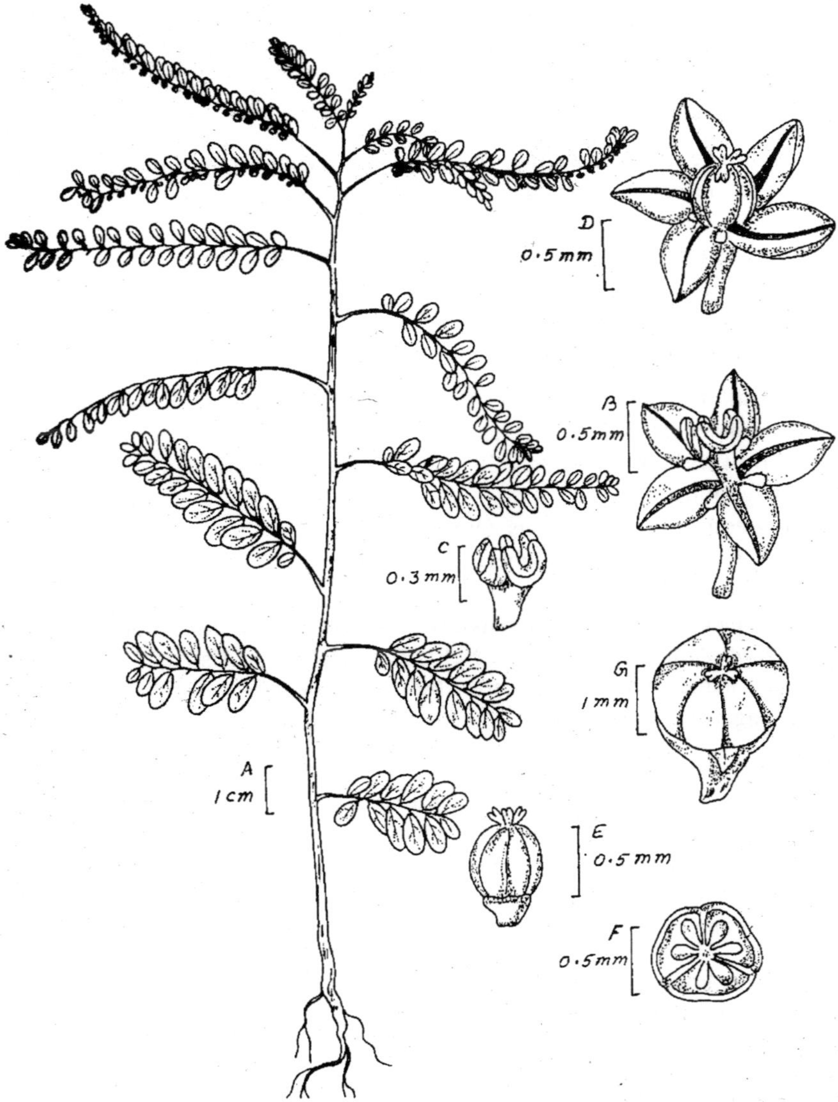


Fig. 68: *Phyllanthus amarus* Schum. & Thonn.
A. Twig; B. Male flower; C. Androecium; D. Female flower; E. Pistil; F. Ovary T.s.; G. Capsule.

Common weed of open waste lands and in cultvated fields.
Fl.& Fr.: Through out the year.
Sanskrit: Bahupatra.
Local names: *Ben*: Bhuiamla, Sadnazur-mani; *Guj*: Bhony ammali; *Hin*: Jaramal, Jangli amli, Bhuinanvalah, Bhonyabali; *Kan*: Nela nelli, Keranelli gida; *Mal*: Kiha nelli; *Mar*: Bhuivali; *Ori*: Bhui aola, Badiaonla; *Tam*: Keera nelli; *Tel*: Nela usiri.
Trade name: Bhuiamla, Kirinelli.
Propagation: By seeds.

Uses: The aqueous extract of leaves has hypoglycemic activity which appears to be higher than than that of tolbutamide.

**Phyllanthus emblica** L.

Syn: *Emblica officinalis* Gaertn.

Family: Euphorbiaceae.

A small deciduous tree, up to 10m tall, branchlets terete. Leaves oblong. Flowers unisexual, in axillary fascicles, male flowers many in upper axils, female flowers few in lower axils. Fruit drupe, depressed globose, fleshy, seeds trigonous.
Common in dry deciduous forests.
Fl. & Fr.: October–December.
Sanskrit: Amlaki.
Local names: *Ben*: Amla, Amlaki; *Guj*: Amali, Ambala; *Hin*: Amla, Amlika, Aohla; *Kan*: Amalaka nelli; *Mal*: Nelli; *Tam*: Nelli; *Tel*: Usiri.
Trade name: Indian gooseberry, Indian mylobalan.
Propagation: by seeds.

Uses: Fruits useful in the treatment of diabetes.Indian gooseberry, with its high vitamin C content, is considered valuable in diabetes. A table spoon of its juice, mixed with a cup of bitter gourd juice taken daily for two months, will stimulate the iselets Langerhans, that is, the isolated group of cells that secrete the hormone insulin in the pancreas. The mixture reduces the blood sugar in diabetes.

**Phyllanthus lawii** Graham ex Muell.–Arg.

Family: Euphorbiaceae

Shrub, up to 1.5m tall. Leaves elliptic–oblong. Flowers axillary, male flowers solitary or few, female flowers solitary. Fruit globose capsule.
Found in Bihar, Orissa, West Bengal and Deccan peninsula.
Local names: *Mal*: Kuruttu nelliuri, *Mar*: Kati, Khad sherni; *Tam*: Vattunelli.

Uses: Aerial parts used in the treatment of diabetes.

**Physalis peruviana** L.

Family: Solanaceae.

Perennial herb, up to 1.5m tall. Leaves alternate, ovate. Flowers yellow. Fruit berry, orange–yellow, overtopped by inflated calyx.

Introduced, grown in U.P., Punjab and Rajasthan.

Fl. & Fr.: Round the year.

Local names: *Ben*: Tipariya; *Guj*: Moti popti; *Hin*: Tipari; *Kan*: Gudde hannu; *Mar*: Phopti.

Trade name: Cape goose berry.

Uses: Whole plant useful in the treatment of diabetes.

**Pimenta officinalis** Lindl.

Syn: *Pimenta dioica* (L.) Merr.

Family: Myrtaceae.

Bushy ever green tree, up to 9m tall. Leaves oblong to oblong-lanceolate, coriaceous. Flowers white, in terminal and axillary trichotomous paniculate cymes. Fruit globose berry, black or purple when ripe, seeds deep brown.

Grown in gardens.

Trade name: All spice tree, Jamaica pepper tree, Pimento tree.

Propagation: By seeds.

Uses: Plant useful in the treatment of diabetes.

**Pinus roxburghii** Sargent

Syn: *Pinus longifolia* Roxb.

Family: Coniferae.

Tall tree. Needles are in bundles of three, 25–30cm long. Male cones small, female cones 10–20cm long, conical.

Found in the lower Himalayas and other hills. It is commonly planted for ornament.

Local names: *Ass*: Tellia; *Ben*: Saralagach; *Hin*: Chir; *Pun*: Chil; *Tam*: Simaidevadari.

Propagation: By seeds.

Uses: Leaves, roots and stem bark useful in the treatment of diabetes.

**Piper cubeba** L.f.

Family: Piperaceae.

Liana–like climber, rooted at the joints. Leaves ovate, oblong, gland–dotted. Flowers unisexual in smooth scaly spikes, female spikes often curved. Fruit subglobose berries.

Cultivated in Karnataka.

Sanskrit: Kankolam

Local names: *Ben* & *Hin*: Kabab chini; *Guj*: Kalabchim, Tadmiri; *Kan*: Bala menasu; *Mal*: Val-milaku; *Tam*: Valmilagu; *Tel*: Chalavamiriyalu, Tokamiriyalu.

Trade name: Cubebs, Tailed pepper, Tailed cubebs, Java pepper.

Uses: Plant useful in the treatment of diabetes.

**Piper longum** L.

Family: Piperaceae.

Slender, aromatic, dioecious, root climbers. Leaves simple, alternate, ovate to oblong, deeply cordate. Flowers minute on axillary spikes, green at first, turning yellow later, unisexual. Fruit berry, red when ripe, and partially sunk in the fleshy axis of the spike.

In the Evergreen forests of Western Ghats as forest undergrowth. Cultivated in Assam and Kerala.

Sanskrit: Pippali, Magadh.

Local names: *Ben*: Piplamor, *Guj*: Pipli; *Hin*: Pipli, Piplamul; *Kan*: Hipli; *Mal*: Tippali; *Mar*: Pimpli; *Tam*: Tippali, Pippili; *Tel*: Pippallu..

Trade name: Long pepper, Pipali.

Propagation: Crop is raised from 3–5-noded rooted stem cuttings planted in nursery beds during early rainy season. It prefers rich, fertile, well drained, acidic organic soils going up to 1000m elevation. It demands long, humid conditions in high rainfall areas (160–200 cm) and prefers partially shady locations. The planted stems establish rooting in a fortnight and rooted plants are ready for field planting in next 2 months. The rooted plants are firmly fixed in soil during monsoon rains. The crop demands heavy nitrogenous fertilizers. Besides organic manure and mulch are applied to the crop twice during second and third year. A dose of N,P and K of 80, 60 and 30 kg/ha produces optimum yield. Weeding and hoeing are given regularly in early summer season. Weekly irrigation is recommended durinmg dry summer. The vines come to bearing in 6 months after planting (January onwards). The spikes are ready for picking after 2 months. An irrigated crop produces 400 kg/ha of dry spikes in the first year and up to 1–1.3 tonnes/ha the third year.

Uses: The ethanolic extract of the plant is useful in the treatment of diabetes.

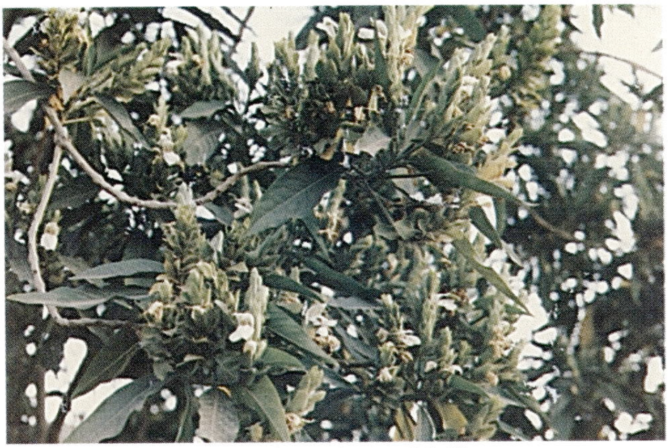

*Adhatoda zeylanica* Medik.

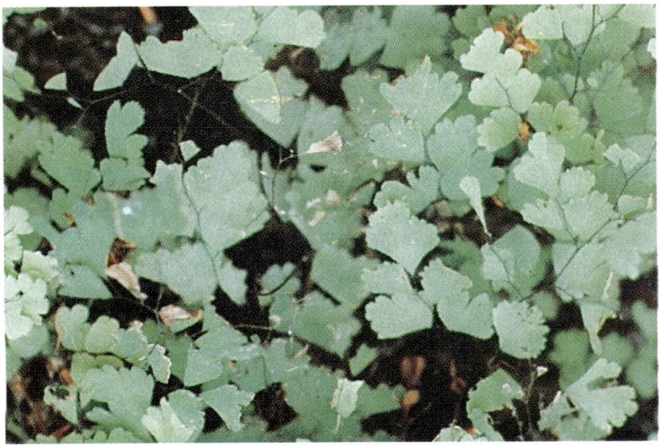

*Adiantum capillus-veneris* L.

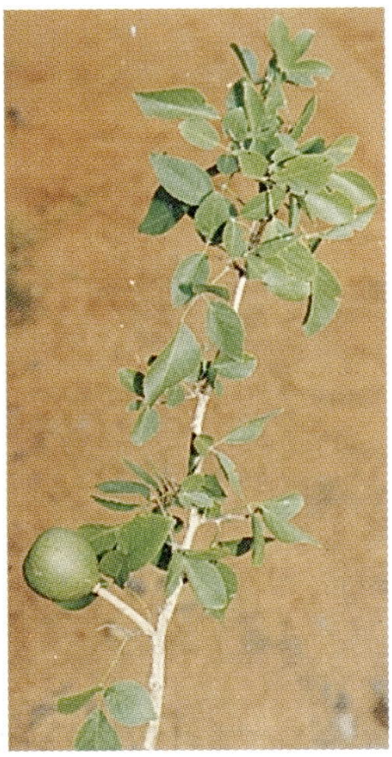

*Aegle marmelos* (L.) Correa

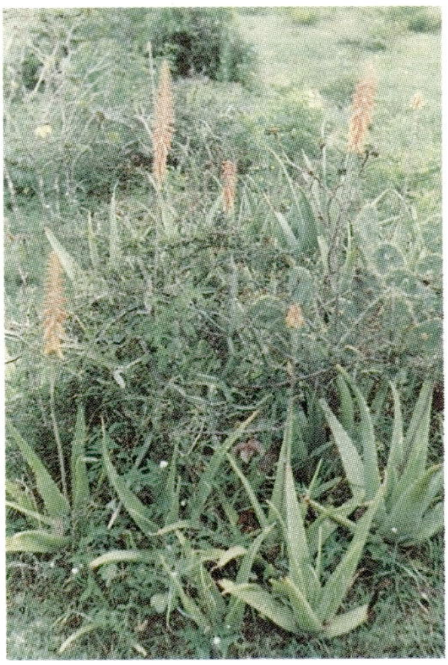

*Aloe vera* (L.) Burm.f.

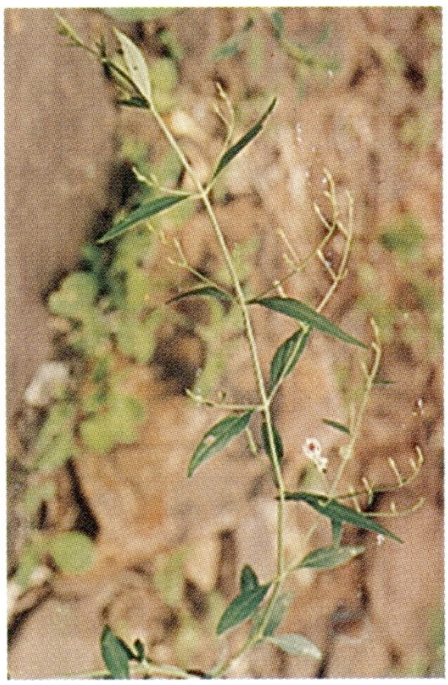

*Andrographis paniculata* (Burm.f.) Nees

**PLATE I**

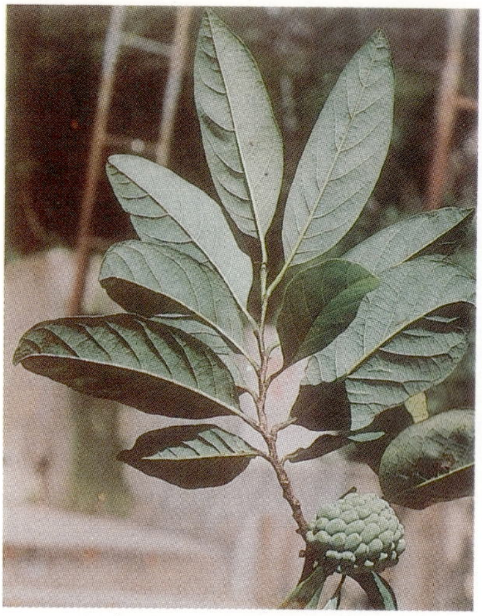

*Annona squamosa* L.

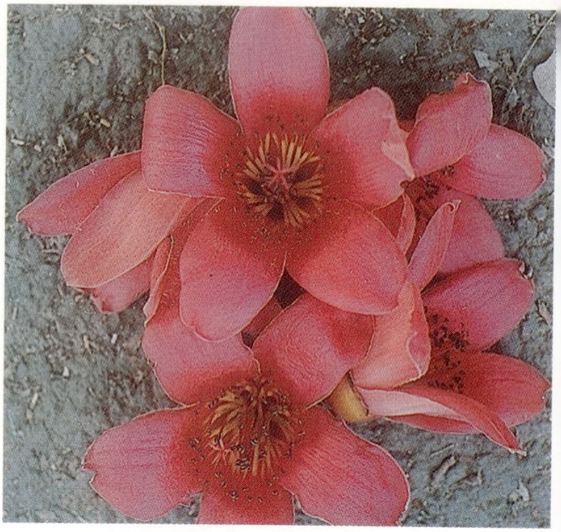

*Bombax ceiba* L.

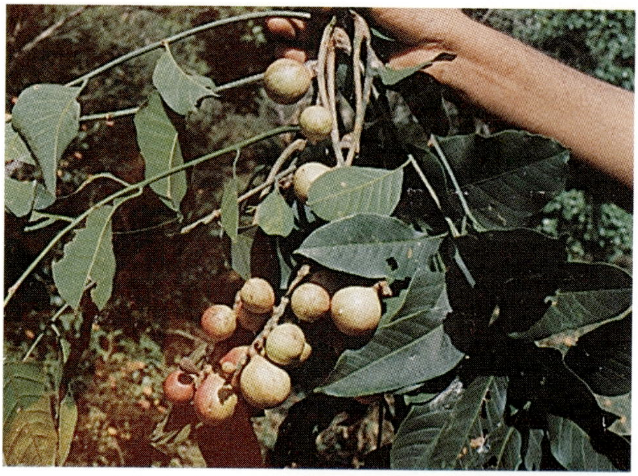

*Aphanamixis polystachya* (Wall.) Parker

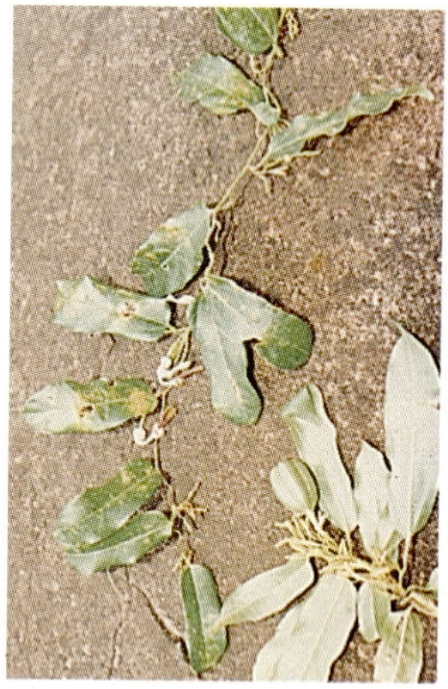

*Aristolochia indica* L.

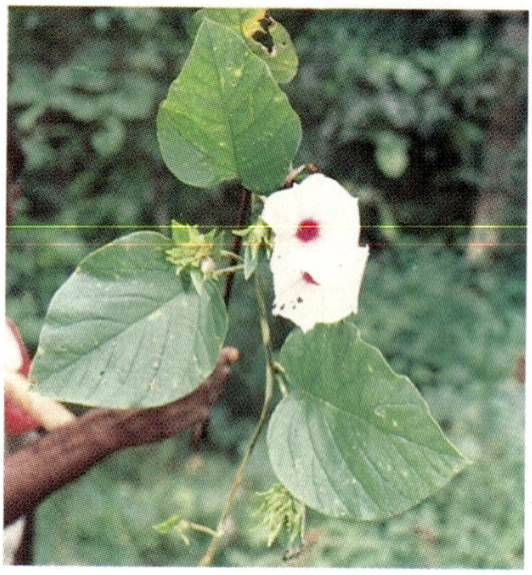

*Argyreia nervosa* (Burm.f.) Bojer

**PLATE II**

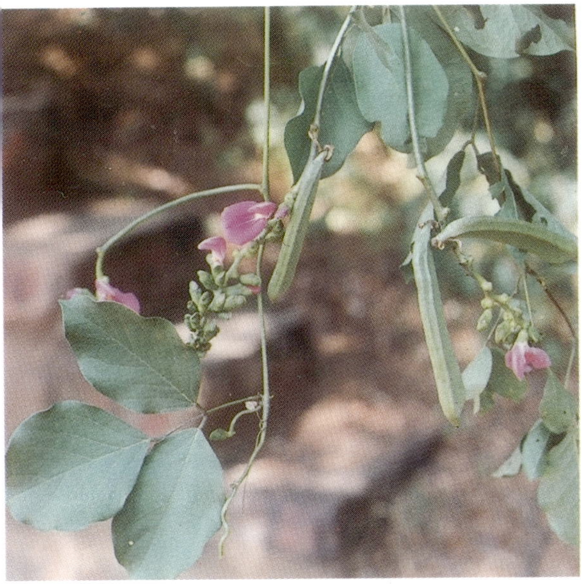

*Canavalia gladiata* (Jacq.) DC.

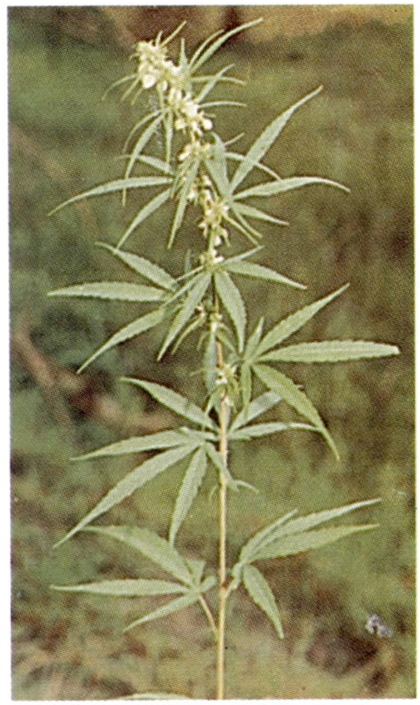

*Cannabis sativa* L.

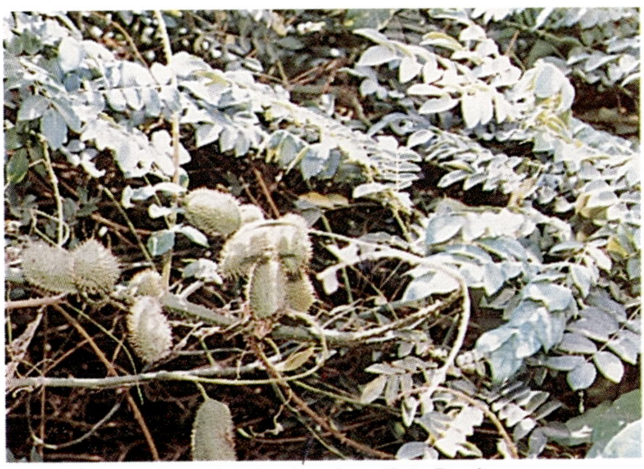

*Caesalpinia bonduc* (L.) Roxb.

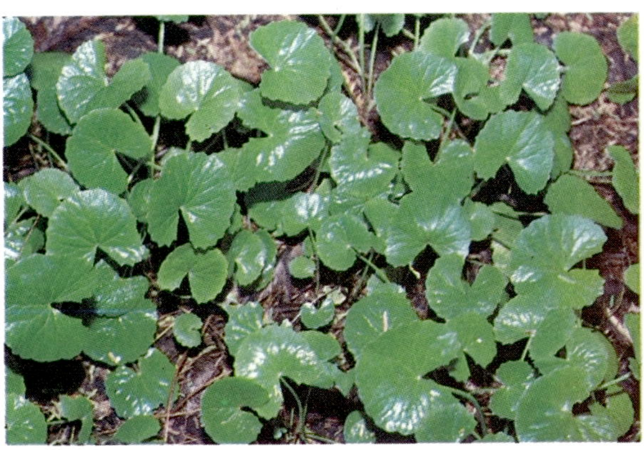

*Centella asiatica* (L.) Urban

**PLATE III**

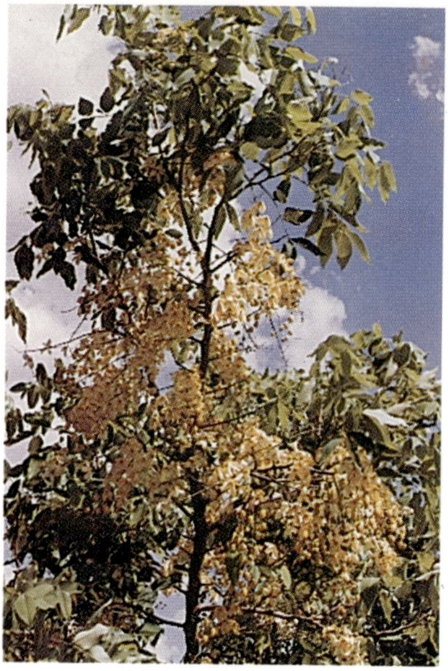

*Cassia fistula* L.

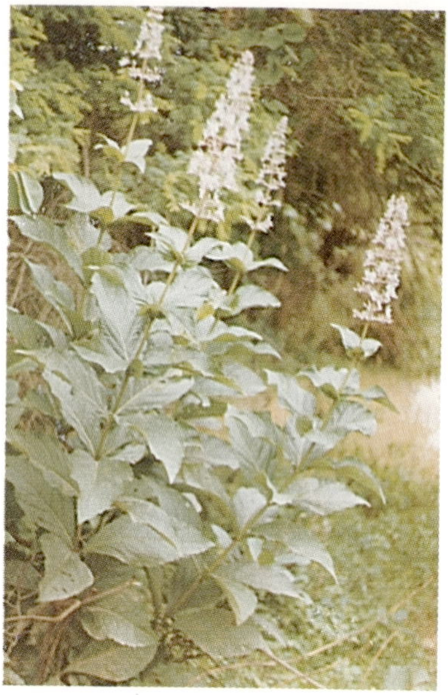

*Clerodendum serratum* (L.) Moon

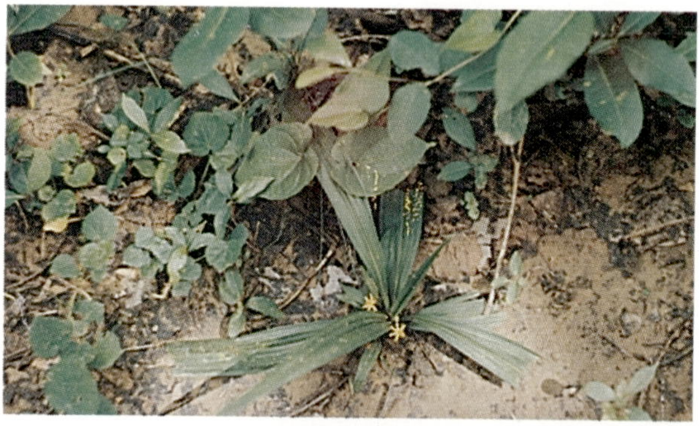

*Curculigo orchioides* Gaertn.

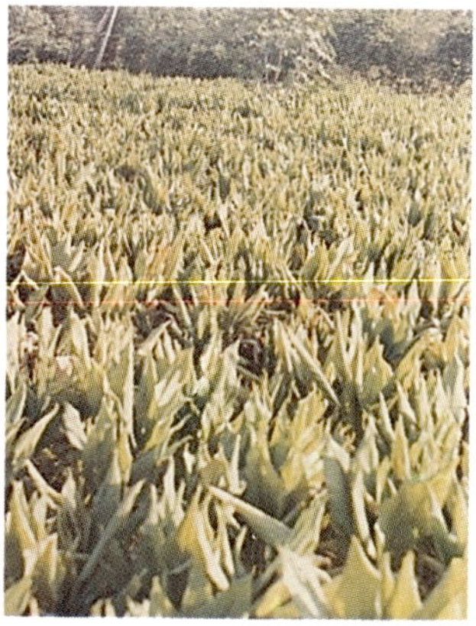

*Curcuma longa* L.

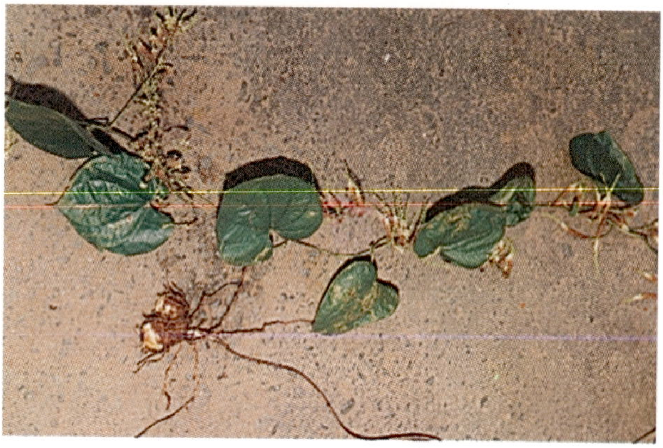

*Dioscorea bulbifera* L.

**PLATE IV**

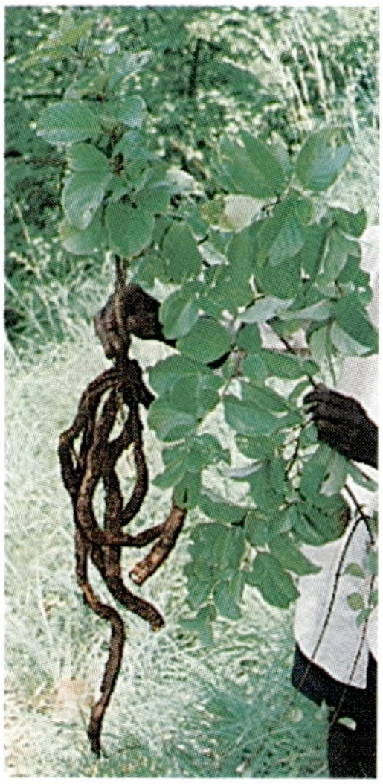

*Decalepis hamiltonii* Wt. & Arn.

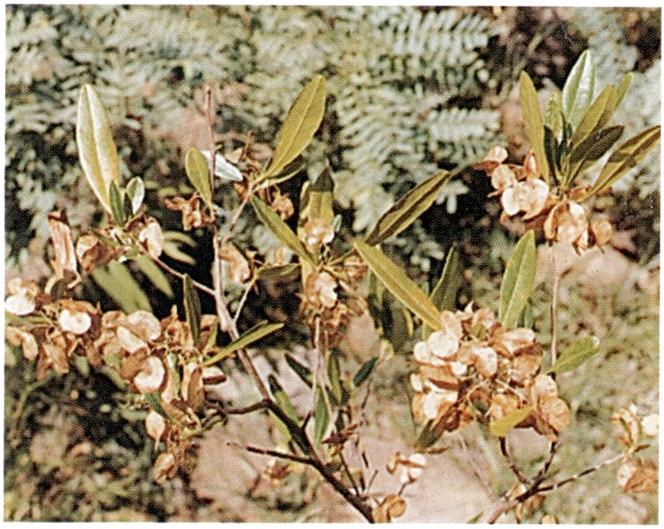

*Dodonea viscosa* (L.) Jacq.

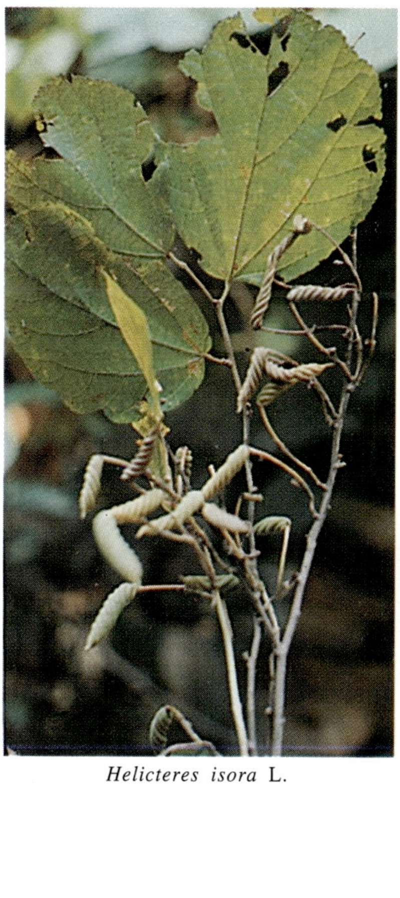

*Helicteres isora* L.

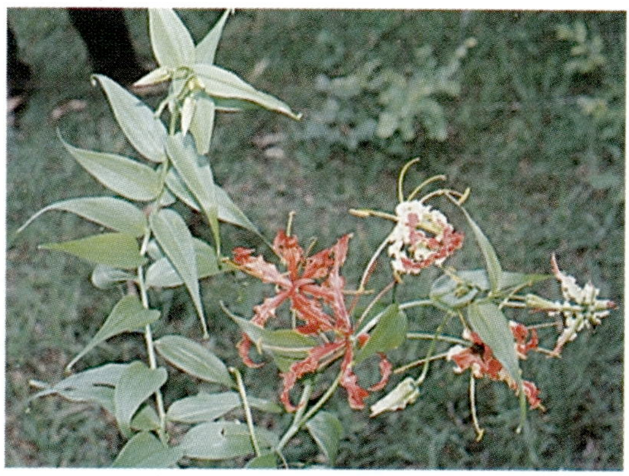

*Gloriosa superba* L.

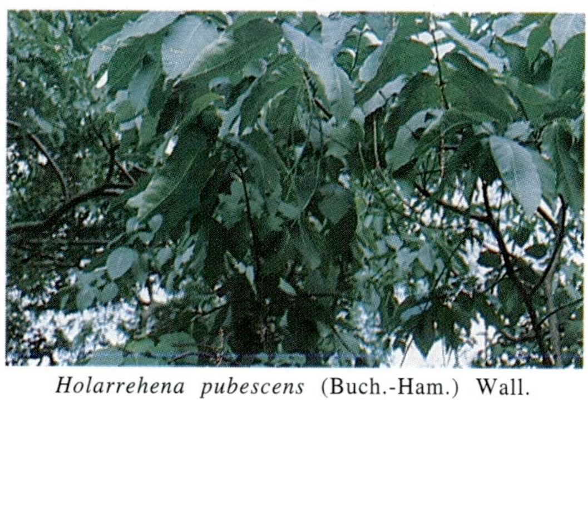

*Holarrehena pubescens* (Buch.-Ham.) Wall.

**PLATE V**

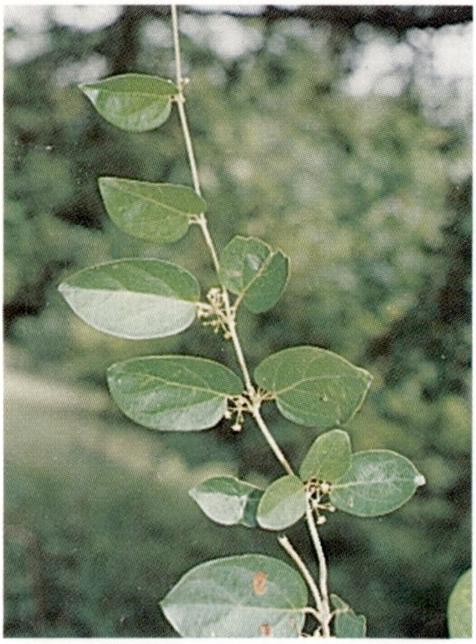

*Gymnema sylvestre* (Retz.) R.Br. ex. Schult.

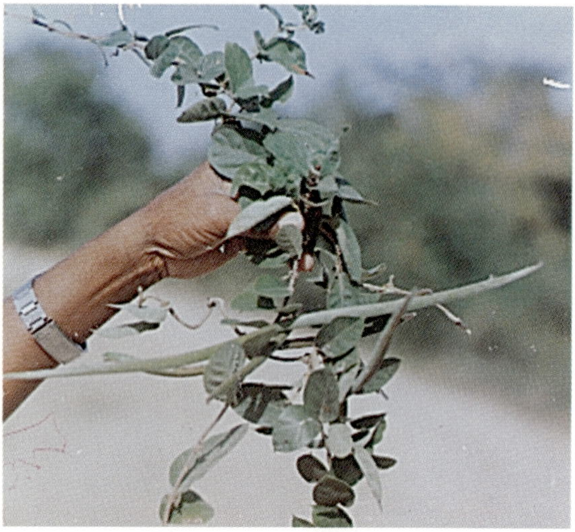

*Holostemma ada-kodien* Schult.

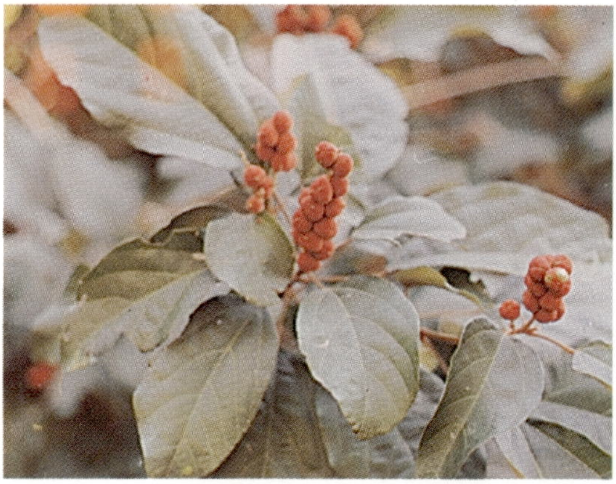

*Mallotus philippensis* (Lam.) Muell-Arg.

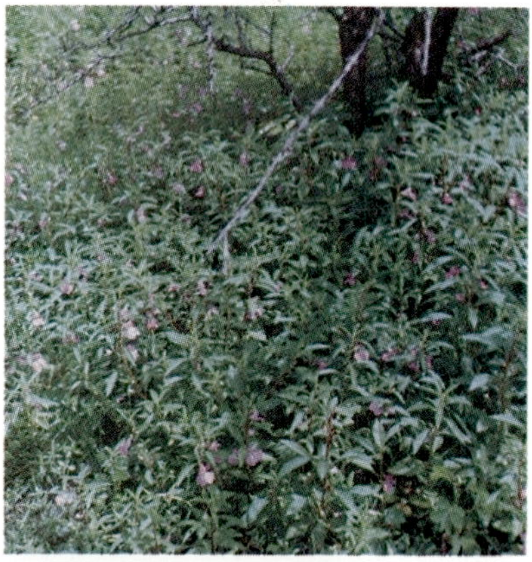

*Impatiens balsamina* (L.) Ait.

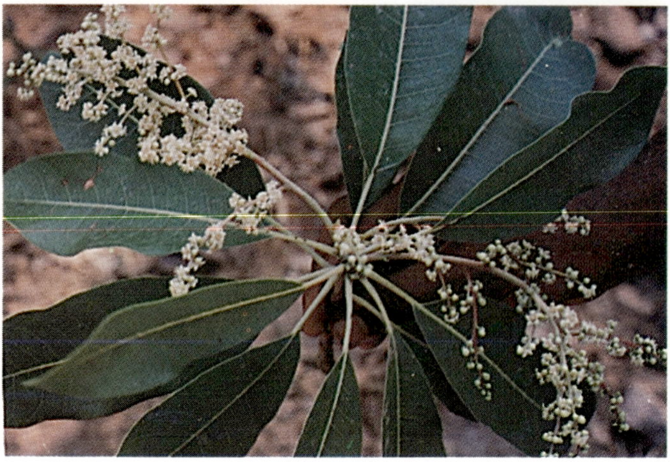

*Mangifera indica* L.

**PLATE VI**

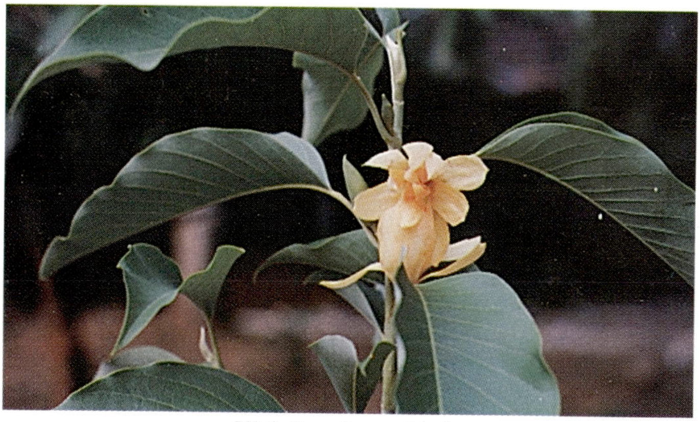

*Michelia champaka* L.

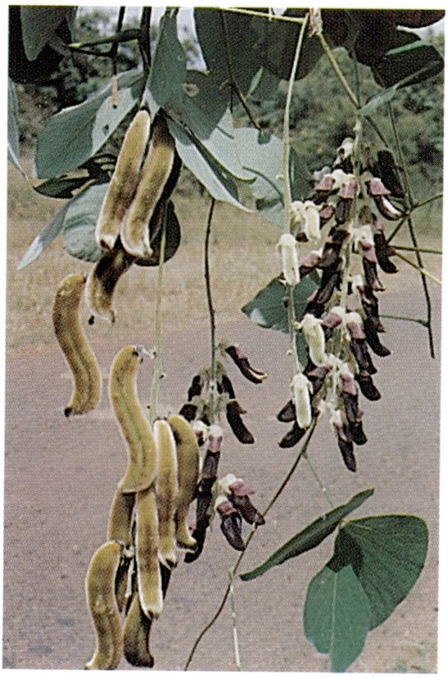

*Mucuna pruriens* (L.) DC.

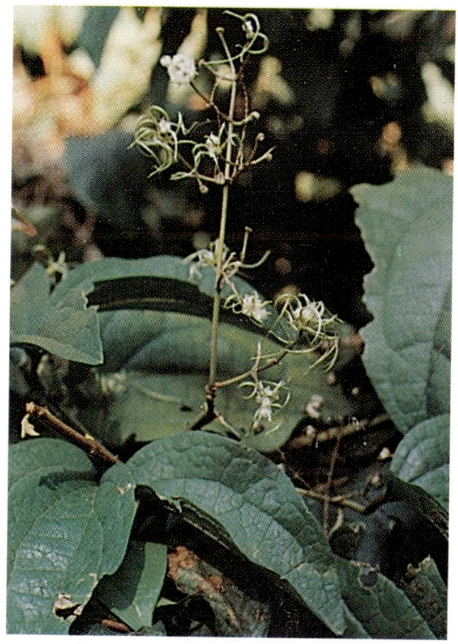

*Naravelia zeylanica* (L.) DC.

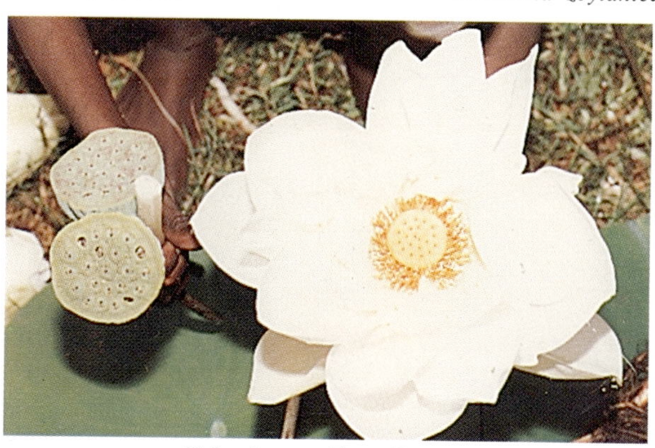

*Nelumbo nucifera* Gaertn.

**PLATE VII**

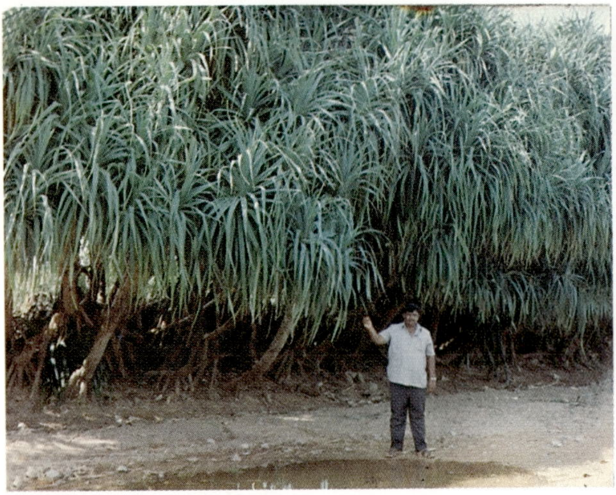

*Pandanus fascicularis* Lam.

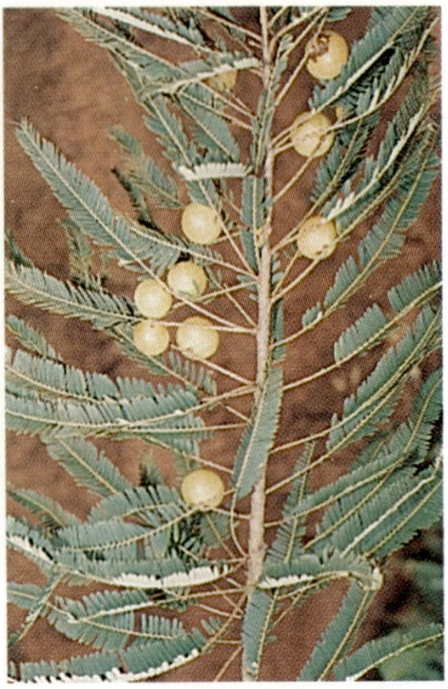

*Phyllanthus emblica* L.

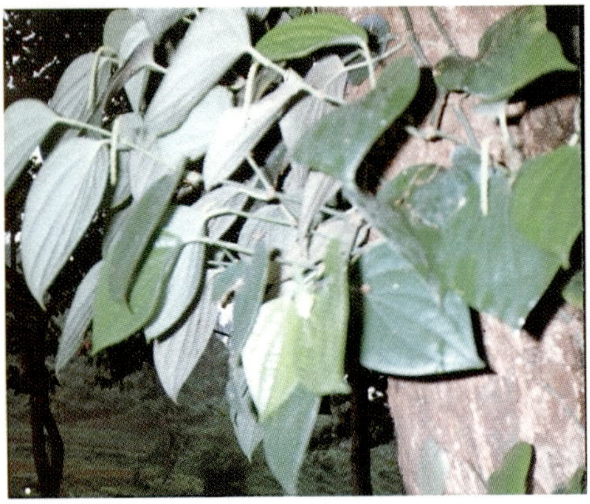

*Piper nigrum* L.

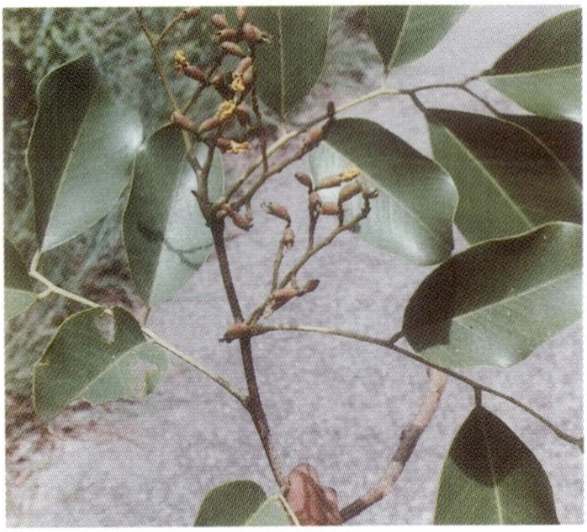

*Pterocarpus marsupium* Roxb.

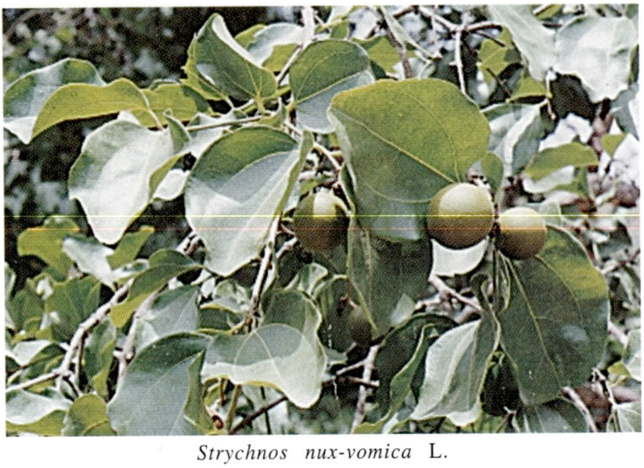

*Strychnos nux-vomica* L.

**PLATE VIII**

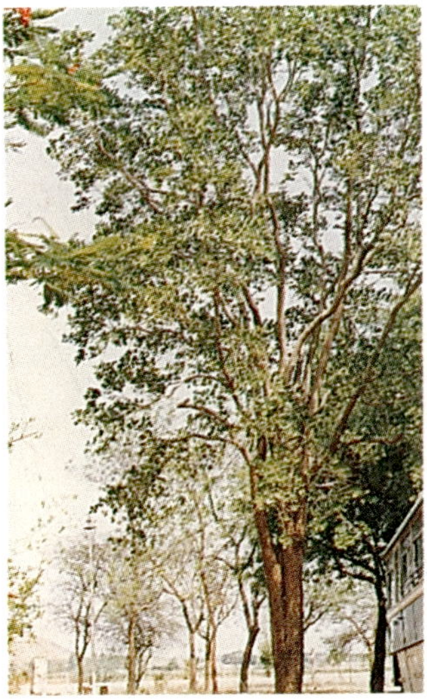

*Pterocarpus santalinus* L.f.

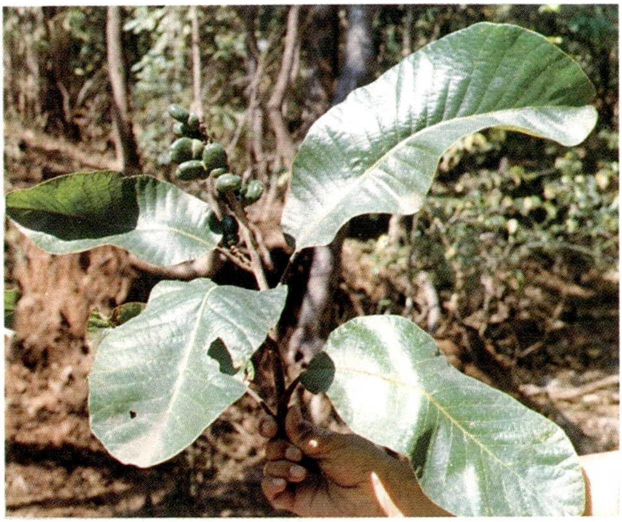

*Semecarpus anacardium* L.f.

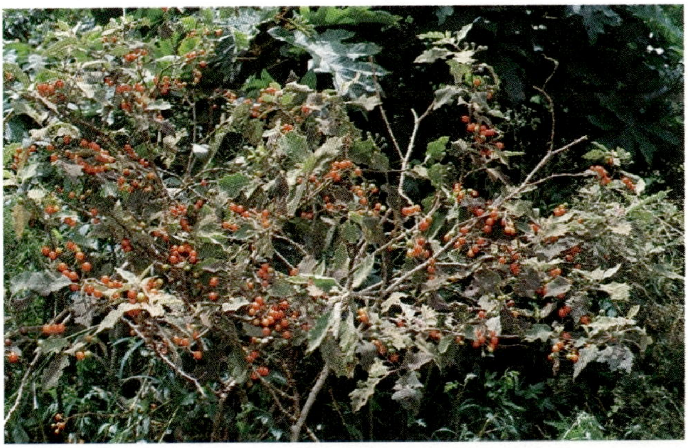

*Solanum anguivi* Lam.

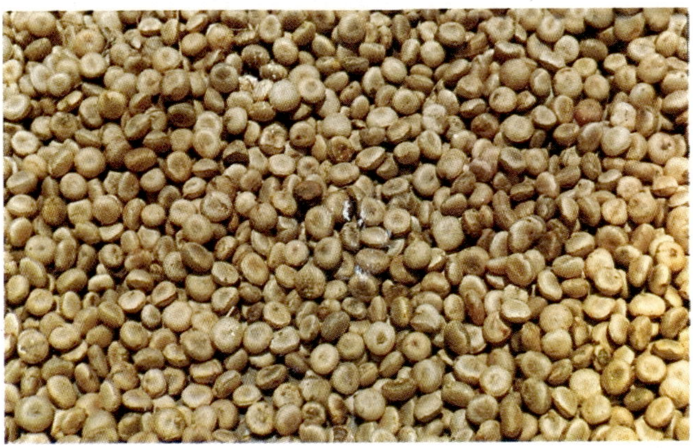

*Strychnos potatorum* L.f. (Seeds)

**PLATE IX**

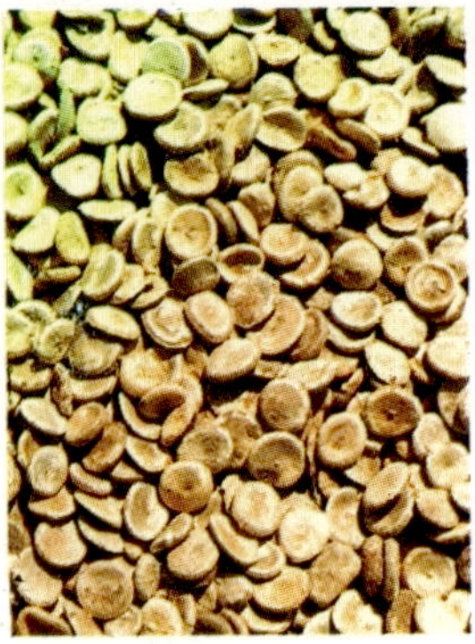

*Strychnos nux-vomica* L (Seeds)

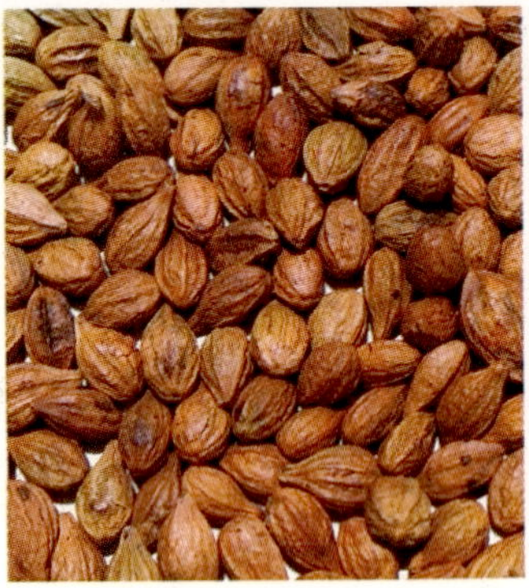

*Terminalia chebula* Retz. (Fruits)

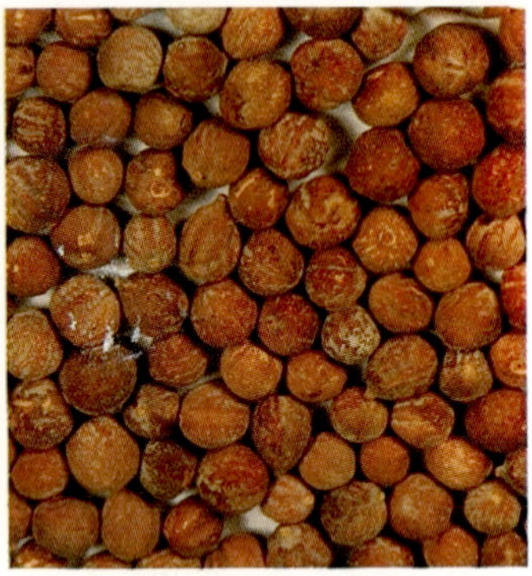

*Terminalia bellerica* (Gaertn.) Roxb. (Fruits)

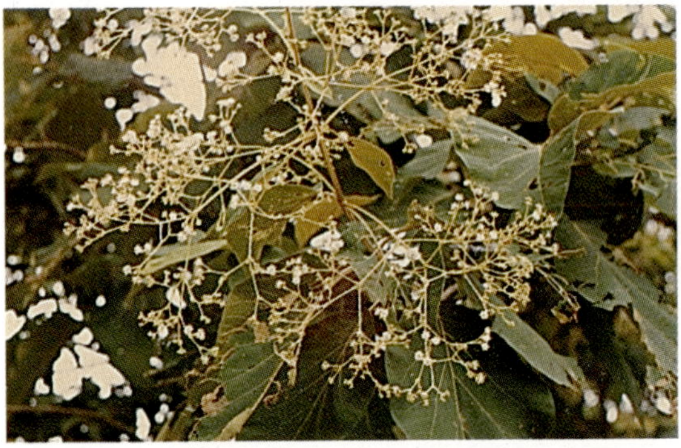

*Tectona grandis* L.f

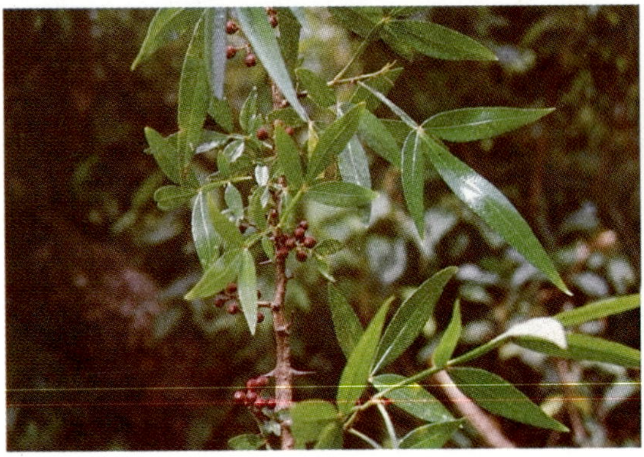

*Zanthoxylum armatum* DC.

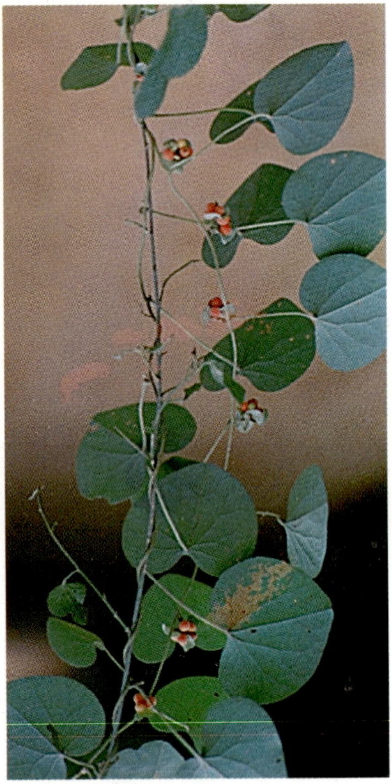

*Tinospora cordifolia* (Willd.) Hook.f. & Thoms.

**PLATE X**

**Piper nigrum** L.

Family: Piperaceae.

A stout, glabrous climber, stems terete. Leaves broadly ovate. Flowers bisexual in axillary spikes. Fruit black when mature.

Mostly found cultivated in the hot and moist parts of India.

Fl. & Fr.: June–April.

Sanskrit: Maricha.

Local names: *Ben* & *Hin*: Kali-mirch, Kalamorich, Golmirch; *Guj*: Kalamari, Kalomirich; *Kan*: Menasu, Ollemenasu; *Mal*: Kurumulaka, Vallijam; *Mar*: Mire, Kalimirch; *Tam*: Milagu, Cevviyam; *Tel*: Miriyalu.

Trade name: Black pepper, common pepper.

Propagation: Stem cuttings.

Uses: Plant useful in the treatment of diabetes.

Active Principle: N-trans-feruloyl piperidine, Feruperine, Dihydroferuperine isoloated from fruits.

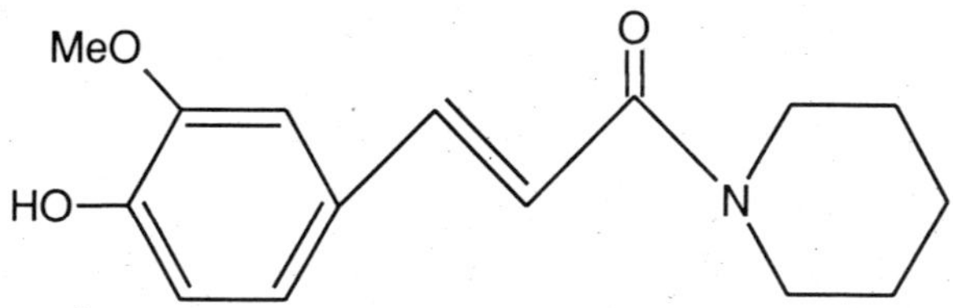


N-trans-Feruloylpiperidine

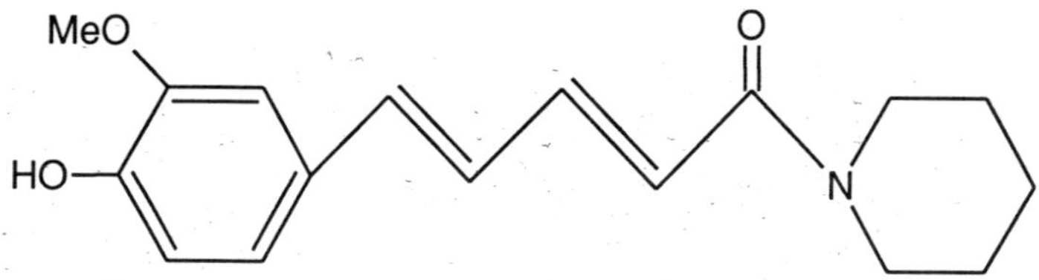


Feruperine

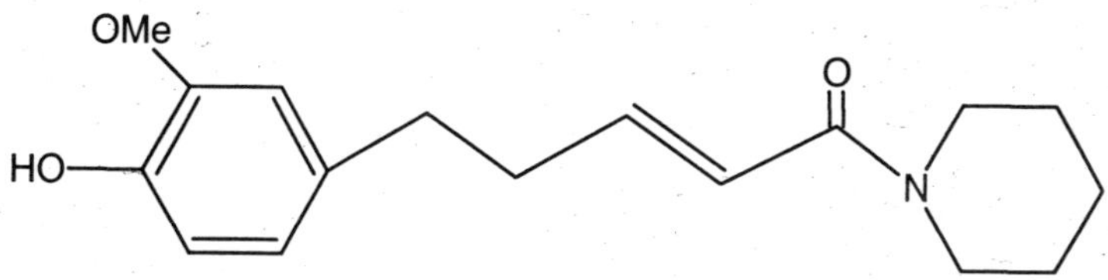


Dihydroferuperine

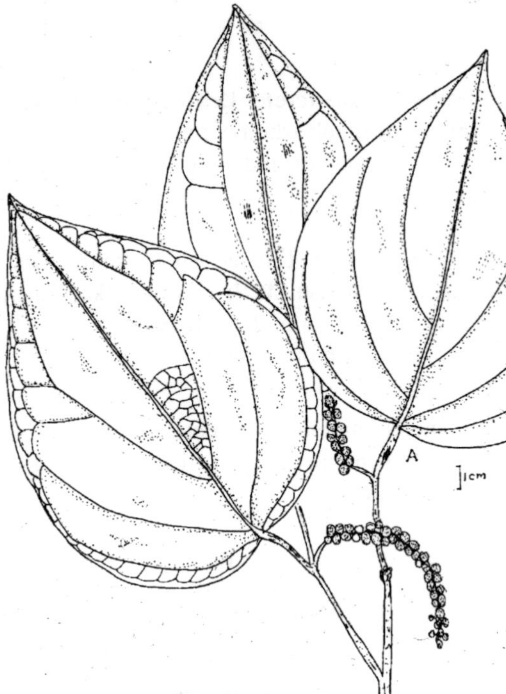


Fig. 69: *Piper nigrum* L.
A. Twig.

**Pistia stratiotes** L.

Family: Araceae.

A floating stemless, stoloniferous, aquatic herb, roots tufted. Leaves sessile, obovate-cuneate, tufted. Flowers minute on a spadix. Fruit ovoid to ellipsoid, crowned by persistent style.

Throughout India, one of the worst weed.

Local names: *Ben*: Takapana, *Hin*: Jalkhumbi, Takapana; *Guj*: Jalashamkhala; *Kan*: Antara gange; *Mal*: Akasa tamarai, Kudapayal; *Mar*: Prasni, Gondala, Jalamandvi; *Ori*: Borajhanji; *Tam*: Akasa tamarai, Koditamarai; *Tel*: Anthara thamara.

Trade name: Tropical duck weed, water lettuce.

Uses: Plant useful in the treatment of diabetes.

•

**Pisum sativum** L.

Family: Fabaceae (Papilionaceae)

Annual, herbaceous tendrillar climber, stems hollow. Leaves pinnately compound with auricled stipules. Flowers white, bluish or purple coloured. Fruit pod, straight or curved, 6–9-seeded.

Cultivated at higher elevations.

Sanskrit: Kalayah.

Local names: *Ben* & *Hin*: Matar; *Guj* & *Mar*: Watani; *Kan*: Batani, *Mal*: Pathanikatala, Pattanippayar; Malankatala; *Tam*: Pattani, Vellaippattani; *Tel*: Batani.

Propagation: By seeds.

Uses: Plant useful in the treatment of diabetes.

**Pithecellobium monadelphum** Kosterm.

Syn: *Pithecellobium bigeminum* auct non Mart.
*Pithecellobium gracile* Bedd.

Family: Mimosaceae.

Small to medium sized tree. Leaves bipinnate, pinnae 1–2 pairs, pinnules elliptic-lanceolate or ovate–oblong. Flowers yellowish white in heads. Fruit pod, flat, twisted.

Found in Eastern Himalayas and Western Ghats.

Local names: *Hin*: Kachlora, *Kan*: Kodakonde; *Mal*: Muthakolappam; *Tam*: Kal pakku.

Uses: Aerial parts and seeds used in the treatment of diabetes.

**Pittosporum napaulense** (DC.) Rehder & Wilson

Syn: *Pittosporum floribundum* Wight & Arn.

Family: Pittosporaceae.

Small tree, up to 10m tall. Leaves apically clustered, lanceolate. Flowers white to cream in much branched terminal corymbs. Fruit globose capsule.

Found in the hills of Peninsular India, and along the foot of outer Himalayas from Punjab eastwards to the hills of Assam.

Fl. & Fr.: May–August.

Local names: *Kan*: Tammata, *Mar*: Vehkali, Vikhari, Vehyenti, Yekaddi, Pisara; *Ori*: Debosundu, Devsan: *Tam*: Kattu sampangi, Nanjundai, Tammata; *Tel*: Rakamuki.

Uses: Aerial parts useful in the treatment of diabetes.

**Plantago ovata** Forssk.

Family: Plantaginaceae.

Softly hairy annual herb, stemless or nearly so. Leaves linear, in a rosette. Flowers minute, in oval or cylindric spikes. Fruit capsule, seeds are boat-shaped, dull white in colour.

Wild in Punjab plains but is largely cultivated elsewhere. India is the largest producer of Isabgol.

Local names: *Ben*: Isabgol, *Hin*: Isabgol; *Tam*: Ishapkol.

Trade name: Isabgol, Psyllium.

Propagation: Isabgol is predominantly grown as cold season crop over medium fertile well drained, loamy soil. It requires cool climate and dry sunny weather. The land should be well prepared to a fine tilth and laid out into small beds of convenient size (8×3m) to facilitate irrigation. It is preferably mixed with 15 cartloads of well-rotten farm yard manure per hectare during land preperation. The seed is sown in November to mid December. Seed (4Kg/ha) mixed with 10 times of sand or sieved farm yard manure should be sown in lines 30 cm apart. The seed should be treated with metalaxyl SD–35 (5g/kg) or mercuric chloride (3g/kg). The seed bed should be covered with thin film of soil by sweeping through by a broom. The seeds germinate 6–7 days after sowing. A light irrigation should be given to facilitate germination. The crop is weeded and hoed 20–25 days and 50–60 days after sowing. The crop needs irrigation at 30 and 70 days age. The basal application of 25–30 Kg each of N and P is sufficient for light and medium fertility sandy soils. The crop matures during March–April 110–130 days after sowing. The weather should be dry and sunny at harvesting. Yellowing of lower leaves is an indicator of maturity which is confirmed by pressing a drying spike between 2 fingers when the mature seeds come out easily. The plants are cut at the ground level after 10 AM, bundled and transported to thrashing shed. These are allowed to dry for 2–3 days and then thrashed with the help of bullocks or a tractor. Average grain yield varied between 800–1000Kg/ha.

Uses: Seeds useful in the treatment of diaetes.

**Plecospermum spinosum** Trecur.

Syn: *Tropis spinosa*

Family: Moraceae

Large thorny shrub or straggler or small tree. Leaves obovate or ovate-elliptic. Flowers unisexual, aggregated in groups of 1–3. Fruit syncarp.

Found in Eastern Himalayas and Deccan.

Local names: *Kan*: Bendaka; *Ori*: Banabana; *Tam*: Achingudi, Daiyal; *Tel*: Koriti, Kodiari.

Uses: Aerial parts useful in the treatment of diabetes.

**Plectranthus barbatus** Andr.

Syn: *Coleus barbatus* (Andr.) Benth.
*Coleus forskohlii* (Willd.) Briq.
*Plectranthus forskohlii* Willd.

Family: Lamiaceae (Labiatae).

Aromatic herb with thick fleshy root stock, stems ascending, slightly branched. Leaves ovate or obovate. Flowers bluish with red glands in spiciform racemes. Fruit nutlets, globose, brown.

Occasional on laterite and rocky soils in Uttar Pradesh, Bihar, Sikkim, Gujarat, Western Ghats and Andhra Peadesh Now extensively cultivated all over India.

Fl. & Fr.: August–March.

Sanskrit: Gandira.

Local names: *Hin*: Pashanabhedi, Pathatchur; *Kan*: Makkadi beru; *Mar*: Garmalu, Mainmul; *Tel*: Pashana bhedi.

Trade name: Coleus.

Uses: Roots contain Forskolin which is used for diabetes.

Active principle: Alkaloid Forskolin present in roots.

**Plumeria rubra** L.

Family: Apocynaceae.

Deciduous, profusely branched tree, up to 10m tall. Leaves broadly obovate-spathulate. Flowers cream with yellow centre. Fruit paired follicles, scarce.

Often planted in temples.

Fl.: April–June Fr.: Scarce.

Sanskrit: Ksirachampaka.

Local names: *Ben*: Dalan phul, Gorur champa; *Guj*: Rhada champo; *Hin*: Golainchi; *Kan*: Devaganigile, Kadu sampenge; *Mal*: Ezha-champakam, Arali; *Mar*: Khair champa, Sonchampa; *Ori*: Kart champa, Golochi, Torato; *Tam*: Arali, Kallimandhara; *Tel*: Devaganneru.

Trade name: Pogado tree.

Propagation: By stem cuttings.

Uses: Stem useful in the treatment of diabetes.

**Poa pratensis** L.

Family: Poaceae.

Perennial stoloniferous grass, up to 30cm tall. Leaves crowded at the base of the stem, linear. Spikelets in panicle, crowded.

In temperate and alpine zones of Himalayas.

Trade name: Smooth-stalked meadow grass, kentucky blue grass.

Uses: Whole plant useful in the treatment of diabetes.

**Polygonatum multiflorum** All.

Family: Liliaceae.

Perennial rhizomatous herb, up to 90cm tall. Rhizome horizontal with scars of annual stems. Leaves oblong-ovate. Flowers white in whorls. Fruit berry, blue black when ripe.

In Western Himalayas from Kashmir to Kumaon.
Trade name: Solomon's seal.

Uses: Plant useful in the treatment of diabetes.

**Polygonum aviculare** L.

Family: Polygonaceae.

Annual prostrate herb. Leaves elliptic or lanceolate. Flowers small, green in axillary clusters. Fruit nut, ovoid.
Distributed from Kashmir to Kumaon.
Local names: *Ben*: Machuties; *Hin*: Machoti, Bannatia, Bannalia; *Pun*: Kesru.

Uses: Roots used in the treatment of diabetes.

**Polygonum bistorta** L.

Syn: *Polygonum paleaceum* Wall. ex Hook.f.

Family: Polygonaceae.

Perennial herb, up to 60cm tall. Leaves radical and cauline with winged petioles, radical ovate-lanceolate, cauline smaller. Flowers white or pink in spikes.
In Himalayas from Kashmir to Sikkim and hills of Assam.
Trade name: Bistort, Snake–root.

Uses: Plant useful in the treatment of diabetes.

**Pongamia pinnata** (L.) Pierre

Syn: *Pongamia glabra* Vent.
*Cytisus pinnatus* L.
*Derris indica* (Lam.) Bennet
*Galedupa indica* Lam.

Family: Leguminosae (Fabaceae).

Small tree, up to 15m tall. Leaves imparipinnate, leaflets 5–9, opposite, thin coriaceous, ovate or ovate-oblong. Flowers pinkish-white in axillary racemes. Pod obliquely-oblong or elliptic, 1 or rarely 2-seeded, seed reddish brown.
Common along river banks and in plains. Planted as avenue tree.
Fl.: May–July, Fr.: December–May.
Sanskrit: Karanjah.
Local names: *Ass*: Karchaw; *Ben*, *Guj*, *Hin* & *Mar*: Karanj, Karanja; *Kan*: Honge; *Mal*: Pungu, Punnu; *Ori*: Koranjo; *Pun*: Sukhchein, Karanj, Paphri; *Tam*: Ponga, Pongam, Pungam; *Tel*: Kanuga chettu.
Trade name: Indian Beech.

Uses: Flowers useful in the treatment of diabetes.

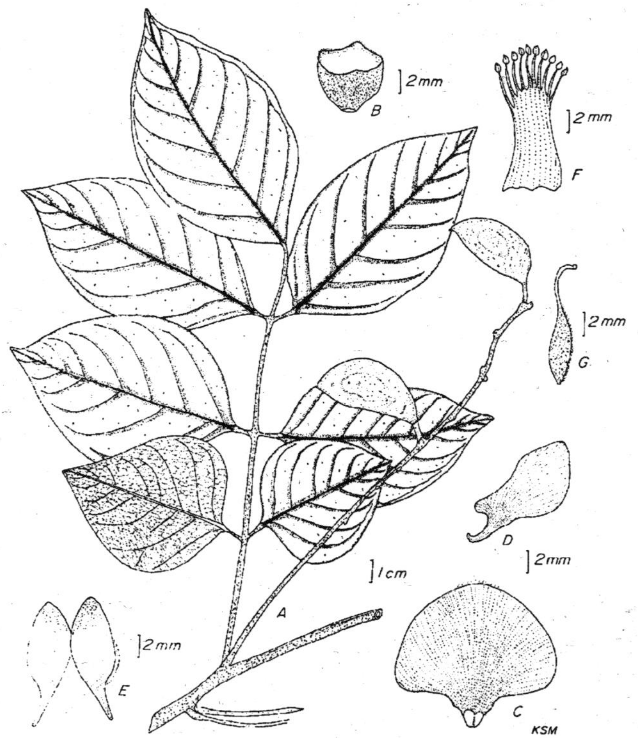


Fig. 70: *Pongamia pinnata* (L.) Pierre
A. Twig; B. Calyx; C. Standard petal; D. Wing petal; E. Keel petal; F. Staminal column; G. Pistil.

**Porana paniculata** Roxb.

Family: Convolvulaceae.

Large woody twiner. Leaves ovate, cordate. Flowers white in dense panicles. Fruit capsule, ovoid–globular.

Found almost throughout northern India.

Trade name: Bridal creeper.

Uses: Aerial parts used in the treatment of diabetes.

**Portulaca oleracea** L.

Family: Portulacaceae.

Annual prostrate, succulent, glabrous herbs. Leaves linear or obovate-oblong, fleshy. Flowers yellow in terminal clusters. Fruit ovoid capsule. Seeds many, black.

Common weed in cultivated fields and wastelands.

Fl.& Fr.: Round the year.

Sanskrit: Ghotika, Lonika.

Local names: *Ben*: Baralonia; *Guj*: Moti loni, Ghol; *Hin*: Khursa, Baralania, Kulfa; *Kan*: Dooddagooni soppu; *Mal*: Kariecheera; *Mar*: Bhuigoli, Kurfah, Mhotigol; *Ori*: Purunisag; *Tam*: Kari keerai, Paruppukiray, Pullikirai; *Tel*: Pedda payali kura, pappukura.

Trade name: Common purslane.

Propagation: By stem cuttings.

Uses: Whole plant and seeds useful in the treatment of diabetes.

**Potamogeton crispus** L.

Family: Potamogetonaceae.

Aquatic submerged herb. Leaves submerged, oblong-elliptic or oblanceolate. Flowers in spikes. Fruit drupelets.

Throughout India.

Fl. & Fr.: September–February.

Uses: Whole plant useful in the treatment of diabetes.

**Premna corymbosa** (Burm.f.) Rottl.

Syn: *Cornutia corymbosa* Burm.f.
*Premna serratifolia* L.
*Premna integrifolia* L.

Family: Verbenaceae.

Small tree, spiny. Leaves elliptic-ovate. Flowers greenish white in terminal corymbs. Fruit drupe, black when ripe.

Rare in forests.

Fl. & Fr.: January–September.

Sanskrit: Agnimatha.

Local names: *Mal*: Munna; *Tel*: Padmaka, Agnimatha.

Trade name: Fire Brand Teak of Deccan.

Propagation: By stem cuttings, seeds.

Uses: Roots and stem bark useful in the treatment of diabetes.

**Premna latifolia** Roxb.

Family: Verbenaceae.

Medium sized tree, up to 6m tall. Leaves ovate. Flowers pale–white in terminal corymbs. Fruit drupe, black when ripe.

Deccan peninsula, Bihar, Orissa and West Bengal.

Fl. & Fr.: April–September.

Local names: *Mal.*: Knappa; *Ori.*: Gondhna; *Tam.*: Pachumullai, Erumai munnai; *Tel.*: Pedda-nelli koora.

Uses: Stem bark useful in the treatment of diabetes.

**Prosopis chilensis** (Molina) Stuntz.

Syn: *Prosopis juliflora* (Sw.) DC
*Mimosa juliflora* Sw.

Family: Mimosaceae.

Armed shrub or small tree, up to 10m tall. Leaves bipinnate, pinnae 1–2 pairs, leaflets 15–17 pairs, oblong. Flowers yellow in axillary spikes. Fruit pod.

Throughout drier parts of India.

Local names: *Hin*: Vilayatikikkar, Vilayati babul; *Tel*: Sarkar Thumma.

Trade name: Mesquite.

Uses: Aerial parts used in the treatment of diabetes.

**Prunus dulcis** (Muller) D.A. Webb.

Syn: *Prunus amygdalus* Batsch.
*Prunus communis* Fritsch.
*Amygdalus communis* L.

Family: Rosaceae.

Medium sized deciduous tree, up to 8m tall. Leaves alternate, oblong-lanceolate. Flowers white tinged with red, showy, appearing before or with the early foliage. Fruit drupe, flesh splitting at maturity exposing the pitted stones, seed flattened.

Cultivated in Kashmir and Punjab.

Sanskrit: Vatadah, Vatamah.

Local names: *Ben*, *Guj* & *Hin*: Badam; *Kan*: Badamu; *Mal*: Badam, Badamkotta; *Tam*: Vadam-kottai; *Tel*: Badam vittulu.

Trade name: Almond.

Uses: Leaves and seeds useful in the treatment of diabetes.

**Prunus persica** Batsch.

Family: Rosaceae.

Small tree, up to 8m tall. Leaves oblong to broad lanceolate. Flowers pink, solitary. Fruit subglobose, fleshy, with a hard and deeply pitted stone.

Found cultivated in Kashmir, Uttar Pradesh, Himachal Pradesh and to a limited extent in Nilgiris.

Fl. & Fr.: January–March.

Local names: *Hin*: Aru, Shaftalu.

Trade name: Peach, Nectarine.

Propagation: By seeds.

Uses: Aerial parts useful in the treatment of diabetes.

**Psidium guajava** L.

Family: Myrtaceae.

Small tree, up to 9m tall, branchlets appressed tomentose. Leaves opposite-decussate, oblong or ovate-lanceolate, coriaceous. Flowers white, axillary, solitary or in pairs. Fruit globose berry, seeds numerous.

Cultivated all over India.

Fl. & Fr.: Round the year.

Sanskrit: Perukah, Mansala.

Local names: *Ben*: Goaachhi, Peyara; *Guj*: Jamrud, Jamrukh, Peru; *Hin*: Amrud, Safed Safari; *Kan*: Gova, Jamaphala, Perala, Sibi, Sebehabbu; *Mal*: Pera, Koyya; *Mar*: Jamba, Tupkel; *Ori*: Bodojamo, Jamo, Julabojamo, Pijuli; *Pun*: Anjirzard; *Tam*: Koyya, Segappugoyya, Sengoyya, Vellaikoyya, Uyyakkondan; *Tel*: Jama; *Urdu*: Amrud.

Trade name: Common Guava.

Propagation: Air layering and by seeds.

Uses: Fruits and leaves useful in the treatment of diabetes. Leaves (4/5) are to be soaked in water overnight, the liquid is filtered and given to the patient for a month daily in the morning.

**Pterocarpus marsupium** Roxb.

Family: Fabaceae (Leguminosae).

Tall deciduous tree, bark thick grey with vertical cracks. Leaves odd pinnate, 5–7-foliolate, leaflets elliptic-oblong, coriaceous. Flowers yellow in terminal panicles. Fruit winged pod.

Common in forests of Peninsular India, Bihar and Uttar Pradesh.

Fl. & Fr.: March–February.

Sanskrit: Asanahm Bijakah.

Local names: *Guj*: Biyo, Hiradakhan; *Hin*: Bijasal, Asan, Bibla, Piasal, Pitasara; *Kan*: Honne bange; *Mal*: Venga; *Mar*: Bibla, Honne; *Ori*: Begsara; *Tam*: Vengai; *Tel*: Yegisa, Yegi.

Trade name: Indian kino Tree.

Propagation: by seeds.

Uses: The decoction of heart wood taken for 10 days or heart wood powder in a dose 5gr. twice daily or extract that gets from overnight soaking of heart wood taken for a month reduces blood sugar level.

**Pterocarpus santalinus** L.f.

Family: Fabaceae (Leguminosae)

Tall, deciduous tree, bark deeply cleft, brownish black. Leaves 3-foliolate,

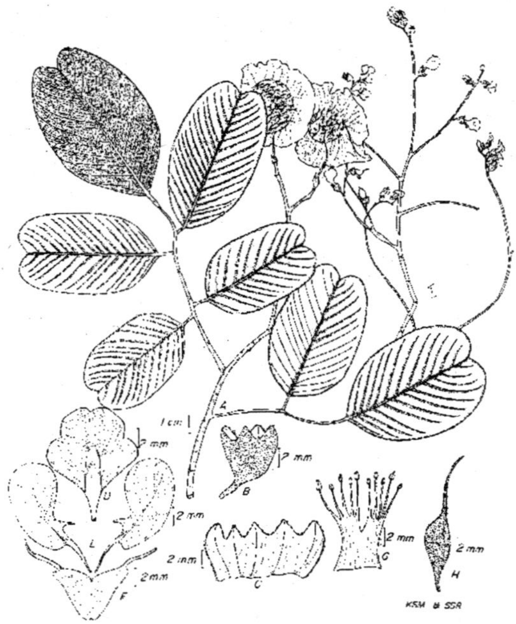

Fig. 71: *Pterocarpus marsupium* Roxb.
A. Twig; B. Calyx split open; D. Standard petal; E. Wing petals; F. Keel petals; G. Staminal column; H. Pistil; I. Flowering twig.

leaflets ovate-orbicular or oblong. Flowers axillary in simple or sparingly branched racemes. Fruit round pods with a broad wing.

Endemic to the hills of Cuddapah, Nellore, Chittoor and Kurnool districts in Andhra Pradesh and Chingelput district in Tamil Nadu.

Fl. & Fr.: April–July.

Sanskrit: Raktachandan.

Local names: *Ben & Hin*: Raktachandan, Lalchandan; *Guj*: Ratanjalli; *Kan*: Agaru, Honne, Kempugandha chekke; *Mal*: Parrangam, Tilaparin; *Mar*: Tambada chandana; *Ori*: Raktachandan; *Tam*: Atti, Sivapu chandan, Chen chandan, Semmarm; *Tel*: Yerrachandanamu, Rakta chandanamu.

Trade name: Red sanders.

Propagation: By seeds and stumps.

Uses: Aqueous extract of wood twice per day useful in the treatment of diabetes.

**Pterospermum acerifolium** Willd.

Family: Sterculiaceae.

Evergreen tree, up to 24m tall. Leaves variable in size and shape, oblong. Flowers large, axillary, solitary or in pairs, white, fragrant. Fruit capsule, oblong.

Found in the sub-Himlayan tract and outer valleys from Yamuna eastwards to West Bengal and in Assam and Manipur, Bihar, Karnataka, A.P. and Andamans.

Local names: *Ben*: Kanak champa, Muskunda; *Hin*: Kanak–Champa, Kaniar, Muchkund, *Tel*: Matsa Kanda; *Ori*: Kanaka-champa.

Uses: Leaves useful in the treatment of diabetes.

**Pueraria lobata** (Willd.) Ohwi

Syn: *Pueraria thunbergiana* (Sieb. & Zucc.) Benth.
*Pueraria hirsuta* Schneid. non Kurz.

Family: Fabaceae (Papilionaceae).

Perennial vine with tuberous roots. Leaves trifoliolate, leaflets entire or shallowly 2–3-lobed. Flowers mauve or violet coloured, in dense pubescent racemes. Fruit pod, flat.

Native of Japan and China, cultivated in India for edible roots.

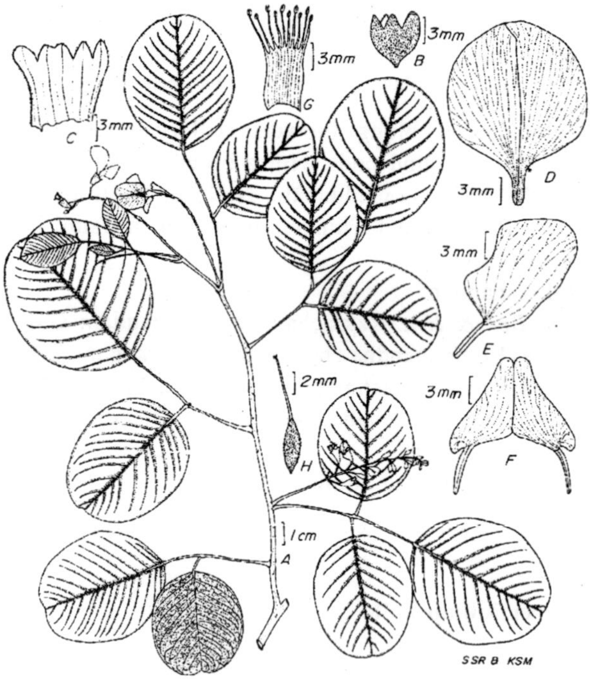


Fig. 72: *Pterocarpus santalinus* L.f.
A. Twig; B. Calyx; C. Calyx split open; D. Standard petal; E. Wing petal; F. Keel petals; G. Staminal column; H. Pistil.

Trade name: Kudzu.

Uses: Flowers used in the treatment of diabetes.

**Pueraria tuberosa** (Roxb. ex Willd.) DC.

Syn: *Hedysarum tuberosum* Roxb. ex Willd.

Family: Fabaceae (Papilionaceae)

A large woody climber, branchlets appressed velvety. Leaves 3-foliolate, leaflets ovate, laterals oblique, inequilateral, thin coriaceous, glabrous above, appressed white silky beneath. Flowers pale violet in panicles. Fruit pod, linear, seeds 3–6.

Occasional in dry deciduous forests.

Sanskrit: Vidari, Kandapalash.

Local names: *Ben*: Shimia, Batraji; *Guj*: Vidarikand, Phagvelo, Khakarvel; *Hin*: Sural, Bilaikand; *Kan*: Gumadi gida, Bidrerakanda; *Mal*: Mutukku,

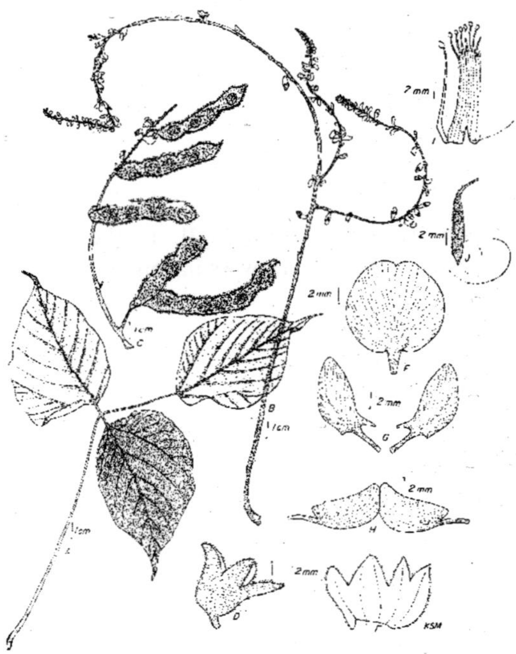

Fig. 73: *Pueraria tuberosa* (Roxb. ex Willd.) DC.
A. Vegetative twig; B. Flowering twig; C. Fruiting twig; D. Calyx; E. Calyx split open; F. Standard petal; G. Wing petals; H. Keel petals; I. Staminal column; J. Pistil.

Palmutukku; *Mar*: Badra, Pithana; *Tam*: Darigummadi; *Tel*: Dhari Gummadi.
Trade name: Indian kudzu.
Propagation: By tuberous roots.

Uses: Tubers useful in the treatment of diabetes.

**Punica granatum** L.

Family: Punicaceae.

Deciduous, small tree, up to 6m tall, bark smooth, branchlets often spine tipped. Leaves oblanceolate or oblong. Flowers bright red, solitary or 2–3 together, terminal. Fruit globose berry, crowned by persistent calyx-lobes, interior septate with membranous wall, pulp pellucid, pinkish.
Cultivated for its edible fruit.
Fl. & Fr.: Through out the year.
Sanskrit: Dadimah.
Local names:*Hin*: Anar; *Kan*: Dhalimbe; *Tam*: Mathulai, Madhulami; *Tel*: Danimma.
Trade name: Pomegranate.
Propagation: By seeds.

Uses: Aerial parts and flowers useful in the treatment of diabetes.

**Quercus lamellosa** Sm.

Family: Fagaceae.

Large evergreen tree, up to 30m tall. Leaves broadly oblong to lanceolate. Flowers unisexual, male flowers in spikes, female flowers solitary or in short spikes.
Found in Eastern Himalayas.

Uses: Stem bark used in the treatment of diabetes.

**Quercus lineata** Blume.

Family: Fagaceae.

Small or medium sized tree. Leaves oblong or ovate-lanceolate. Flowers unisexual, male and female in spikes.
Found in Eastern Himalayas Khasi and Naga hills of Assam.

Uses: Stem bark used in the treatment of diabetes.

**Quassia amara** L.

Family: Simaroubaceae.

Erect shrub, up to 3m tall, bark light coloured. Leaves unequally pinnate with broadly winged rachis, leaflets obovate. Flowers purple in terminal racemes. Fruit drupe, purple black when ripe, seeds globular.

Grown in gardens.

Propagation: By seeds, by cuttings or layers.

Uses: Plant useful in the treatment of diabetes.

**Quercus infectoria** Olivier

Family: Fagaceae.

Shrub or small tree. Leaves alternate, very rigid, apical galls are formed by gall wasp. Flowers unisexual in catkins. Fruit cupula covered by scales.

Native of Greece, Asia minor, Syria and Iran. The galls of this plant are imported into India.

Local names: *Ben*: Maju-phal; *Hin*: Maju-phal, Mazu, Muphal; *Kan*: Machikai; *Mal*: Majakam, *Tam*: Machakai; *Tel*: Machi kaya.

Trade name: Gall oak, Dyer's oak.

Uses: The leaf galls are astringent because they contain tannins. The dry extract exhibits hypoglycemic efficacy.

**Raphanus sativus** L.

Family: Brassicaceae.

Annual or biennial herb, up to 1m tall. Root tuberous. Lower leaves are lyrately pinnatisect. Cauline leaves simple. Flowers in loose racemes. Fruit inflated, with long tapering beak, seeds 2–8, globose.

Cultivated throughout India.

Sanskrit: Mulaka.

Local names: *Ben*, *Guj*, *Hin* & *Mar*: Muli, Mula, Mura muri; *Kan*, *Mal*, *Tam* & *Tel*: Mullangi.

Uses: Whole plant useful in the treatment of diabetes.

**Rauvolfia serpentina** (L.) Benth. ex Kurz.

Syn: *Ophioxylon serpentinum* L.

Family: Apocynaceae.

Small erect, perennial undershrub, up to 1m tall. The root system consists of a prominent tuberous, soft tap root, up to 6 cm in diameter having a corky outer bark. Leaves in whorls of 3, oblanceolate, glabrous. Flowers pink or white in corymbose cymes. Fruit drupe, purplish black when ripe.

Occasional in moist deciduous forests of Sub-Himalayan tracts from Himachal Pradesh to Arunachal Pradesh, Western Ghats and Eastern Ghats; also cultivated occasionally.

Fl. & Fr.: March–May.

Sanskrit: Sarpagandha.

Local names: *Ben*: Chandra; *Hin*: Chhotachand, Sarap-gandha; *Kan*: Sarpagandha, Sutranabhi; *Mal*: Amalpori, Tulunni; *Mar*: Harki, Sapasanda; *Ori*: Patal garur, Sanochado; *Tam*: Sarpakanta, Covannamilpodi; *Tel*: Sarpagandha, Pathalagaridi.

Trade name: Serpentine root.

Propagation: The plant grows well in hot humid climate, but prefers shady habitats of forest. It requires very high rainfall ranging from 250 cm to 500 cm and a temperature range of 10–30° C. It can grow in different kinds of soils ranging from red, laterite loam to sandy alluvial loam, but thrives best in well-drained humus-rich clayey soils.

It is propagated by seeds, roots, root stumps and cuttings. As the collection of seeds from wild resources is both laborious and costly, vegetative propagation has been advocated for raising plantation. Root cuttings of 3 to 5 cm long are planted in holes in June and July and are almost completely covered with earth leaving only 1 cm above the surface. The cuttings sprout with in 3 weeks if good moisture is maintained in this period. A success of 50 to 80% has been obtained by various workers in India. About 100 kg of root cuttings are required to plant an hectare of land. The crop propagated by seed is better as yields by this method is larger. About 5 kg of seeds are required per hectare. All seeds are not viable and hence seeds should be used in surplus. Seeds are sown in nursery beds in April–May at a distance of 15–25 cm in rows. The seeds germinate in 4–8 weeks. When the seedlings are three months old they are transplanted into the fields with a spacing of 30×45 cm. The field before transplantation is ploughed and 45–50 tons of Farm Yard manure is added. NPK fertilizers at the rate of 80, 40, 40, are applied. The weeds are removed periodically.

Roots (and rhizomes) of the plant constitute the crude drug. As recommended by the Indian Pharmacopoeia the drug is fully formed when the plant is 4 years old. The plants are uprooted carefully during October–November and root parts are seperated. The bark of root is retained in tact. They are thoroughly washed. The roots are sun-dried till they retain a moisture content of 12%. The roots are stored away from light. They are cut into pieces (2–15 cm long and 3–20mm in diameter). The roots are cylindrical and almost unbranched. Their colour ranges from light brown to greyish below. The pieces of old roots posses longitudinal ridges while those of young ones wrinkles. The average yield of roots in 1200 kg per hectare.

Uses: Roots useful in the treatment of diabetes.
Active constituent: Reserpine present in roots.

**Rhizophora mucronata** Poir.

Syn: *Rhizophora mangle* Roxb.

Family:Rhizophoraceae

Evergreen large shrub or small tree. Leaves elliptic. Flowers creamy white in cymes. Fruit ovoid–conical.
Tidal shores and creeks of India.
Fl. & Fr.: March–October.
Local names: *Ben*: Kamo, Bhora; *Kan*: Kandaale; *Mal*: Paniccha kandal, Pinkandal, Venkankal; *Mar*: Kandal; *Ori*: Rai, Rohi; *Tam*: Kandal, Sorapinnai; *Tel*: Uppuponna, Adavi-ponna.

Uses: Aerial parts and stem bark used in the treatment of diabetes.

**Rhododendron campanulatum** D. Don

Family: Ericaceae.

Evergreen shrub or small tree, up to 6m tall. Leaves elliptic or ovate. Flowers white, in various shades of purple and pink, in few-flowered corymbs. Fruit capsule.
Found throughout Himalayas.
Local names: *Ben*: Ghentaboras; *Hin*: Cherailu.

Uses: Aerial parts used in the treatment of diabetes.

**Rhus chinens** Mill.

Family: Anacardiaceae.

Deciduous tree, up to 11m tall. Leaves imparipinnate, leaflets 5–13, very variable in shape. Flowers white or pale yellowish green in terminal tomentose panicles. Fruit drupe, orbicular, red when ripe.
Found in temperate Himalayas, Assam and Nagaland.
Local names: *Hin* & *Pun*: Arkhar, Chechar, Dudla, Tetri.

Uses: Plant is used to treat Diabetes millitus.

**Rhus wallichii** Hook.f.

Syn: *Rhus vernicifera* DC.

Family: Anacardiaceae.

Deciduous tree, up to 15m tall. Leaves imparipinnate, leaflets 5–9, elliptic, oblong or ovate. Flowers greenish yellow in axillary panicles. Fruit globose drupe.

Found in temperate Himalayas from Kashmir to Nepal.

Local names: *Pun*: Kambal, Gadambal.

Uses: Aerial parts useful in the treatment of diabetes.

**Ricinus communis** L.

Family: Euphorbiaceae.

A tall glabrous annual or perennial shrub, stem hollow or pithy, often brittle. Leaves palmately 7–11-lobed, long petioled. Flowers greenish in terminal panicles, unisexual. Fruit a capsule or schizocarp, 2–3-valved, pericarp warty, seeds mottled.

Cultivated all over India for its oil seed.

Sanskrit: Erandah.

Local names: *Hin & Mar*: Erandi, Arandi; *Kan*: Eranda, Haralu, Avudala; *Tam*: Andagam, Sitta-manakku, Amanakku, Attagam, Vattamam; *Tel*: Amudamu.

Trade name: Castor oil plant.

Propagation: By seeds.

Uses: Roots and aerial parts useful in the treatment of diabetes.

**Rivea ornata** Choisy

Family: Convolvulaceae.

A climbing or straggling shrub. Leaves orbicular, glabrous above, white silky beneath. Flowers white, fragrant, 3-or more-flowered axillary cyme. Fruit capsule, subglobose, brown.

Found in Konkan, Deccan and South India.

Fl. & Fr.: May–November.

Sanskrit: Phanji.

Local names: *Guj*: Phang nijat; Mar: Phand; *Tam*: Muchuddai; *Tel*: Boddi Teega.

Propagation: By branch cuttings.

Uses: Sap useful in the treatment of diabetes.

**Rosmarianus officinalis** L.

Family: Lamiaceae.

Evergreen branched subshrub, up to 1.5m tall. Leaves linear, coriaceous. Flowers few in axillary racemes, bluish or white or pale violet. Fruit nutlets, brown.

Grown in gardens for ornament purpose.
Local names: *Hin*: Rusmari.
Trade name: Rosemary.
Propagation: By seeds or rooted cuttings.

Uses: Plant useful in the treatment of diabetes.

**Rourea minor** (Gaertn.) Alston

Syn: *Rourea santaloides* Wight & Arn.
*Rourea commutata* Planch.
*Rourea pulchella* Planch.
*Rourea acuminata* Hook.f.

Family: Connaraceae.

Stout evergreen liana. Leaflets very variable. Flowers small, white, in axillary racemes. Fruit oblique–ellipsoid, brown with orange-coloured or red arils.

Western part of peninsula, West Bengal, Assam, Manipur and Andaman & Nicobar Islands.

Local names: *Ben*: Vidhadaki, Vitaraka; *Guj*: Varadharo; *Hin*: Kalavidhara; *Kan*: Hulee-Chalaballa, Kake soppu; *Mal*: Kuriel; *Tel*: Chadrapudi.

Uses: Roots and twigs are employed in the treatment of diabetes.

**Rubia cordifolia** L.

Syn: *Rubia munjista* Roxb.

Family: Rubiaceae.

A rugose vine or herb, branches 4-angled. Leaves whorled, 4 at the node, cordate. Flowers white in terminal and axillary dichasial cymes. Fruit globose drupe, fleshy.

Rare in moist deciduous forests throughout India.
Fl. & Fr.: June–October.
Sanskrit: Manjistha, Kala-Meshika, Yojanavalli.
Local names: *Ass*: Majathi, Majeti; *Ben*: Majith, Manjisthe, Manjit; *Hin*: Manjit; *Kan*: Manjustha; *Mal*: Manjetti, Manipur-Moyun; *Mar*: Manjestha; *Ori*: Manjistha; *Pun*: Khuri, Kukaraphali, Manjit, Majit, Mitu, Munzat, Runa, Runang, Sheni, Tiuru; *Tam*: Manjitti, Shevelli; *Tel*: Tamravalli, Manjestatiga, *Urdu*: Manjithe.
Trade name: Indian Madder.
Propagation: By seeds.

Uses: Aerial parts useful in the treatment of diabetes.

**Rubus fruticosus** L.

Syn: *Rubus discolor* Weihe & Nees

Family: Rosaceae.

Large erect shrub, stems with short stout prickles. Leaves with white stellate tomentum beneath. Flowers pink. Fruit with fleshy drupes, black when ripe.

Found in Kashmir.

Trade name: Alish, Akhi, Kanachi.

Uses: Leaves used in the treatment of diabetes.

**Rubus idaeus** L.

Family: Rosaceae.

Perennial shrub, up to 2m tall, roots with suckers, stems armed with prickles. Leaves pinnate, leaflets 3–5 or 7. Flowers white in axillary and terminal cymes. Fruit red, aggregate.

Cultivated in a small scale in South Indian Hill Stations.

Trade name: European raspberry.

Uses: Leaves useful in the treatment of diabetes.

**Rubus paniculatus** Sm.

Family: Rosaceae.

Found in Temperate Himalayan regions from Punjab to Assam.

Local names: *Pun*: Kalaakhi

Uses: Aerial parts used in the treatment of diabetes.

**Ruellia tuberosa** L.

Family: Acanthaceae.

Erect herb, up to 50cm tall, roots tuberous. Leaves obovate to lanceolate. Flowers blue to violet in axillary dichasial cymes. Fruit oblong capsule.

Fl. & Fr.: September–May.

Cultivated for its flowers, often as an escape.

Uses: Plant useful in the treatment of diabetes.

**Rumex acetosa** L.

Family: Polygonaceae.

Erect, perennial herb, up to 75cm tall. Radical leaves ovate-oblong. Flowers unisexual, dioecious, in long terminal panicles. Fruit nut.
Found in Western Himalayas from Kashmir to Kumaon.
Local names: *Ben*: Chukapalam: *Hin*: Khatta palak.
Trade name: Garden sorrel.

Uses: Leaf and stem useful in the treatment of diabetes.

**Rumex nepalensis** Spreng.

Family: Polygonaceae.

Tall, robust, annual or perennial herb, up to 1.2m tall. Leaves oblong-ovate. Flowers bisexual, green, in whorls on leafless racemes.
In temperate Himalayas from Kashmir to Bhutan.
Local names: *Ben*: Pahari Palang.

Uses: Whole plant useful in the treatment of diabetes.

**Rumex patientia** L.

Syn: *Rumex orientalis* Bernh.

Family: Polygonaceae.

Erect perennial herb, up to 2m tall. Leaves elliptic-ovate. Flowers in lax or dense panicles. Fruit nut.
Found in the western Himalayas from Kashmir to Kumaon.
Trade name: Patience Dock.

Uses: Plant useful in the treatment of diabetes.

**Rumex vesicarius** L.

Family: Polygonaceae.

Annual erect herb, up to 30cm tall. Leaves elliptic-ovate or oblong. Flowers white or pink in terminal and leaf-opposed racemes. Fruit nut.
Cultivated throughout India.
Trade name: Bladder Dock.
Local names: *Hin*: Chuka, Palak, Plang sag, *Kan*: Sukki Soppu, Jussi, Soppu; *Tam*: Shakkan Kirai; *Tel*: Chukka kura.

Uses: Seeds useful in the treatment of diabetes.

**Salacia chinensis** L.

Syn: *Salacia prinoides* DC.
*Salacia latifolia* Wall. ex Laws.

Family: Hippocrateaceae.

Small, erect or straggling tree or large woody climbing shrub. Leaves ovate to lanceolate. Flowers 2–6, clustered together on axillary tubercles, yellowish. Fruit small, globose, red when ripe, one-seeded.

Found throughout India.

Local names: *Ben*: Dimal, Modhuphal; *Mal*: Cherukuranti; *Mar*: Ingli, Nisul-bondi.

Uses: Roots have been used as an antidiabetic drug in the indigenous system of medicine and clinical tests are said to have substantiated their efficacy.

**Salacia macrosperma** Wight

Family: Hippocrateaceae.

A diffuse rambling or scandent shrub. Fruit globose, orange coloured.

Found in Western Ghats from Konkan Southwards.

Local names: *Mal*: Anakoranti; *Mar*: Lendphal.

Uses: The ethanolic extract showed hypoglycemic activity. It also showed reduction of blood sugar level.

**Salacia reticulata** Wight

Family: Hippocrateaceae.

Climbing shrub. Leaves elliptic or subovate. Flowers 6 in each axil. Fruit tuberculate.

Found in southern Orissa and Kerala.

Sanskrit: Etanayakam.

Local names: *Mal*: Koranti; *Tel*: Anukudu chettu.

Uses: Root bark used in the treatment of diabetes.

**Salvadora persica** L.

Family: Salvadoraceae.

Large much branched, evergreen shrub or small tree, up to 10m tall. Leaves elliptic-oblong. Flowers greenish-yellow in axillary and terminal panicles. Fruit fleshy drupe, spherical, red when ripe.

Commonly planted in Mosques and Muslim burial grounds.

Fl. & Fr.: November–April.

Sanskrit: Pilnh.

Local names: *Ben*: Jhal; *Guj*: Kharijal, Kharjar, Pilu, Moti Jalya, Piludi; *Hin*: Jhak, Kharjal; *Kan*: Goni mara; *Mar*: Khakhin, Kickni, Miraj, Mirajoli,

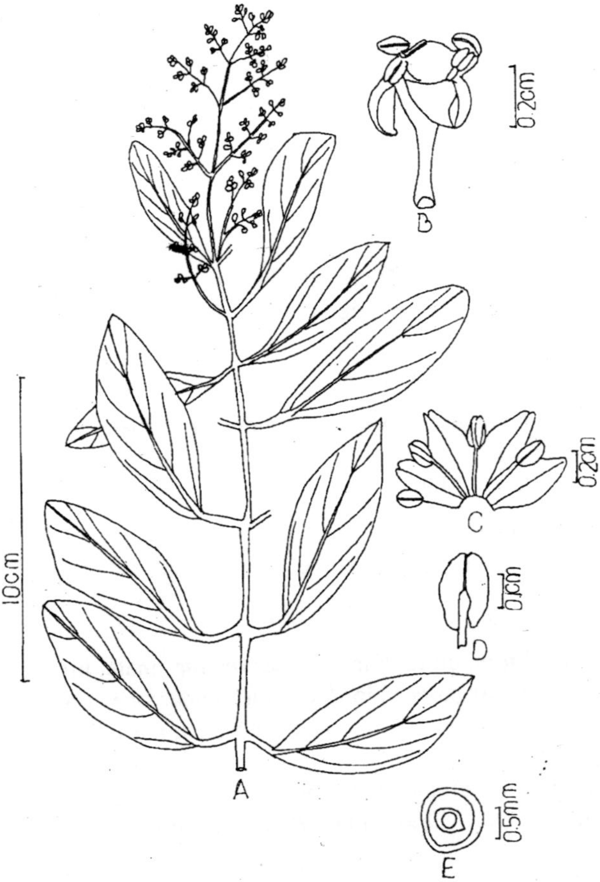


Fig. 74: *Salvadora persica* L.
A. Twig; B. Flower; C. Corolla; D. Stamen; E. T.S. of ovary.

Pelu, Pilva, Rhakhan, Thorapilu; *Ori*: Kotungo, Toboto, Oilu; *Tam*: Kalaua, Karkol, Perungoli, Ughaiputtai, Vivay; *Tel*: Gogu Gunia, Wargu.

Trade name: Salt Bush Tree, Tooth Brush Tree, Meshwak.

Propagation: By seeds.

Uses: Roots useful in the treatment of diabetes.

**Salvia officinalis** L.

Family: Lamiaceae (Labiatae).

Sub-shrub, up to 60cm tall, stems white woolly. Leaves oblong or oblong-lanceolate, aromatic. Flowers blue, purple or white in simple racemes.

Often cultivated.

Local names: *Hin*: Salvia sefakuss.
Trade name: Sage, garden sage.
Propagation: By stem cuttings.

Uses: Leaves useful in the treatment of diabetes.

**Salvia plebeia** R. Br.

Family: Lamiaceae (Labiatae).

Stout, annual herb, up to 50cm tall. Leaves oblong-lanceolate. Flowers white or lilac in paniculate–spicate racemes. Fruit nutlets.
Common weed throughout India.
Fl. & Fr.: September–March.

Uses: Whole plant used in the treatment of diabetes.

**Samanea saman** (Jacq.) Merr.

Syn: *Mimosa samanea* Jacq.
*Enterlobium saman* (Jacq.)Prain

Family: Mimosaceae.

Large unarmed tree, up to 20m tall. Leaves bipinnate, pinnae 2–4 pairs, leaflets 6–7 pairs, basal pairs oblong-elliptic, upper ones obovate. Flowers pinkish-brown in terminal or axillary corymbose panicles. Pod linear-oblong, brownish-black.
Frequently planted along roadsides.
Local names: *Ori*: Chakunda; *Tam*: Thoongumoonjimaram; *Tel*: Nidraganneru.

Uses: Aerial parts useful in the treatment of diabetes.

**Sambucus nigra** L.

Family: Caprifoliaceae.

Shrub or small tree, up to 6m tall. Leaves odd pinnate, leaflets 3–7, ovate or oblong. Flowers creamy white in terminal corymbose cymes, scented. Fruit globose, purple or black when ripe.
Grows wild in Kangra and Simla hills in Himachal Pradesh.
Trade name: European elder, Black Elder.

Uses: Plant used in the treatment of diabetes mellitus.

**Santalum album** L.

Family: Santalaceae.

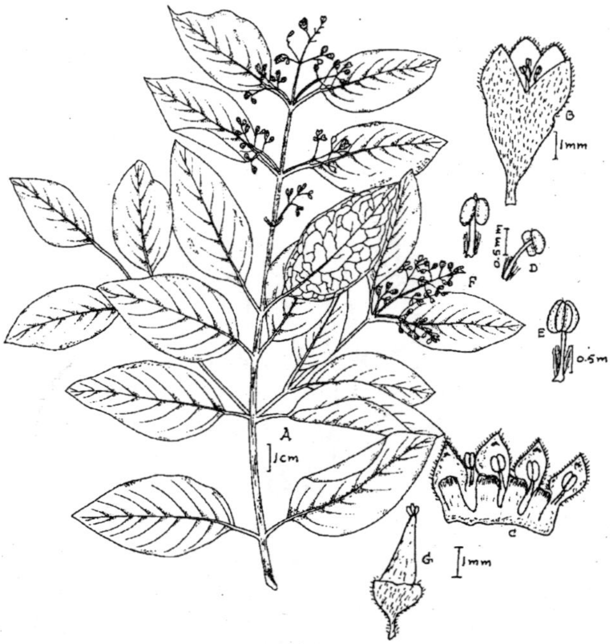


Fig. 75: *Santalum album* L.
A. Twig; B. Flower; C. Corolla split open; D.-F. Stamens; G. Pistil.

Small evergreen tree with slender drooping branches. The sapwood white and odorless, the heartwood yellowish brown, strongly scented. Leaves elliptic ovate to lanceolate. Flowers in terminal and axillary paniculate cymes.

Common in forests of Karnataka,Tamil Nadu and Southern Andhra Pradesh; planted elsewhere.

Fl. & Fr. January–October.

Sanskrit: Chandana.

Local names: *Ben*: Chandan, Peetchandan, Srikhanda, Sufaid chandan; *Guj*: Sukhad, Sukhet; *Hin*: Safed chandan, Chandan; *Kan*: Gandada, Sreegandha; *Mal*: Chandanam,Maleyam; *Mar*: Chandan, Safed chandan; *Ori*: Chondono; *Tam*: Chandanam, Sandhanam; *Tel*: Chandanamu, Sreegandhamu, Gandhapuchekka.

Trade name: Sandal tree.

Propagation: By seeds.

Uses: Wood useful in the treatment of diabetes.

**Saraca asoca** (Roxb.) de Wilde

Syn: *Jonesia asoca* Roxb.
*Saraca indica* auct non L.

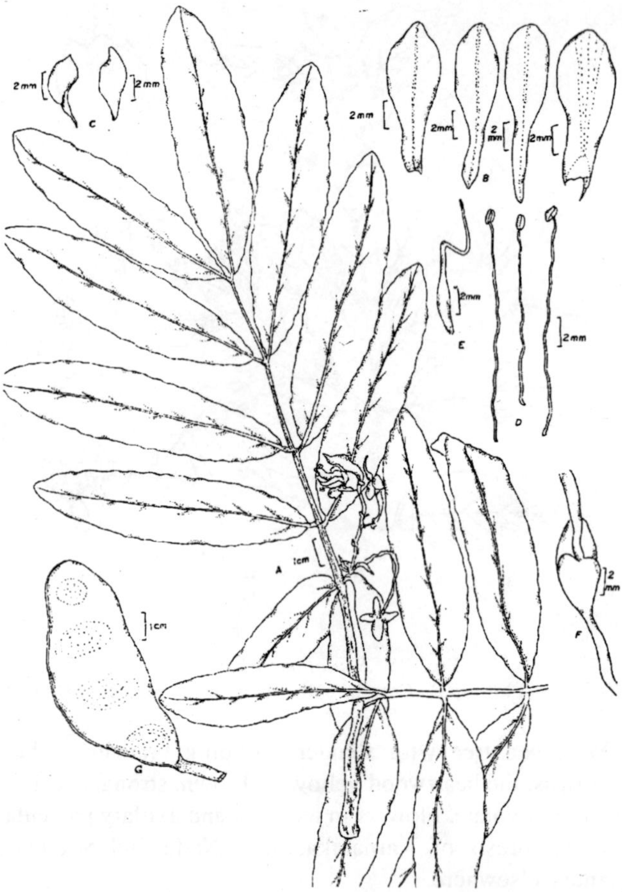


Fig. 76: *Saraca asoca* (Roxb.) de Wilde
A. Twig; B. Sepals; C. Bracts; D. Stamens; E. Pistil; F. Bracts entire; G. Pod.

Family: Caesalpiniaceae.

Ever green tree, up to 5m tall. Leaves even pinnate, leaflets 4–6 pairs, oblong, coriaceous. Flowers brilliant orange-yellow, pink with age in short dense corymbose panicles. Fruit oblong pod, compressed, flat.

Western and Eastern Ghats, Uttar Pradesh, Bihar, West Bengal, Orissa and North-Eastern States.

Fl. & Fr.: All seasons.

Sanskrit: Ashoka.

Local names: *Ben*: Asok, Ashoka; *Guj*: Ashopalava, Asupala; *Hin*: Asok, Asoka; *Kan*: Ashoka mara, Seethe mara; *Mal*: Asokam, Asjogam; *Mar*: Ashoka, Jasundi; *Ori*: Oshoko; *Tam*: Asoka, Asoka pattai; *Tel*: Ashoka, Vanjulamu.

Trade name: Ashoka.

Uses: Aerial parts and flowers useful in the treatment of diabetes.

**Saussurea heteromalla** (D.Don) Raizada & Saxena

Syn: *Saussurea candicans* C.B. Clarke
*Carduus heteromallus* D. Don

Family: Asteraceae (Compositae).

Robust annual herb, up to 1.5m tall. Leaves cottony below, oblong or ovate-oblong. Flowers pale red in terminal heads. Fruit achene, 5-angled.
Himalayas from Kashmir to Bhutan.

Uses: Whole plant is used to treat diabetes mellitus.

**Scindapsus officinalis** (Roxb.) Schott.

Syn: *Pothos officinalis* Roxb.

Family: Araceae.

Climbing shrub. Leaves ovate, elliptic or nearly orbicular. Flowers greenish yellow in spadix enclosed in an oblong spathe. Fruit berry.
In Sub Himalayan tract, West Bengal, Orissa, Andhra Pradesh and Andaman Islands.
Fl. & Fr.: November–January.
Sanskrit: Gaja pippali, Kari-pippali, Kapivalli.
Local names: *Ben*: Gaja pipal, *Hin*: Gajapipal, Pippal-jhanca; *Kan*: Dodda–hippali; Gaja–hippali; *Mal*: Anatti pipili, *Mar*: Thorapimpli; *Tam*: Anaitippili; *Tel*: Enugupippalu, Gaja–pippalu.

Uses: Fruit useful in the treatment of diabetes.

**Scleria levis** Retz.

Syn: *Scleria hebecarpa* Nees.

Family: Cyperaceae.

Perennial, rhizomatous herb, up to 80cm tall. Leaves linear. Flowers in terminal panicles. Fruit nut, ovoid–globose, white.
Found almost throughout India.
Fl. & Fr.: March–October.

Uses: Whole plant useful in the treatment of diabetes.

**Scoparia dulicis** L.

Family: Scrophulariaceae.

Annual erect herb, up to 90cm tall. Leaves lanceolate. Flowers small, white. Fruit capsule, globose.

Weed in many parts of India.

Trade name: Sweet broom weed, Goat weed.

Uses: Whole plant useful in the treatment of diabetes.

**Securinega leucopyrus** (Willd.) Muell.–Arg.

Syn: *Fluggea leucopyrus* Willd.

Family: Euphorbiaceae.

Shrub, up to 5m tall. Leaves obovate. Flowers in axillary clusters. Fruit capsule, globose, white when ripe.

Fl. & Fr.: June–October.

Local names: *Tel*: Tella purugudu.

Uses: Aerial parts useful in the treatment of diabetes.

**Securinega virosa** (Willd.) Baill.

Syn: *Phyllanthus virosus* Roxb. ex Willd.
*Fluggea microcarpa* Bl.

Family: Euphorbiaceae.

Shrub, to 5m tall. Leaves elliptic-obovate. Flowers in axillary cymes, unisexual, dioecious. Fruit capsule, globose.

Fl. & Fr.: June–December

Local names: *Tel*: Sulamunata.

Uses: Seeds useful in the treatment of diabetes.

**Semecarpus anacardium** L.f.

Family: Anacardiaceae.

Moderate sized deciduous tree with red blaze exuding resin which blackens on exposure. Leaves very large, crowded at the ends of branches. Flowers greenish-white in terminal panicles. Fruit oblong-ovoid drupe, shining black when ripe.

Occasional in dry deciduous forests throughout warm parts and tropical outer Himalayas.

Fl. & Fr.: May–December.

Sanskrit: Bhallataka.

Local names: *Ass*: Bholaguri; *Ben*: Bhela, Bhalatuki, Nelama; *Guj*: Bhilamu; *Hin*: Belatak, Bhela, Bheyla, Bhilwa, Bilaran; *Kan*: Agnimukhi, Bhallataka,

Geru, Gerubija, Gerkayi, Goddugeru, Karigeru, Cheru, Keru, Kerubija; *Mal*: Chera, Herkkuru; *Mar*: Bibha, Bibba; *Tam*: Seranlottai, Shenkottai; *Tel*: Nalla Jidi, Bhallatakamu.

Trade name: Marking nut, Oriental Cashew.

Propagation: By seeds.

Uses: Fruit useful in the treatment of diabetes.

**Senecio tenuifolius** Burm.f.

Family: Asteraceae (Compositae).

Annual erect, glabrous herb, up to 50 cm tall. Leaves pinnatifid or bipinnatifid. Flowers yellow, in terminal heads, heterogamous. Fruit achene, obovate, ribbed, hairy between ribs.

On the dry hills of the Western Ghats from Konkan southwards to Kerala up to an altitude of 1500m.

Fl. & Fr.: September–December.

Local names: *Tel*: Katimera chamanthi.

Propagation: By seeds.

Uses: Whole plant useful in the treatment of diabetes.

**Sesamum orientale** L.

Syn: *Sesamum indicum* L.

Family: Pedaliaceae.

An annual erect, pubescent herb. Lower leaves lobed or deeply divided, upper ones undivided, linear-oblong. Flowers axillary, solitary, pink or rosy. Fruit capsule.

Cultivated for oil seed.

Fl. & Fr.: Through out the year.

Sanskrit: Tila.

Local names: *Hin* & *Mar*: Til; *Guj*: Tal; *Kan* & *Tam*: Ellu; *Mal*: Karuthi ellu; *Ori*: Khasa, Rasi; *Tel*: Nuvvulu.

Trade name: Sesame, Gingelly.

Propagation: By seeds.

Uses: Plant useful in the treatment of diabetes. Laddus are prepared with seeds (handful) and given to patient, one laddu daily for seven days for curing diabetes.

**Sida spinosa** L.

Family: Malvaceae.

Woody, much branched, erect herbs-undershrubs, stems and branches rough with spiny tubercles at the nodes below the petioles. Leaves ovate-elliptic or oblong. Flowers yellow with red tinge, axillary, solitary or 2–5 in clusters. Fruit schizocarp, wrinkled, mericarps 5, seeds ovoid.

Occasional weed of waste places and forests throughout India.

Fl.& fr.: September–March.

Sanskrit: Mahabala.

Local names: *Ben*: Gorakchaulia, Pila-barella, Bon methi; *Guj*: Kantolobal, Nagbala, Gangeti, Khareti; *Hin*: Gulsa kari, Jangli-methi, Bharigar, Gangeram; *Kan*: Kaadu menthya; *Mal*: Kattuventiyam; *Mar*: Ganded hamam, Gangeti, Kanteritukati, Tukati-khareti; *Tam*: Arivalmanaippundu, Mayirmanikkam; *Tel*: Nagabala.

Trade name: Prickly Sida.

Propagation: By seeds.

Uses: Whole plant useful in the treatment of diabetes.

**Siegesbeckia orientalis** L.

Family: Asteraceae.

Annual, erect, viscid pubescent herb, up to 80cm tall. Leaves ovate. Flowers yellow in terminal heads. Fruit achene, ribbed.

Throughout India.

Local names: *Guj*: Pilibadkadi; *Tam. & Tel.*: Katampam, Kadambi.

Uses: Whole plant useful in the treatment of diabetes.

**Silybum marianum** (L.)Gaertn.

Syn: *Cardus marianum* L.

Family: Asteraceae (Compositae).

Erect, annual or biennial herb, up to 1.3m tall. Leaves pinnatifid to ovate, lobes spiny. Flowers purple or white in globose heads, involucral bracts spiny. Fruit cypsela.

Weed in Kashmir, Punjab and other north-west parts of India.

Local names: *Kan*: Pavitramullina Gida.

Trade name: Milk Thistle, Holy thistle.

Uses: Plant useful in the treatment of diabetes.

Active constitutent: Silymarin.

**Sisymbrium brassiciformis** C.A.Mey.

Syn: *Sisymbrium columnae* Hook.f. & T. Anders.

Family: Brassicaceae.

Erect, stout, annual herb. Leaves runcinate or sometimes almost entire, segments ovate-oblong to lanceolate. Flowers pale yellow in racemes. Fruit siliqua, very slender.
Found in Himalayas from Kashmir to Kumaon.

Uses: Whole plant used to treat diabetes mellitus.

**Smithia conferta** Smith

Syn: *Smithia geminiflora* Roth

Family: Fabaceae (Papilionaceae).

Spreading herb, up to 45cm long. Leaves paripinnate, leaflets 5–9 pairs, linear–oblong. Flowers yellow in axillary capitate racemes. Fruit pod, moniliform.
Throughout India.
Fl. & Fr.: September–November.
Local names: *Mal*: Elakanni, Thiruthali; *Mar*: Naichi bhaji; *Tam*: Elakanni.

Uses: Whole plant used in the treatment of diabetes.

**Solanum anguivi** Lam.

Syn: *Solanum indicum* auct non L.

Family: Solanaceae.

Annual, diffuse, much branched undershrub, up to 1.5m tall, prickly with sharp, yellowish spines. Leaves ovate, shallowly lobed. Flowers blue-purple in racemose cymes, extra-axillary. Fruit berry, globose, yellow when ripe.
Throughout warmer parts of India.
Fl. & Fr.: August–December..
Sanskrit: Vrihati, Bhantaki.
Local names: *Ben*: Byakura, Gurkamai; *Hin*: Barhanta, Birhatta; *Mal*: Cheruchunda, Cheruvazhudhena; *Mar*: Ringani dorli, Inoti ringini; *Tam*: Mulli, Pappara mulli; *Tel*: Kakamunchi, Mulla vankaya, Tell-mulaka.
Trade name: Poison berry.

Uses: Fruits useful in the treatment of diabetes.

**Solanum nigrum** L.

Family: Solanaceae.

An annual, erect, much branched, unarmed herb, up to 1m tall. Leaves ovate, glabrous. Flowers white, in extra axillary cymes. Fruit globose berry,

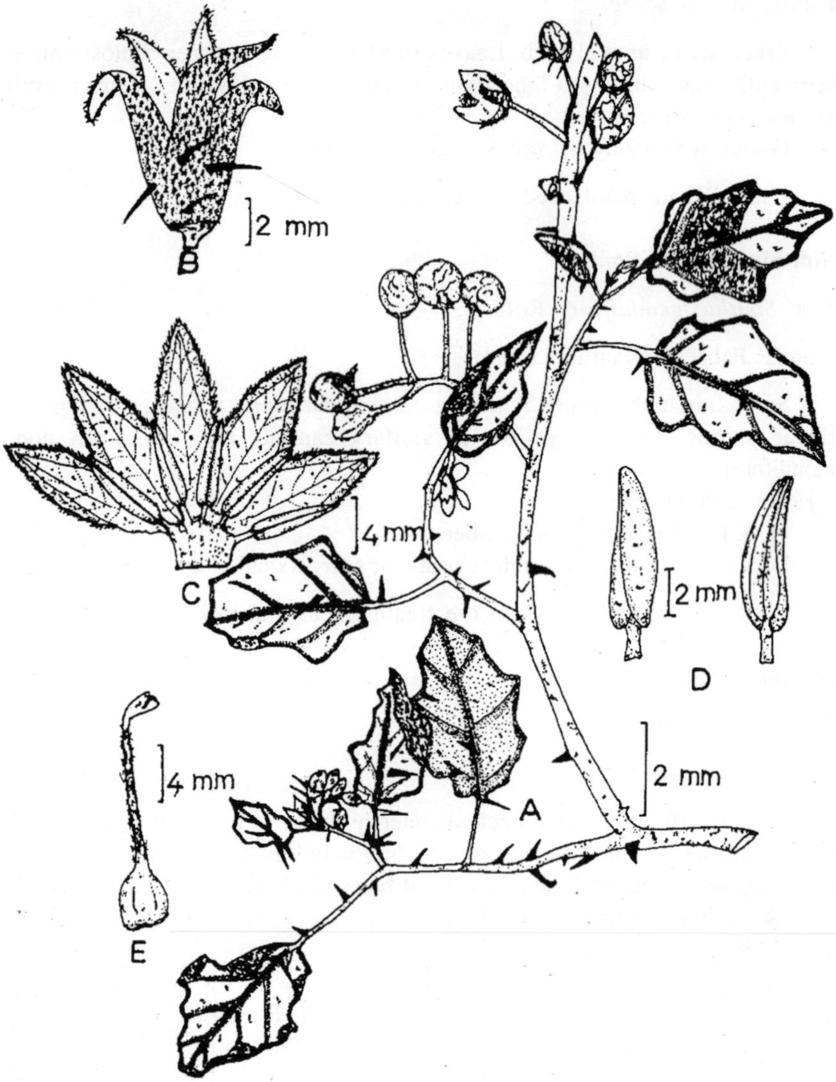


Fig. 77. *Solanum anguivi* Lam.
A. Twig, B. Calyx, C. Corolla split open with stamens, D. Stamens, E. Pistil

glabrous, purplish red when ripe, seeds many, ovate-reniform.

Common weed of waste places, road sides and cultivated fields.

Fl. & Fr.: Round the year.

Propagation: By seeds.

Sanskrit: Kakamaci.

Local names: *Ben*: Gurkamai, Kakmachi, Tulidun; *Guj*: Piludi; *Hin*: Makoi; *Tam*: Munatakali; *Tel*: Kamanchi.

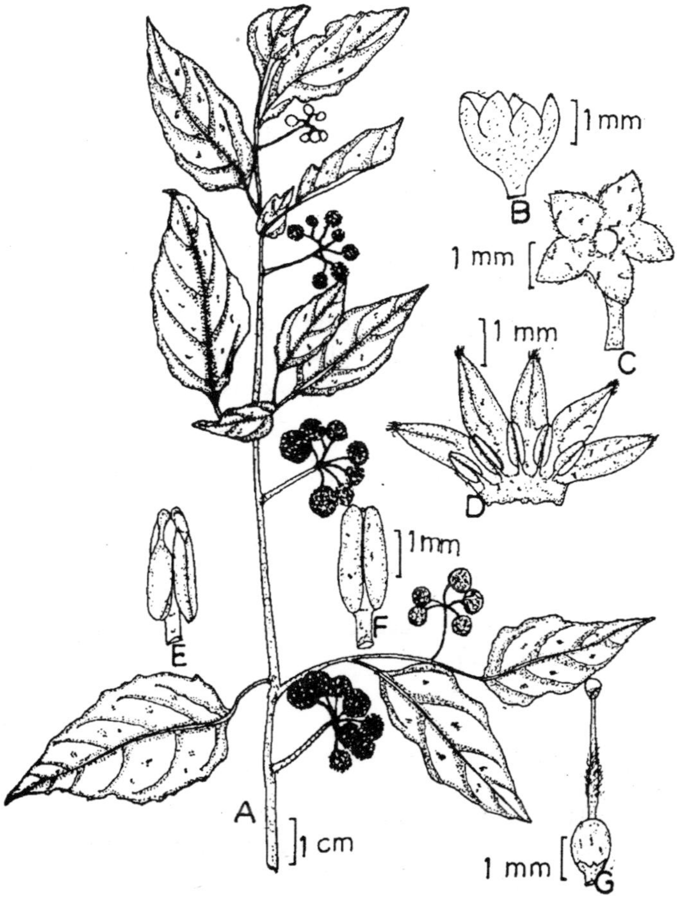


Fig. 78. *Solanum nigrum* L.
A. Twig; B & C. Calyx; D. Corolla split open with stamens; E & F. Stamens; G. Pistil.

Trade name: Black Night-Shade.

Uses: Plant useful in the treatment of diabetes.
Active constituent: Lupeol.

**Solanum torvum** Sw.

Family: Solanaceae

Armed, erect undershrub, up to 2.5m tall. Leaves ovate, shallowly lobed. Flowers white in dense cymes. Fruit berry, yellowish when ripe.

Throughout the tropical parts of India.

Local names: *Ben*: Gota Begum; *Kan*: Kadusunde, Sondaegida,

Sundakkayi; *Mal*: Kaatuchunta; *Tam*: Sundaikai; *Tel*: Chundaikai, Kottuvastu, Ustekaya.

Fl. & Fr.: September–January.

Uses: Fruit useful in the treatment of diabetes.

Active constituent: Lupeol.

**Solanum trilobatum** L.

Family: Solanaceae.

Armed, climbing undershrub. Leaves ovate-angular, prickly. Flowers violet, in extra-axillary cymes. Fruit globose berry, seeds circular.

Occasional in plains especially on the coast.

Fl. & Fr.: December–March.

Sanskrit: Alarka.

Local names: *Kan*: Mullumusta, Habbusundae-gida; *Mal*: Tutavalam; *Ori*: Nabhiankuri; *Tam*: Tudhuvelum, Toothuvilai; *Tel*: Vuschinta ush.

Trade name: Climbing brinjal.

Propagation: By seeds.

Uses: Fruit useful in the treatment of diabetes.

Active constituent: Lupeol.

**Solanum tuberosum** L.

Family: Solanaceae

Much branched, bushy shrub, up to 1m tall, underground stems bearing edible tubers. Leaves pinnately lobed, lobes ovate or ovate-oblong. Flowers white in cymose panicles. Fruit globose berry, seeds many, flattened.

Cultivated in hill stations.

Local names: *Ben & Hin*: Alu; *Guj & Mar*: Batata; *Kan*: Batate, Alugidde; *Mal*: Urulan kizhangi; *Tam*: Uralakilangu, Wallaraikilangu; *Tel*: Bangaladumpa, Urlagadda.

Trade name: Potato.

Uses: Tuber useful in the treatment of diabetes.

Active constituent: Lupeol.

**Sonneratia apetala** Buch.–Ham.

Family: Sonneratiaceae–Lythraceae

Small to moderate sized tree, up to 10m tall. Leaves oblong or narrow–elliptic. Flowers white, solitary or 2–3 in a terminal cluster. Fruit globose capsule.

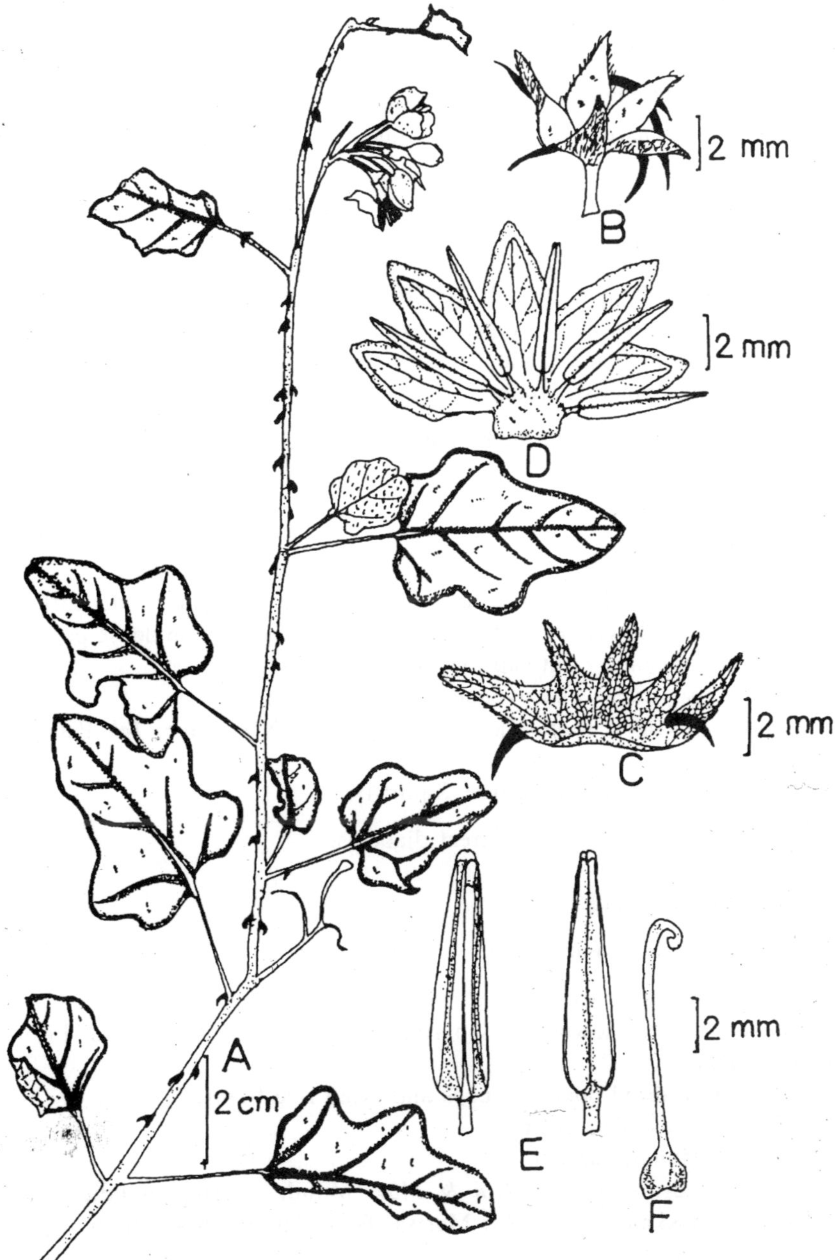


Fig. 79: *Solanum trilobatum* L.
A. Twig; B. Calyx; C. Calyx split open (dorsal side);
D. Corolla split open with stamens; E. Stamens; F. Pistil.

Found in tidal forests of West Bengal and Peninsular India.
Local names: *Ben*: Keora; *Mar*: Kandal, Undi; *Ori*: Keora, Kerna; *Tam*: Marama; *Tel*: Kyalanki.

Uses: Aerial parts used in the treatment of diabetes.

**Spartium junceum** L.

Family: Fabaceae (Leguminosae).

Aromatic shrub, up to 3m tall. Leaves simple, linear–lanceolate. Flowers yellow, in terminal racemes, fragrant. Fruit pod.
Grown in Punjab and Simla.
Trade name: Spanish broom.

Uses: Plant used in the treatment of diabetes.

**Spathodea campanulata** Beauv.

Family: Bignoniaceae.

Tall tree, up to 20m tall. Leaves imparipinnately compound, leaflets elliptic or ovate. Flowers bell-shaped, scarlet red or orange in dense pendulous, terminal raceme. Fruit capsule, seeds winged.
Planted in gardens and avenues.
Local name: *Hin*: Rugtoora; *Kan*: Lujjekaya, Neerukaye; *Tel*: Patade, Patadiya.
Trade name: African tulip tree, Squirt tree.

Uses: Stem bark is used to treat diabetes.

**Sphaeranthus indicus** L.

Family: Asteraceae (Compositae).

Annual diffuse or suberect aromatic herb, stems winged. Leaves obovate or spathulate. Flowers pink-purple in sessile, terminal heads. Fruit oblong achene.
Common in dried ponds, ditches and dried rice fields.
Fl. & Fr.: November–April.
Sanskrit: Mundi, Sarvani.
Local names: *Ben*, *Guj*, *Hin* & *Mar*: Mundi, Gorakh mundi; *Mal*: Mirangani, Adakkamaniyan; *Ori*: Murisa, Buikadamba, Bokashungi; *Tam*: Kottaranthai; *Tel*: Bodasaramu.
Trade name: East Indian Globe Thistle.
Propagation: By seeds.

Uses: Whole plant useful in the treatment of diabetes.

**Spinacia oleracea** L.

Family: Chenopodiaceae.

Annual, erect herb, up to 60cm tall. Leaves ovate-oblong, variously lobed. Flowers unisexual, greenish, male flowers in terminal leafless spikes, female flowers in axillary clusters. Fruit capsule.

Cultivated all over India for leafy vegetable.

Local names: *Ben*: Palang; *Hin*: Isfanaj; *Guj. & Mar*: Palak; *Kan*: Spinachsoppu; *Ori*: Palaksag, Mithapalanga; *Tam*: Vasayleykiray; *Tel*: Dumpavachli.

Uses: Aerial parts used in the treatment of diabetes.

**Stephania glabra** Miers

Syn: *Stephania rotunda* Hook.f. & Thoms.

Family: Menispermaceae.

Dextrorse twiner.

Uses: Roots useful in the treatment of diabetes.

**Stereospermum suaveolens** (Roxb.) DC.

Syn: *Bignonia suaveolens* Roxb.

Family: Bignoniaceae.

Large deciduous trees. Leaves 1-pinnate, leaflets 5–9, elliptic. Flowers dull crimson in large panicles. Fruit capsule, straight.

Occasional in forests of drier localities, often planted.

Fl. & Fr.: September–February.

Sanskrit: Patala, Patali.

Local names: *Ben*: Parlu, Ghunta, Mug; *Hin*: Paral, Padaria; *Kan*: Hude, Hulave; *Mal*: Vedankorana, Puppatiri; Parul, Padal; *Ori*: Patoli; *Tam*: Padiri, Appu; *Tel*: Kokkesa, Patala.

Trade name: Paarul mool.

Propagation: By seeds.

Uses: Roots useful in the treatment of diabetes.

**Striga gesnerioides** (Willd.) Vatke

Syn: *Buchnera gesnerioides* Willd.
*Striga orobanchoides* Benth.

Family: Scrophulariaceae.

A total parasite on *Lepidagathis cristata* with reddish brown stem, up to 25cm tall. Leaves reduced to linear scales. Flowers pink in terminal spikes. Fruit capsule.

Fl. & Fr.: August–January.

Uses: Whole plant useful in the treatment of diabetes.

**Strychnos nux-vomica** L.

Family: Loganiceae.

Deciduous tree, up to15m tall, often with short, strong axillary spines. Leaves elliptic-orbicular, coriaceous. Flowers greenish-white, fragrant, in terminal compound cymes. Fruit globose berry, thick shelled, orange when ripe, slightly rough, but shining, seeds many.

Common in deciduous forests of West Bengal, Bihar, Orissa, Central India, Maharashtra and Peninsular India.

Fl. & Fr.: March–August.

Sanskrit: Karaskara, Chipita.

Local names: *Ben*: Kuchila, Thakesur; *Guj*: Kuchla; *Hin*: Bailewa, Chibbinge, Kajra, Kuchla, Nirmal; *Kan*: Hemmushti, Ittangi, Itti, Kajavara, Kanjira, Kasara; *Mal*: Kannirakkuru, Kanniram, Kairram, Tettamperahmaram; *Pun*: Kagnhala, Kajra, Kuchila, Hubul garab; *Tam*: Etti kagodi, Kalam, Kanjiga, Kanjirai, Kanjiram; *Tel*: Mushti, Mushini; *Urdu*: Azaraki, Kuchala.

Trade name: Snake wood, poison nut.

Uses: Fruit used in the treatment of diabetes.

**Strychnos potatorum** L.f.

Family: Loganiaceae.

Medium sized deciduous tree, bark black, cracked and scaly. Leaves ovate-elliptic, glabrous. Flowers white in axillary sessile cymes. Fruit globose berry, black when ripe.

Common in dry deciduous forests of Central, Eastern and Peninsular regions.

Fl. & Fr.: April–November.

Sanskrit: Kataka, Ambu-Prasada.

Local names: *Ben*: Nirmali; *Hin*: Nirmali, Nelmal; *Kan*: Chilli-bija, Chali; *Mal*: Tettemparal, Thetham; *Mar*: Nirwali, Chilhara; *Ori*: Kotaku; *Tam*: Ttetan-kottai, Terran; *Tel*: Chilla.

Trade name: Clearing nut tree.

Uses: Leaf, stem bark and seed are used in the treatment of diabetes.

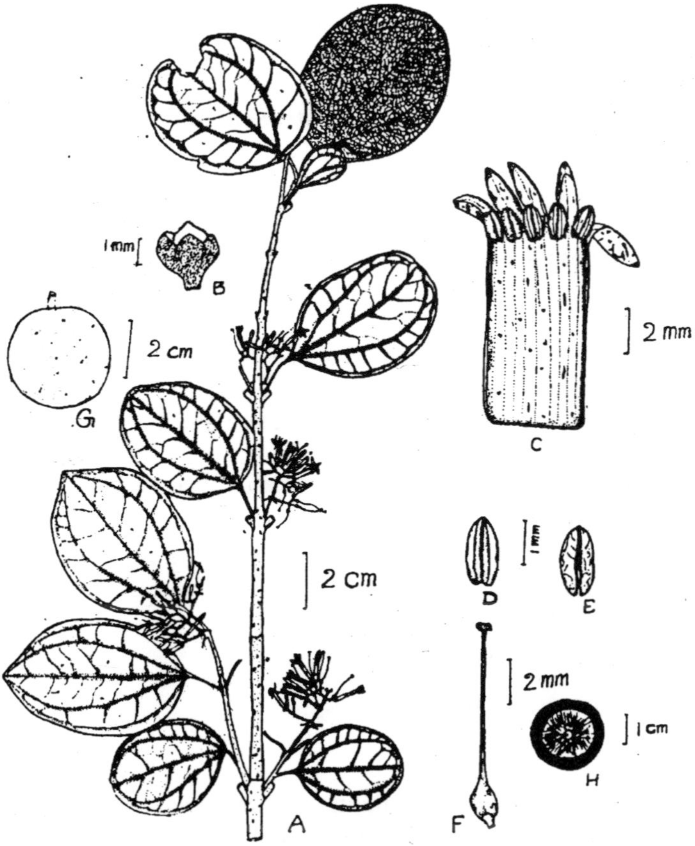


Fig. 80: *Strychnos nux-vomica* L.
A. Twig; B. Calyx; C. Corolla spread out; D. & E. Anthers; F. Pistil; G. Fruit; H. Seed.

Seeds (3/4) are to be dried and grinded to powder. One tea spoon of the powder is to be given with water for curing diabetes. Green leaves of jamun (4/5) are ground and given to the patient empty stomach for a few days to cure diabetes.

**Swertia chirayita** (Roxb. ex Flem.) Karst.

Syn: *Swertia chirata* (Wall.) Clarke
*Gentiana chirayita* Roxb. ex Flem.
*Ophelia chirata* Griseb.

Family: Gentianaceae.

Annual herb, up to 1.5m tall. Leaves opposite, sessile. Flowers pale green, tinged with purple. Fruit ovoid.

It occurs in temperate Himalayas between 1200 and 3000m from Kashmir to Assam.

Sanskrit: Kirata–tikta.

Local names: *Ben*: Chirata; *Hin*: Chirayata, *Kan*: Nelabeva; *Mar*: Chirayita; *Tam & Tel*: Nila vembu.

Uses: Whole plant useful in the treatment of diabetes.

**Symplocos racemosa** Roxb.

Family: Symplocaceae.

A small tree, about 6m tall. Leaves coriaceous, dark green. Flowers white or pale yellow, in small axillary clusters. Fruit purplish black when ripe.

It occurs in plains and lower hills of Eastern and Central India.

Sanskrit: Lodhra.

Local names: *Ass*: Lapong–dong, Dieng Lamaki; *Ben*: Lodhi; *Guj*: Lodhra; *Hin*: Lodh; *Mar*: Lodhra; *Tel*: Loddugu.

Propagation: By seeds.

Uses: Aerial parts useful in the treatment of diabetes.

**Syzygium alternifolium** (Wight) Walp.

Syn: *Eugenia alternifolia* Wight

Family: Myrtaceae.

Deciduous trees, bark greyish, slightly fissured. Leaves ovate-elliptic to suborbicular, thick coriaceous. Flowers cream or yellowish white, sweet scented, in axillary cymes. Fruit globose berry, dark purple, crowned with persistent calyx tube.

Common in Nallamalais and Seshachalam hill ranges of Eastern Ghats.

Fl & Fr.: March–June.

Local names: *Tam*: Manchi-moyadi, Mogi; *Tel*: Mogi. Movi, Manchi, Moyadi.

Uses: The seeds contain sapogenins, quercetin and Kaempferol. Seed powder 3 times a day reduces glucose level in blood.

**Syzygium aromaticum** (L.) Merr. & Perry

Syn: *Eugenia caryophyllata* Thunb.
*Eugenia aromatica* Kuntze
*Caryophyllus aromaticus* L.

Family: Myrtaceae

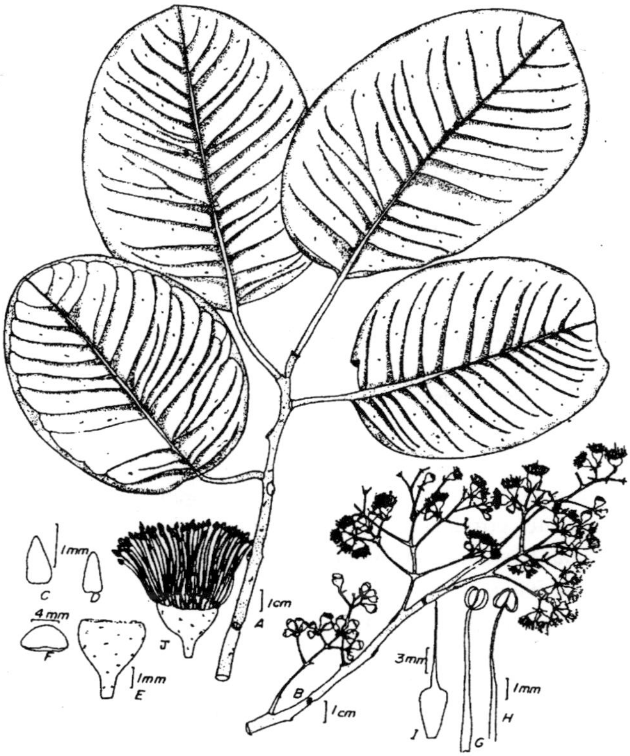


Fig. 81: *Syzygium alternifolium* (Wight) Walp.
A. Twig; B. Flowering branch; C. Bract; D. Bracteole; E. Calyx; F. Calyptra; G. & H. Stamens; I. Pistil; J. Flower.

Pyramid-shaped ever green tree, up to 12m tall. Leaves elliptic to lanceolate, coriaceous. Flower buds borne in small clusters at the ends of branches, greenish, turning pink at maturity, aromatic. Fruit drupe, fleshy, dark pink, 1-seeded.

Grown in Tamil Nadu and Kerala

Local names: *Ben*, *Guj*, *Hin* & *Mar*: Laung; *Kan*: Lavanga; *Mal*: Karayampu; *Tam*: Kirambi; *Tel*: Lavanga.

Propagation: By seeds.

Uses: Shoot and aerial parts useful in the treatment of diabetes.

**Syzygium cerasoideum** (Roxb.) Raizada

Syn: *Eugenia operculata* Duthie

Family: Myrtaceae.

Small or medium-sized, evergreen tree, up to 10m tall. Leaves broadly elliptic or obovate. Flowers white, sessile in trichotomous panicles. Fruit berry, globose or ellipsoid.

Found in Sub Himalayan tracts from Yamuna to Assam and Bihar and Orissa.

Local names: *Hin*: Dugdugia, Piaman; *Ori*: Pita Jam, Monisiagamo.

Uses: Aerial parts useful in the treatment of diabetes.

**Syzygium cumini** (L.) Skeels

Syn: *Syzygium jambolanum* (Lam.) DC.
*Myrtus cumini* L.
*Eugenia jambolana* Lam.

Family: Myrtaceae.

Tall tree, bark ashy brown, smooth. Leaves opposite decussate, elliptic-oblong or lanceolate, coriaceous, glabrous. Flowers pale greenish white in axillary or terminal trichotomous panicles. Fruit berry, ovate or oblong, shining bright to dark when mature, 1-seeded.

Common in forests throughout India.

Fl. & Fr.: April–June.

Sanskrit: Jambuh.

Local names: *Ben*: Jam, Kalajam; *Guj*: Jambu; *Hin*: Jamun, Jabava; *Kan*: Neeram Nerula; *Mal*: Perinnaral; *Mar*: Jambul; *Ori*: Jamo; *Pun*: Jammu; *Tam*: Neredam, Naval, Sambal; *Tel*: Neredu.

Trade name: Jaman, Black Plum.

Uses: The seeds are hypoglycemic. Jambul fruit is regarded in traditional medicine as a specific against diabetes because of its effect on the pancreas. The fruit as such, the seeds and fruit juice are all useful in the treatment of this disease. The seeds contain a glusoside 'jamboline' which is believed to have the power to check the pathological conversion of starch into sugar in cases of increased production of glucose. The seeds should be dried and powdered. One teaspoon of this powder should be mixed in one cup of milk or water or half a cup of curd, and taken twice daily.

The inner bark is also used in the treatment of diabetes. The bark is dried and burnt. It will produce an ash of white colour. This ash should be pestled in mortar, strained and bottled. The diabetic patient should be given ten grams of this ash on an empty stomach with water in the morning and twenty grams in the afternoon, and in the evening an hour after taking meals.

An equal quantity of Indian gooseberry powder, Jaman powder and bitter gourd powder also makes a very useful remedy for diabetes. A teaspoon of this mixture once or twice a day would be effective in checking the progress of this disease (Bakhru, 1998).

**Syzygium jambos** (L.) Aeston

Syn: *Eugenia jambos* L.

Family: Myrtaceae.

Evergreen spreading tree, up to 9m tall. Leaves lanceolate. Flowers greenish white in short, terminal racemose cymes. Fruit globose, pale yellow or pinkish white, seeds grey in succulent pericarp.

Cultivated in most parts of India for ornament.

Local names: *Ben*: Gulabjamb, Jamrul; *Hin* & *Mar*: Gulabjaman; *Kan*: Pannerale; *Mal*: Jambavam, Malakkachampa; *Ori*: Golabjamli; *Tam*: Perunaval; *Tel*: Jambuneredu.

Trade name: Rose apple.

Uses: In Brazil, a decoction of the dry leaves is taken in diabetes.

**Talinum portulacifolium** (Forsk.) Asch. & Schweinf.

Syn: *Orygia portulaciflia* Forsk.
*Talinum cuneifolium* (Vahl) Willd.
*Portulaca cuneifolia* Vahl

Family: Portulacaceae.

Annual erect, robust herb, up to 75cm tall. Leaves obovate, fleshy. Flowers pink in terminal lax panicles. Fruit globose capsule, seeds black.

Rajasthan southwards into the Peninsular region.

Fl. & Fr.: August–November.

Uses: Plant useful in the treatment of diabetes.

**Tamarindus indica** L.

Family: Caesalpiniaceae.

Tree, about 15–30m tall, bark fissured. Leaves even pinnate, leaflets 12–16 pairs, oblong. Flowers yellow with pink striations in terminal few-flowered racemes. Pod linear-oblong, falcate, with brittle epicarp, pulpy mesocarp and leathery endocarp, seeds 1-many, quadrangular, brown, shining.

Common both in forests and plains, also planted in topes and avenue tree.

Fl. & Fr.: March–September.

Sanskrit: Chincha, Tintrini.

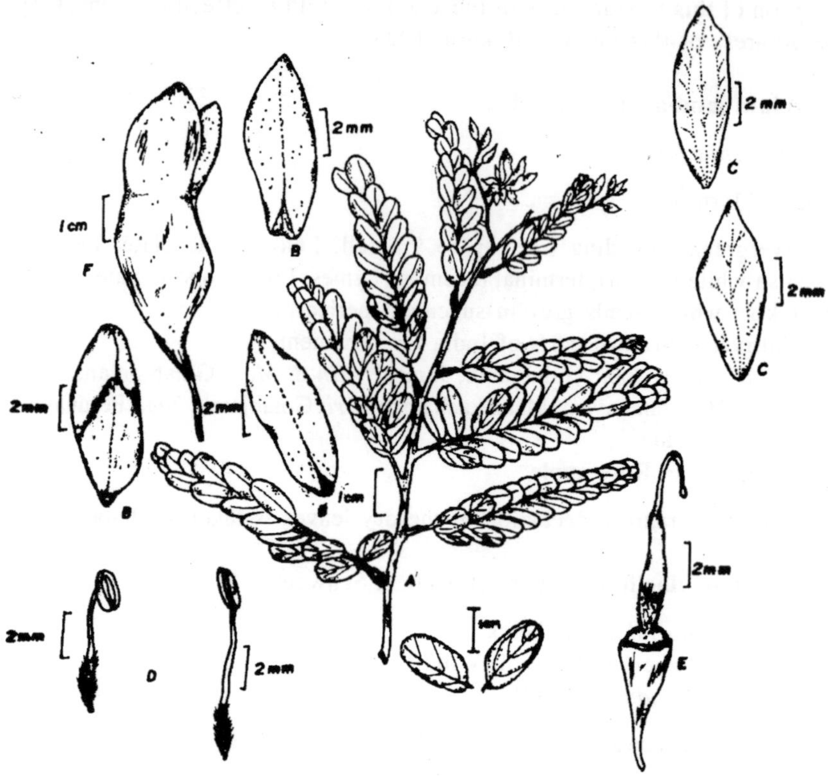


Fig. 82: *Tamarindus indica* L.
A. Twig; B. Sepals; C. Petals; D. Stamens; E. Pistil; F. Pod.

Local names: *Ben*: Ambli, Nuli, Tentul, Tetai, Tintil, Tintiri, Tinturi; *Guj*: Ambli, Amli; *Hin*: Imoli, Amli, Amlica; *Kan*: Amla, Amli, Amlike, Gotu, huli, Hunase, Hunis, Madhrapulli, Puli, Sinja, Tintrini, Sukram, Valampuri; *Mal*: Puli, Valampuli; *Mar*: Ambali, Amli, Chicha, Chinch; *Ori*: Koina, Koyna, Koya, Omlika, Tentuli, Tintidi; *Pun*: Imli; *Tam*: Ambilam, Puli, Amilam; *Tel*: Chintachettu; *Urdu*: Imli.

Trade name: Tamarind tree.

Propagation: By seeds.

Uses: Plant useful in the treatment of diabetes.

**Taraxacum officinale** Webber ex Wiggers

Family: Asteraceae (Compositae).

Scapigerous perennial herb with thick rhizome, latex milky. Leaves radical, sessile, narrowly oblong, irregularly pinnatifid. Flowers golden yellow in terminal heads. Fruit achene with soft, white, copious pappus.

Found throughout temperate Himalayas, in Khasi hills of Meghlaya, Mishmi hills of Arunachal Pradesh and in the hills of South India at altitudes 3000–5400m.

Local names: *Ben*: Pitachumki; *Hin*: Dulal, Barau, Kanphul; *Guj*: Pathardi; *Kan*: Kaadu seventhi; *Mar*: Undarkani, Kashmiri: Hand; *Pun*: Dudli, Baran, Radam, Kanphul, Shamukei.

Trade name: Taraxacum, Dandelion.

Uses: Whole plant useful in the treatment of diabetes.

**Tecoma stans** (L.) H.B.K.

Syn: *Bignonia stans* L.
*Stenolobium stans* (L.) Seem.

Family: Bignoniaceae.

A large shrub or small tree. Leaves imparipinnate, leaflets dentate, lanceolate. Flowers yellow, in terminal panicle. Fruit capsule, linear, seeds winged.

Cultivated and naturalized.

Propagation: By seeds.

Local names: *Kan*: Koreneklar; *Tam*: Sonapatti; *Tel*: Pachagotla.

Uses: The leaves are given in diabetes. An aqueous extract of the stem and leaves when administered to anesthetized dogs, produces an immediate fall of arterial blood pressure and a transient hyperglycemia followed by slow decrease in blood sugar level.

Chemistry: An indole-metabolizing enzyme, Indole-oxygenase has been isolated from the leaves. The leaves contain alkaloids Tecomine, tecostanine and tecostidine.

**Tectona grandis** L. f.

Family: Verbanaceae.

Large deciduous trees, branchlets quadrangular, stellate tomentose. Leaves very large, broadly elliptic, glabrous above, stellate pubescent below. Flowers yellowish in terminal dichotomous, large panicles. Fruit drupe, enclosed in enlarged calyx.

Common through out Southern India, south of Godavari river.

Fl. & Fr.: June–January

Sanskrit: Saka.

Local names: *Ass*: Ching-jagu; *Ben*: Segum; *Guj*: Sagach; *Hin*: Sagwan; *Kan*: Jadi, Sagwani, Tega, Tyagadamara; *Mal*: Thekku, Tekka; *Mar*: Saga; *Ori*: Singuru; *Tam*: Tekkumaram; *Tel*: Teku.

Trade name: Teak.

Propagation: By seeds, stumps and bud grafting.

Uses: Leaves useful in the treatment of diabetes.

**Tephrosia purpurea** (L.) Pers.

Syn: *Cracca purpurea* L.

Family: Fabaceae

Glabrescent, erect undershrubs. Leaves imparpinnate, leafleats 9–19, obovate. Flowers bluish pink to purple in leaf-opposed pseudoracemes. Fruit pod, downy-puberulous, slightly falcate, 5–7-seeded.

Common in waste lands and road sides.

Fl. & Fr.: Through out the year.

Sanskrit: Sharapunkha.

Local names: *Hin*: Sarpanka; *Kan*: Empali; *Mal*: Kozhejil; *Mar*: Sirapakha, Udhadi; *Tam*: Kavali; *Tel*: Vempali.

Propagation: By seeds.

Uses: Seeds useful in the treatment of diabetes.

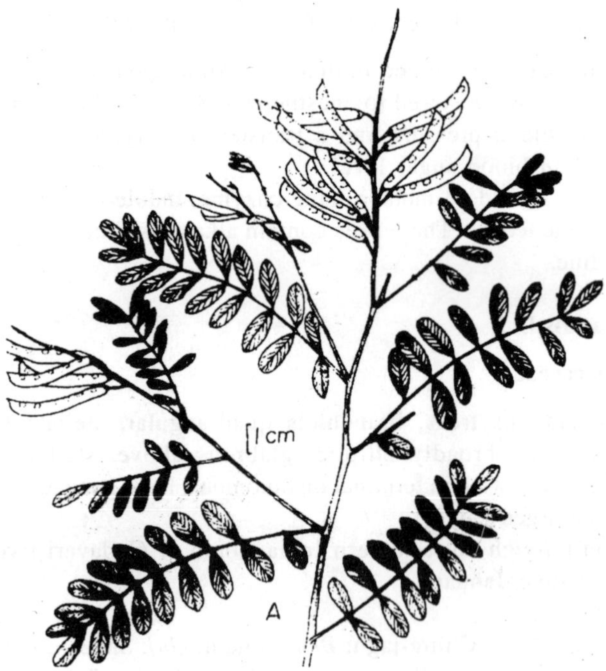


Fig. 83: *Tephrosia purpurea* (L.) Pers.
A. Twig.

**Tephrosia villosa** (L.) Pers.

Syn: *Galega villosa* L.
*Tephrosia hitra* (Buch.-Ham.) Benth.
*Galega hitra Buch.*-Ham.

Family: Fabaceae (Papilionaceae).

Erect, silky-villous undershrubs. Leaves imparipinnate, leaflets 5–7 pairs, obovate-oblanceolate. Flowers pink in axillary racemes. Fruit pod, seeds 6–8, strophiolate.

Common in waste lands and road sides.

Fl. & Fr.: June–October.

Local names: *Guj*: Runchalisarpankho; *Ori*: Sroetokolothiya; *Tam*: Vaykkavalai, Punaikkaivettalai; *Tel*: Nooguvempali.

Uses: The fresh root is credited with hypoglycemic properties. The leaves are used to treat diabetes.

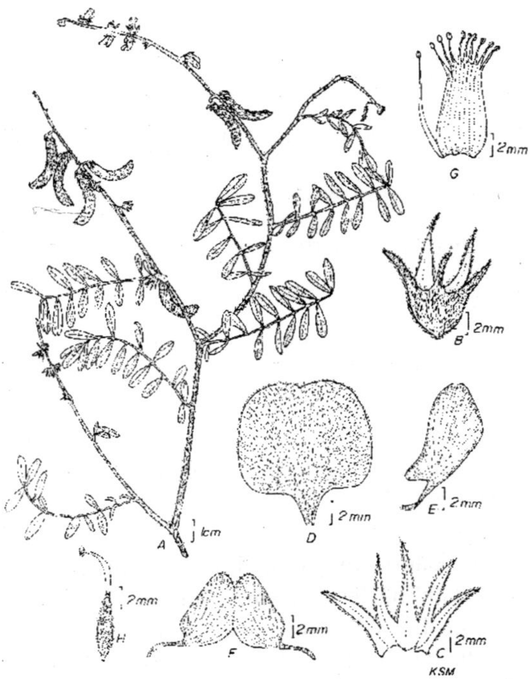


Fig. 84: *Tephrosia villosa* (L.) Pers.
A. Twig; B. Calyx; C. Calyx split open; D. Standard petal; E. Wing petal.

**Teramnus labialis** (L.f.) Spreng.

Syn: *Glycine labialis* L.f.

Family: Fabaceae (Papilionaceae).

Slender twing herb. Leaves 3-foliolate, obovate-lanceolate. Flowers pink, in axillary racemes. Fruit pod, compressed.
Throughout India.
Fl. & Fr.: November.
Local names: *Hin*: Mahoni, Mashpurai; *Ben*: Mashani; *Gui*: Valiyavelo; *Tam*: Kattualandu.

Uses: Whole plant used in the treatment of diabetes.

**Terminalia arjuna** (Roxb. ex DC.) Wight & Arn.

Syn: *Pentaptera arjuna* Roxb. ex DC.

Family: Combretaceae.

Large deciduous tree, up to 30m tall. Leaves oblong or obovate-oblanceolate. Flowers dull yellow in panicles of spikes. Fruit drupe, 5-angled, 5-winged, woody.
Fl. & Fr.: April–December.
Local names: *Tel*: Tellamaddi, Nirmaddi.

Uses: Plant useful in the treatment of diabetes.

**Terminalia bellirica** (Gaertn.) Roxb.

Syn: *Myrobalanus bellirica* Gaertn.

Family: Combretaceae.

Large deciduous tree, bark bluish-grey with vertical cracks. Leaves crowded at the ends of branches, coriaceous, broadly elliptic or obovate. Flowers cream coloured, scented, in axillary spikes. Fruit ovoid drupe, with grey-velvety woolly hairs.
Common in deciduous forests throughout India.
Fl. & Fr.: April–December.
Sanskrit: Vibhitaka.
Local name: *Ass*: Bauri, Bhaṃosa, Hulluch, Silli; *Ben*: Badam, Bahera, Boira, Bhill; *Guj*: Badamlili, Deshibadam, Lilibada; *Hin*: Badami, Himbadam, Bahera, Bhaira, Bahirda, Vibhitaka; *Kan*: Badami, Santi, Thari, Thani, Kadubadami, Natubadambi; *Mal*: Tanni, Tusham; *Mar*: Bangalibadam, Hiranibadam, Baheda, Beda Berda, Nat Badam; *Ori*: Bodamo, Desiyabadam, Bohera; *Pun*: Balela, Birha; *Tam*: Amandi, Nattubadumai, Tani, Tyhandri, Pinga, Siruppinga, Vedumai; *Tel*: Tani, Thandra, Tadi.

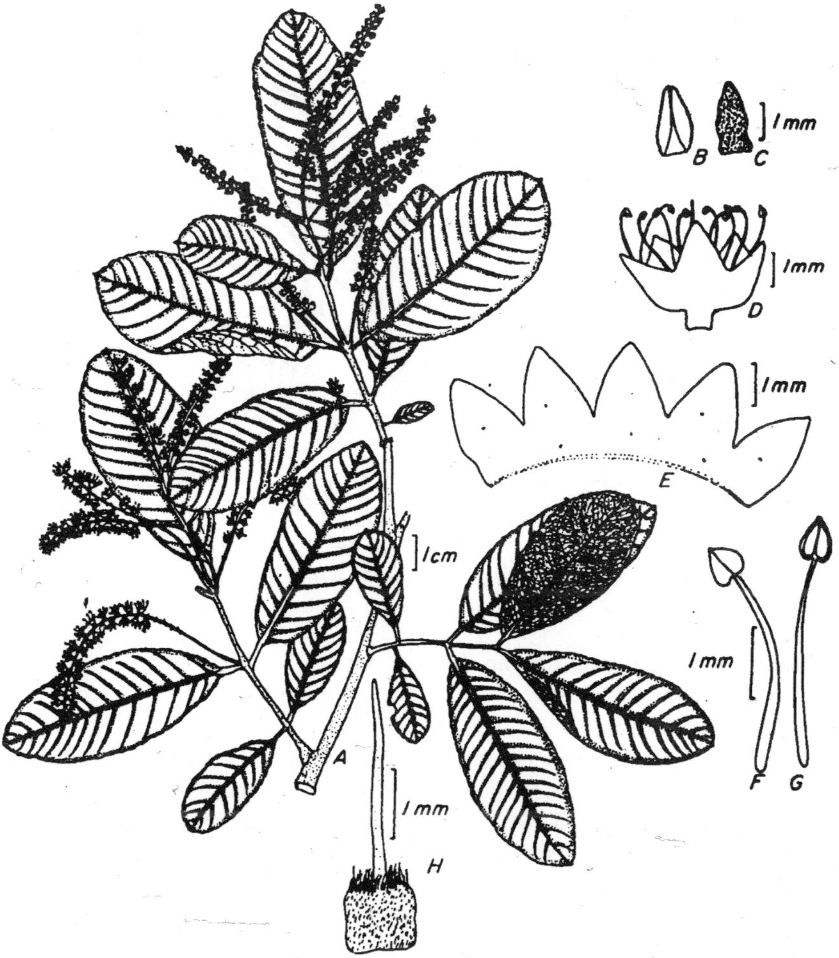


Fig. 85: *Terminalia arjuna* (Roxb. ex DC.) Wight & Arn.
A. Twig; B. & C. Bracteoles; D. Flower; E. Calyx split open; F. & G. Stamens; H. Pistil.

Trade name: Beleric Myrobalan.
Propagation: By seeds.

Uses: Plant useful in the treatment of diabetes.

**Terminalia catappa** L.

Family: Combretaceae.

Deciduous tree, up to 1.5m tall. Leaves densely clustered at the ends of branchlets, alternate, obovate. Flowers cream-coloured in axillary spikes. Fruit ellipsoid, 2-ridged.

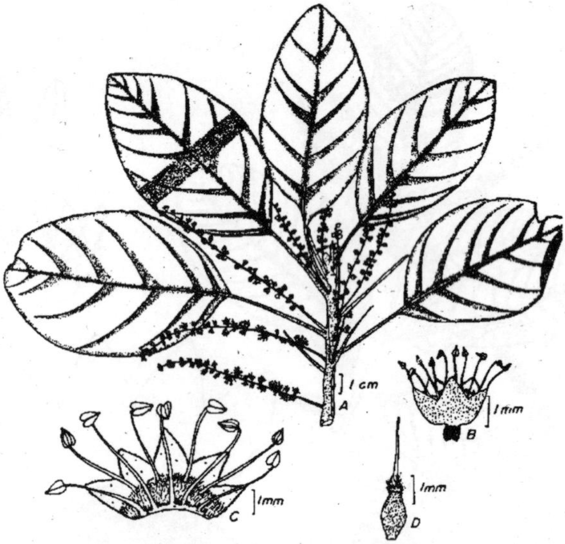


Fig. 86: *Terminalia bellirica* (Gaertn.) Roxb.
A. Twig; B. Flower; C. Calyx with stamens; D. Pistil.

Planted in gardens and as an avenue tree.

Fl. & Fr.: September–June.

Sanskrit: Grahadruma.

Local names: *Ben*: Bangla badam, Kath badam; *Guj*: Badamlili, Lilibadam; *Hin*: Deshibadam, Janglibadam, Patel badam, Hijji badam; *Kan*: Taree; *Mal*: Adamaram; *Ori*: Badamo, Sesiyo badamo; *Tam*: Natvadom, Amani, Pinga, Sirruppinga, Vatta kottai; *Tel*: Badam.

Trade name: Indian Almond Tree.

Propagation: By seeds.

Uses: Plant useful in the treatment of diabetes.

**Terminalia chebula** Retz.

Syn: *Myrobalanus chebula* (Retz.) Gaertn.

Family: Combretaceae.

A moderate sized deciduous tree, up to 20m tall. Leaves subopposite, ovate, with two glands near base. Flowers dull white in simple spikes, fragrant. Fruit ovoid drupe, yellowish-green.

Occasional in deciduous forests of Himachal Pradesh, Karnataka, Kerala, Tamil Nadu,. Andhra Pradesh, Uttar Pradesh and West Bengal.

Fl. & Fr.: March–December.

Sanskrit: Haritaki, Harra, Harada, Abhaya.

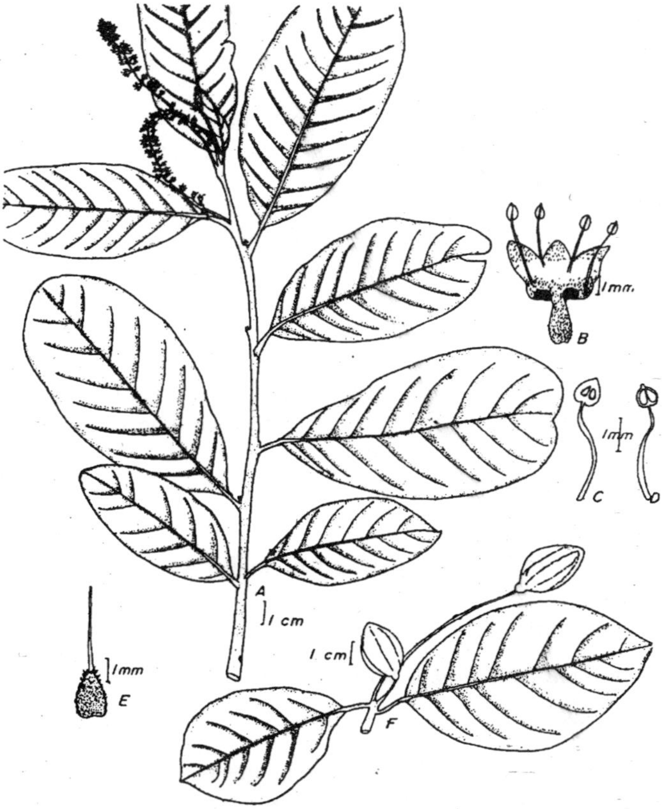


Fig. 87: *Terminalia chebula* Retz.
A. Twig; B. Part of Calyx with stamens; C. & D. Stamens; E. Pistil; F. Fruiting branch.

Local names: *Ass*: Hilikha; *Ben*: Haritaki; *Guj*: Hirdo; *Hin*: Har, Harara, Harra; *Kan*: Aralaikai, Halli, Arile, Harade, Haritaki; *Mal*: Kattuka, Kadukka; *Mar*: Habra, Hirada, Hirda; *Ori*: Horida, Horiroki, Janthi horida, Karedha; *Pun*: Halela, Har, Harrar, Huch; *Tam*: Amagola, Arabi, Aridabi, Attan, Kadu, Kadukkay; *Tel*: Karakkaya; *Urdu*: Haegarad.

Trade name: Chebulic Myrobalan, Ink tree.

Propagation: By seeds.

Uses: Powder of the seed is in use in the treatment of diabetes.

**Thymus serpyllum** L.

Syn: *Thymus linearis* Benth.

Family: Lamiaceae (Labiatae).

Variable, aromatic, prostrate, evergreen shrub, up to 25cm tall. Leaves small, elliptic or oblong-ovate or lanceolate. Flowers polygamous, in whorls. Fruit nutlet.

Found in Himalayas from Kashmir to Nepal.

Local names: *Hin*: Banajwain, *Pun*: Kalandar zatar, Masho, Rang sbur.

Trade name: Wild Thyme.

Uses: Plant useful in the treatment of diabetes.

**Thymus vulgaris** L.

Family: Lamiaceae (Labiatae).

Low, perennial undershrub, up to 30cm tall. Leaves oblong-lanceolate, coriaceous. Flowers purplish or bluish to almost white in verticillasters. Fruit nutlets, brown.

Cultivated in Nilgiris.

Trade name: Common Thyme, Garden thyme.

Uses: Plant useful in the treatment of diabetes.

**Tinospora cordifolia** (Willd.) Hook. f. & Thoms.

Syn: *Menispermum cordifolium* Willd.

Family: Menispermaceae.

Woody climber, with succulent stems throwing aerial roots. Leaves cordate, glabrous. Flowers unisexual, male flowers in axils of bracts, female solitary. Fruit globose, red when ripe, sessile.

Common in South India and Arunachal Pradesh.

Fl. & Fr.: Through out the year.

Sanskrit: Guduchi, Amrita.

Local names: *Ben*: Golancha; *Guj*: Gulvel; *Hin*: Gulancha, Giloe; *Kan*: Yuganiballi, Amrutoballi, Madhuparne, Phalani; *Mal*: Cittamrtu, Amrtu; *Mar*: Guloe, Giroli; *Tam*: Cintil, Amirtakkoti, Amudem chindil,; *Tel*: Tippateega.

Trade name: Gulonga, Tinospora.

Propagation: By seeds.

Uses: Dried powder of leaf or whole plant taken three times a day for over 20 days keeps glucose level normal.

**Tinospora crispa** (L.) Miers ex Hook.f. & Thoms.

Syn: *Tinospora tuberculata* (Lam.) Beumee ex K. Heyne.
*Tinospora rumphii* Boerl.

Family: Menispermaceae.

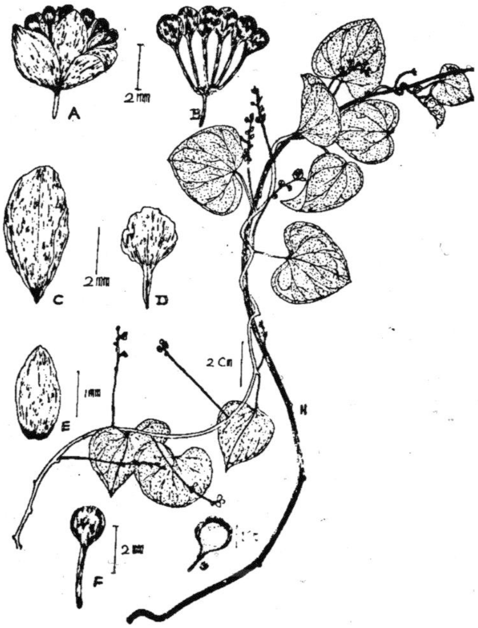

Fig. 88: *Tinospora cordifolia* (Willd.) Hook. f. & Thoms.
A. Flower; B. Androecium; C. Sepal; D. Petal; E. Bract; F. Stamen; G. Fruit; H. Twig.

Large climber. Leaves ovate-oblong. Flowers small, yellowish green, unisexual, in solitary or fascicled racemes. Fruit drupe, oblong.

Found in Assam.

Uses: The stems are used against diabetes.

**Toddalia asiatica** (L.) Lam.

Syn: *Toddalia aculeata* Pers.

Family: Rutaceae.

Armed straggler, branchlets glandular-tomentose, terminal prickles recurved. Leaves 3-foliolate, sessile. Flowers in axillary panicles, unisexual. Fruit berry, 1-5-seeded.

Common in forests throughout India.

Fl. & Fr.: July–February.

Sanskrit: Tikshanakshi, Kanchan.

Local names: *Ben*: Kada-tadali; *Hin*: Jangli-kalimirch; *Kan*: Kadumenagu, Mukkamastige; *Mal*: Kaka-toddali; *Tam*: Milagarnai, Kattumilagu, Milagu charanai; *Tel*: Kondakasinda, Mirapakandra, Kondamirapa.

Trade name: Forest pepper, Lopez Tree, Wild orange Tree.
Propagation: By seeds.

Uses: Aerial parts used for the treatment of diabetes.

**Toona ciliata** Roem.

Syn: *Cedrela toona* Roxb. ex Rottl.

Family: Meliaceae.

Trees, up to 25m tall. Leaves imparipinnate, leaflets 6–9 pairs, lanceolate or ovate-lanceolate. Flowers white, in terminal or axillary panicles. Fruit capsule, seeds winged.
Fl. & Fr.: December–March.

Uses: Leaves used in the treatment of diabetes.

**Tragia involucrata** L.

Family: Euphorbiaceae.

Climbing or twining hispid herb with stinging hairs. Leaves linear-lanceolate or linear-elliptic. Flowers in axillary and terminal racemes, unisexual, male flowers many from middle above, female flowers few, near the base. Fruit capsule, hispid.
Rare in forests in coastal and Rayalaseema districts.
Fl. & Fr.: December–March.
Sanskrit: Dhusparsha, Vrischikali.
Local names: *Kan*: Kiriturachi, Sannaturachi; *Mal*: Cherukodithura; *Tam*: Cherukunjuru, Eirrukancharivaya; *Tel*: Theegaduradagunta, Chinnaduradagunta.
Trade name: Indian stinging nettle.
Propagation: By seeds.

Uses: Aerial parts useful in the treatment of diabetes.

**Trema orientalis** Blume

Syn: *Trema amboinensis* auct.
*Celtis orientalis* L.

Family: Ulmaceae.

Evergreen tree, up to 10m tall. Leaves obliquely ovate-oblong. Flowers monoecious, minute, whitish or greenish, axillary in clusters, male cymes more compact than the female. Fruit drupe, globose, black when ripe.
Throughout India.

Local names: *Ben*: Chikan, Jibon; *Guj*: Gol; *Hin*: Gio; *Kan*: Gorklu, Koruhale; *Mal*: Ama, Malantotali, Rathi; *Ori*: Kahrkas, *Tam*: Ambarathi, Chenkolam; *Tel*: Budamuru; Chakamanu, Gaddanelli.

Uses: Aerial parts useful in the treatment of diabetes.

**Tribulus terrestris** L.

Family: Zygophyllaceae.

A prostrate spreading herb, up to 40 cm long. Leaves paripinnate, leaflets 4–7 pairs, oblong. Flowers yellow, solitary, axillary or leaf-opposed. Fruit globose, spiny. Seeds many in each of the 5 parts.

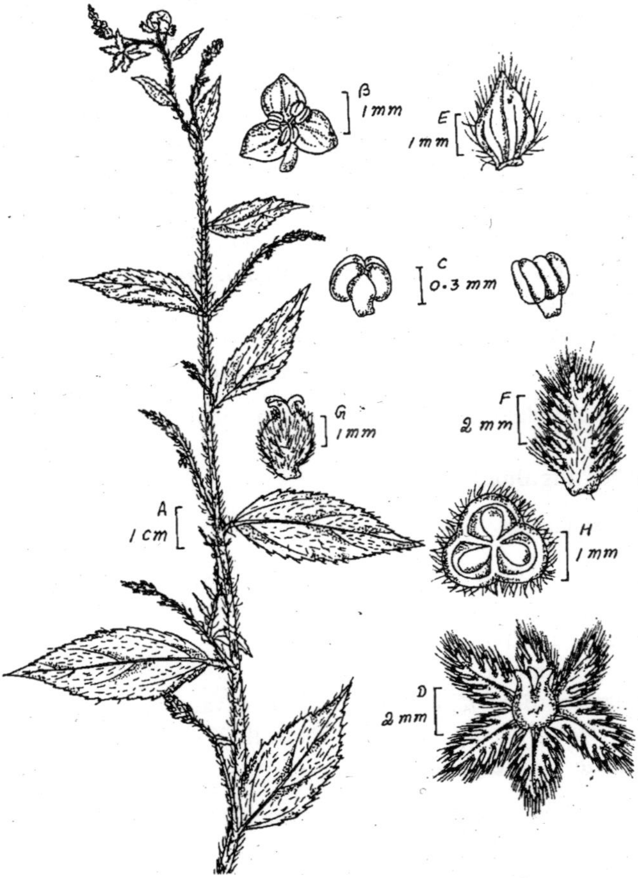


Fig. 89: *Tragia involucrata* L.
A. Twig; Male: B. Flower; C. Anthers; D. Flower; E. Bract; F. Involucre lobe; G. Pistil; H. Ovary T.S.

Common weed of waste lands, road sides and open forests all over India.

Sanskrit: Gokshura, Ikshugangha.

Local names: *Ben. & Ori*: Gakhura, Gokshra; *Guj*: Betagokhru, Mitha gokhru, Nahana gokhru; *Hin*: Gokshri, Hussuk; *Kan*: Neggilu, Sanna neggilu, Negalu; *Mal*: Nerinni, Nerungil; *Mar*: Sharatte. Sarata; *Tam*: Neruncil, Kamaraci; *Tel*: Palleru.

Trade name: Land Caltrops, Puncture vine.

Porpagation: By seeds.

Uses: Seeds of *Tribulus terrestris* and seeds of guar in equal quantitities are crushed and ground. It is kept inside the leaf of wheat or vegetable. After 3 days it is taken out and eaten, one tea spoon in the morning for 4–5 days.

**Trichodesma zeylanicum** (Burm.f.) R. Br.

Syn: *Borago zeylanica* Burm. f.

Family: Boraginaceae.

Annual, erect, hispid herb, up to 1m tall. Leaves opposite, elliptic-lanceolate. Flowers pale blue, axillary, solitary. Fruit nutlets.

Peninsular India.

Fl. & Fr.: November–February.

Local names: *Hin*: Hetenuria, Jalasirasa; *Mar*: Jalashirasi.

Uses: Whole plant useful in the treatment of diabetes.

**Trichosanthes anguina** L.

Family: Cucurbitaceae.

Annual creeper, tendrils 2–3-fid. Leaves of various shapes, lobed, deeply cordate. Flowers monoecious, male in axillary racemes, female solitary, axillary. Fruit up to 2m long, pale green.

Sanskrit: Ckachinda.

Local names: *Ben*: Ckichinga, *Guj*: Padavali; *Hin*: Ckachinda; *Kan*: Padavlakayi; *Mal*: Patavalanga; *Mar*: Padwal; *Tam*: Pudal; *Tel*: Potlakaya.

Trade name: Snake gourd.

Uses: Whole plant used in the treatment of diabetes.

**Trichosanthes bracteata** (Lam.) Voigt.

Syn: *Trichosanthes palmata*

Family: Cucurbitaceae.

Grows in moist localities all over India.

Sanskrit: Shvetapushipi.

Local names: *Ben*: Makal; *Hin*: Lal Indrayan, Mahakal; *Guj*: Ratanindrayan; *Kan*: Avaguda-hannu; *Mal*: Kakatonti; *Mar*: Kauandala; *Tam*: Koratti; *Tel*: Avaduta.

Uses: Whole plant used in the treatment of diabetes.

**Trichosanthes cucumeriana** L.

Family: Cucurbitaceae.

Annual climber, branches sparsely puberulous, tendrils slender, branched. Leaves orbicular-reniform or broadly ovate, angular or 5–7-palmately lobed, densely glandular pubescent below. Flowers white, male flowers in racemes, female flowers solitary. Fruit berry, glabrous, green and striped when fresh, scarlet or orange when ripe, seeds many, flattened.

Occasional throughout India.

Sanskrit: Amritaphala, Kashtbanjan.

Local names: *Ben*: Banpatol; *Guj*: Kadwamparwal; *Hin*: Jangli chachinda; *Kan*: Bettada-Padawala; *Mal*: Pepatolam; *Mar*: Ranacha Padwal; *Tam*: Paeypuda; *Tel*: Chetipotla.

Propagation: By seeds.

Uses: Plant useful in the treatment of diabetes.

**Trichosanthes dioica** Roxb.

Family: Cucurbitaceae.

Dioecious climber with a perennial root stock. Leaves cordate or ovate-oblong. Flowers unisexual, male peduncles paired, both 1-flowered, female solitary. Fruit globose, red when ripe.

Found wild in north India, also cultivated.

Sanskrit: Putulika.

Local names: *Ben*: Potol; *Guj & Ori*: Patal; *Hin & Pun*: Parwal; *Kan*: Kaadu-padvla; *Mal*: Patolam; *Tel*: Kommupotla; *Tam*: Kombupudalai.

Trade name: Pointed gourd.

Uses: Aerial parts, roots and seed are used to treat diabetes.

**Trifolium pratense** L.

Family: Fabaceae (Papilionaceae)

Small, perennial herb. Leaves 3-foliolate, leaflets ovate or oblong. Flowers purple, in long stalked heads. Fruit pod.

Found from Kashmir to Garhwal.

Trade name: Purple clover, broad leaved clover.

Uses: Whole plant used in the treatment of diabetes.

**Trigonella foenum-graecum** L.

Family: Fabaceae (Papilionaceae).

An annual aromatic herb. Leaves pinnately 3-foliolate, leaflets oblanceolate-oblong. Flowers white or creamish, axillary, solitary. Fruit pod, 10–20-seeded, seeds greenish brown, oblong, with a deep groove across on corner.

Cultivated for its seeds and also as leafy vegetable.

Sanskrit: Methika, Chandrika, Asumodhagam.

Local names: *Ben*: Menthi-shak, Methuka, Hoemgreeb; *Hin* & *Ori*: Methi, Muthi; *Kan*: Menthya, Mentesoppu, Menk-palle, Mente; *Mal*: Uluva, Vanthiam; *Mar*: Methi; *Tam*: Vendayam; *Tel*: Menthulu (seeds), Menthiaku (leaves).

Trade name: Fenugreek.

Propagation: By seeds.

Uses: Seeds and aerial parts useful in the treatment of diabetes.The seeds of fenugreek have been found effective in the treatment of diabetes. Seed powder or seeds taken internally two times per day for 30 days or more helps in lowering blood glucose. Levels of serum cholesterol, and triglycerides significantly reduced in the diabetes patients when the seeds were consumed.

**Tripsacum laxum** Nash.

Family: Poaceae.

Perennial tufted grass, up to 4m tall. Leaves broadly lanceolate. Spikes 3, monoecious, male terminal and axillary, falling entire, female basal.

Occasional in Deccan.

Uses: Aerial parts used in the treatment of diabetes.

**Triticum aestivum** L.

Syn: *Triticum sativum* Lam.

*Triticum vulgare* Vill.

Family: Poaceae.

Annual tufted erect grass, up to 1.5m tall. Leaves linear-lanceolate. Spikelets in terminal spikes, awned or awnless. Fruit caryopsis, oblong with blunt ends, with a shallow groove on one face.

Commonly cultivated for its grain.

Local names: *Ben*: Giun, Gom, Gam; *Hin*: Gehun, Giun, Kanak,Gandham; *Kan*: Godhi; *Mal*: Gendum, Kotanpam, Godamba; *Mar*: Gahum, Gahung; *Tam*: Godumai, Godumbayarisi; *Tel*: Godhumalu.

Trade name: Common wheat, Bread wheat.

Uses: Leaf and seed useful in the treatment of diabetes.

**Uraria picta** (Jacq.) Desv.

Syn: *Hedysarum pictum* Jacq.

Family: Fabaceae (Papilionaceae)

Annual erect undershrub. Upper leaves 5–9-foliolate, leaflets linear-oblong. Flowers purple in terminal long cylindrical racemes. Fruit indehiscent pod, 3–6-jointed.

Occasional in forests.

Fl. & Fr.: August–November.

Sanskrit: Prasniparni.

Local names: *Ben*: Salkarjata; *Guj*: Pilavan pithavan, Pilosamarveo; *Hin*: Dabra; *Mar*: Prisniparni; *Ori*: Ishworojota; *Tam*: Sittirappaladai; *Tel*: Pingerragadda.

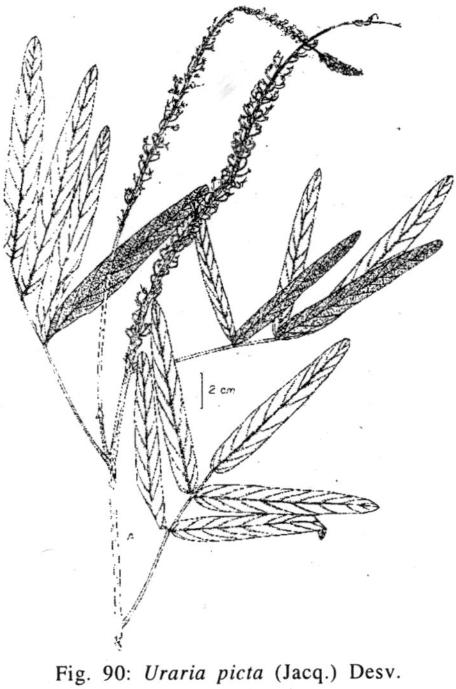


Fig. 90: *Uraria picta* (Jacq.) Desv.
A. Twig.

Propagation: By seeds.

Uses: Whole plant useful in the treatment of diabetes.

**Urtica dioica** L.

Family: Urticaceae.

Robust, dioecious herb, up to 20cm tall, abundantly armed with stinging hairs. Leaves ovate or lanceolate. Flowers greenish in axillary cymes.
Found in Himalayas from Kashmir to Kumaon.
Local names: *Hin*: Bichhu booti.
Trade name: Stinging nettle.

Uses: Whole plant useful in the treatment of diabetes.

**Urtica urens** L.

Family: Urticaceae.

Erect branched annual herb, up to 65cm tall, stem quadrangular with sparse stinging hairs. Leaves ovate or elliptic-ovate. Flowers small in dense axillary cymes. Fruit nut.
Weed in Dehradun and Udhampur district of Jammu.
Trade name: Small nettle.

Uses: Plant useful in the treatment of diabetes.

**Uvaria narum** Blume

Family: Annonaceae.

Large woody climber. Leaves oblong-lanceolate. Flowers reddish or dingy-green, solitary, terminal or leaf-opposed.
In Forests of Western Ghats.
Local names: *Tam*: Pulichan; *Kan*: Kariballi; *Mal*: Narumpal.

Uses: Aerial parts used to treat Diabetes mellitus.

**Valeriana officinalis** L.

Family: Valerianaceae.

Perennial herbs, up to 1m tall, root stock thicker. Leaves opposite, odd pinnate, leaflets lanceolate. Flowers bright pink to white in panicled cymes. Fruit ovate-oblong, yellow, indehiscent.
In temperate Himalayas in Kashmir at 2500m.
Local names: *Hin*: Billioltan, Badrangboya, Jalakan; *Mar*: Kalavala
Trade name: Common Vallerin, Garden Heliotrope.

Propagation: By seeds or through rootstock.

Uses: Root useful in the treatment of diabetes.

**Vanda testacea** (Lindl.) Reichb.f.

Syn: *Aerides testacea* Lindl.
*Vanda parviflora* Lindl.

Family: Orchidaceae.

Epiphyte with a non-pseudobulbous stem, up to 20cm long. Leaves linear-lorate. Flowers cream–yellow in racemes. Fruit capsule.

From Uttar Pradesh to Assam extending southwards to Kerala.

Local names: *Tel*: Vajnika.

Uses: Whole plant useful in the treatment of diabetes.

**Vateria indica** L.

Family: Dipterocarpaceae.

Large, elegant, evergreen tree, up to 30m tall, bark rough. Leaves coriaceous, ovate or oblong. Flowers white, fragrant in terminal corymbose panicles. Fruit ovoid capsule, seeds reddish white or cream coloured.

Evergreen forests of Western Ghats from North Kanara to Kerala.

Sanskrit: Ajakarna.

Local names: *Ben*: Chundrus, Safed damr; *Hin*: Safed damar; *Kan*: Dhupada-mara, Hoogadamara, Munda-dhupa, Saldhupa, Maddi-dhupa; *Mal*: Vellakunturukkum, Peinimarum, Perumpiney, Payani; *Tel*: Telladamaru; Dhupadamaru; *Tam*: Vellaidamaru, Vellaikuntricum, Pineymaram, Dhupmaram.

Trade name: White Dammar, Indian Copal-Tree, Piney Varnish Tree.

Uses: Aerial parts useful in the treatment of diabetes.

**Vatica chinensis** L.

Syn: *Vatica roxburghiana* Blume

Family: Dipterocarpaceae.

Large evergreen tree. Leaves ovate to oblong. Flowers white, fragrant in erect, axillary panicles. Fruit globose.

In South India from Andhra Pradesh to Kerala.

Local names: *Mal*: Adakapyin, Vallepayin, Charupiney.

Uses: Aerial parts used in the treatment of diabetes mellitus.

**Verbena officinalis** L.

Syn: *Verbena spuria* L.
*Verbena sororia* D. Don

Family: Verbenaceae.

Perennial erect or decumbent herb with woody root stock, up to 1.5m tall, stems quadrangular. Leaves oblong or ovate, usually 3-partite, pinnatifid or variously lobed. Flowers in terminal spikes, lilac. Fruit pyrenes, 3-ribbed.

In Himalayas, Kashmir, Bihar, West Bengal and Andhra Pradesh.

Local names: *Hin*: Pamukh.

Trade name: Vervain.

Uses: Whole plant useful in the treatment of diabetes.

**Viburnum foetens** Decne.

Family: Caprifoliaceae.

Large deciduous shrub. Leaves elliptic or oblong. Flowers white or pink. Drupes ellipsoid, red when ripe.

Found in North–West Himalayas.

Uses: Aerial parts used in the treatment of diabetes mellitus.

**Vicia faba** L.

Syn: *Faba vulgaris* Moench

Family: Fabaceae (Papilionaceae).

Hardy, erect, annual herb. Leaves pinnate, leaflets 1–3 pairs, elliptic to oblong. Flowers white with large purplish blotches, in small racemes. Fruit pod, seeds brown or black.

Cultivated all over the country.

Local names: *Hin*: Bakla, Anhuri, Kala matar; *Kan*: Kadu Huralikaya; *Pun*: Chas-tang, Kabli bakla, Raj-rawan; *Urdu*: Raj-rawam.

Trade name: Broad bean, Field bean.

Uses: Plant useful in the treatment of diabetes.

**Vigna mungo** (L.) Hepper

Syn: *Phaseolus mungo* L.
*Phaseolus radiatus* Roxb.

Family: Fabaceae (Papilionaceae).

Erect herbs, up to 30 cm, branches strigose. Leaves 3-foliolate, leaflets oblong-lanceolate or ovate. Flowers yellow, in axillary or leaf-opposed racemes. Fruit pod, hairy, about 10-seeded.

Cultivated for its seeds.

Fl. & Fr.: August–December.

Sanskrit: Masha.

Local names: *Ben*: Mash-kalai; *Guj*: Adad-arad; *Hin*: Urd; *Mar*: Udid, Maga; *Kan*: Uddu; *Mal*: Uzhunnu; *Tam*: Ulundu; *Tel*: Minumulu.

Trade name: Black gram.

Propagation: By seeds.

Uses: Seeds useful in the treatment of diabetes. For a milder type of diabetes, two tablespoons of germinated black gram, taken with half a cup of fresh bitter gourd juice and a table spoon of honey, is said to be useful. It should be taken once daily for three to four months. A restriction should be placed on the intake of carbohydrates. Even in severe cases, regular use of this combination, with other precautions, is useful as a health-giving food for the prevention of various complications that may arise due to malnutrition in diabetics.

10 grams of black gram is soaked in one glass of milk overnight and in the morning it is to be taken with milk for about a week.

**Vigna radiata** (L.) Wilczek. var. **radiata**

Syn: *Phaseolus radiatus* L.
*Phaseolus aureus* Roxb.

Family: Fabaceae (Papilionaceae).

Annual, erect or suberect herb. Leaves trifoliolate, leaflets entire, rarely trilobed and ovate in outline. Flowers yellow or yellowish green and crowded in clusters. Fruit pod, seeds more or less globular, mostly green in colour, but sometimes marbled black and green, yellow, brown or purple brown.

Cultivated throughout India.

Local names: *Ben*: Mung: *Hin*: Mung, *Guj*: Mag; *Kan*: Hesaru; *Mal*: Cherupayaru, *Mar*: Mug; *Tam*: Pasi-payaru, Putcha pesaru; *Tel*: Pesalu, Patchapesalu.

Trade name: Green gram.

Uses: Seeds useful in the treatment of diabetes.

**Vinca major** L. var**. elegantissima** Hort.

Family: Apocynaceae.

Perennial, woody sub-shrub, up to 1m tall. Leaves ovate or broadly ovate to lanceolate. Flowers blue-purple, white or violet, solitary, axillary. Fruit follicles, slightly curved, seeds brown.

Grown in gardens in hills like Nilgiris, Palni hills, Mussorie and Simla.
Trade name: Greater periwink

Uses: Whole plant useful in the treatment of diabetes.

**Vinca minor** L.

Family: Apocynaceae.

Creeping perennial. Leaves lanceolate or elliptic, often ovate, variegated. Flowers typically blue-violet, but varying from pale blue and reddish purple to white. Fruit follicles.
Grown in gardens.
Trade name: Running myrtle, Lesser periwinkle

Uses: Plant useful in the treatment of diabetes.
Active constituent: Akuammidine, isoreserpiline, reserpiline, vincoamine, vicanidine, vinervine, vinsumine.

**Viscum album** L.

Syn: *Viscum costatum* Gamble

Family: Viscaceae.

Yellowish green, dichotomously branched, semiparasitic, evergreen shrub. Leaves lanceolate or elliptic. Flowers in terminal fascicles, male and female on different plants. Fruit pseudoberry, ellipsoid, white.
Found in Himalayas from Kashmir to Nepal at elevations 1200–2700m.
Local names: *Hin*: Ban, Banda; *Kan*: Hasurubadanika; *Pun*: Bhangra, Kabh-bhang, Ahalu, Rini, Reori.
Trade name: Europaean mistletoe.

Uses: Aerial parts useful in the treatment of diabetes.

**Vitex trifolia** L.

Family: Verbenaceae.

A slender bushy shrub or small tree, tender parts softly pubescent. Leaves 1–3-foliolate, leaflets obovate-rhomboid. Flowers bluish in terminal panicles. Fruit drupe, purplish-black when ripe.
Occasional along streams.
Fl. & Fr.: Through out the year.
Sanskrit: Jala Nirgundi.
Local names: *Ben*: Panisamalu; *Hin*: Sufed-sanbhalu; Pani-ke-sanbhalu; *Kan*: Niralakki-gida, Nochhi; *Mal*: Nirnoschi; *Mar*: Indrani, Lingur; *Ori*: Begundia; *Tam*: Nirnocci, Kotiynanirakkunni; *Tel*: Vavili, Niruvavili.

Uses: Aerial parts useful in the treatment of diabetes.

**Withania coagulans** (Stocks) Dunal

Family: Solanaceae.

Rigid, grey under shrub, up to 1.2m tall. Leaves lanceolate-oblong, tomentose. Flowers yellow, in axillary cymose clusters. Fruit globose berry, red or brownish, enclosed in leathery calyx, seeds dark brown.

Found in north-west India, Simla, Garhwal and Kumaon.

Local names: *Ben*: Ashvagandha; *Hin*: Akri, Punir; *Kan*: Asvagandhi; *Tam*: Ammukkura; *Tel*: Panneru-gadda.

Propagation: From seeds.

Uses: Plant useful in the treatment of diabetes.

**Withania somnifera** (L.) Dunal

Syn: *Physalis sommnifera* L.

Family: Solanaceae.

An erect, branched under shrub, stellate tomentose, up to 1m tall. Leaves ovate. Flowers greenish yellow in axillary fascicles. Berry globose, overtopped by the inflated, accrescent calyx, red when ripe. The seeds are small, light, flat and light yellow.

Occasional weed in cultivated fields and waste lands throughout drier parts of India. Also cultivated in Madhya Pradesh and Rajasthan for its roots.

Sanskrit: Aswangandha.

Local names: *Ben*: Ashvagandha; *Guj*: Ghodakun, Ghoda, Asoda, Asan; *Hin*: Punir, Asgandh; *Kan*: Hiri maddina-gadday, Amangura; *Mal*: Amukkuram, Pevetti; *Mar*: Tlli, Kanchuki; *Pun*: Asgand, Isagand; *Tam*: Amukkara, Amukkira; *Tel*: Aswagandha, Pannerugadda.

Trade name: Aswagandha.

Uses: Whole plant useful in the treatment of diabetes.

Propagation: Seeds are sown or broadcast in the nursery just before the onset of rainy season. Five kgs of seeds are sufficient to provide seeds for one hectare. The seedlings are trasplanted when they are 6 weeks old, during late rainy season, in 60 cm spaced rows. Hand weeding at 30 days interval, in order to control the weeds, is necessary. Annual rainfall of 600 to 750mm is best suited for its growth. Sandy loam or light red silts and good drainage is conducive for its growth. The plant flower and fruit during November–December. Harvesting starts in January and continues till March. The entire plant is uprooted for its roots, which are seperated from the aerial parts by cutting the stem 1–2 cm above the ground. They are then trans-

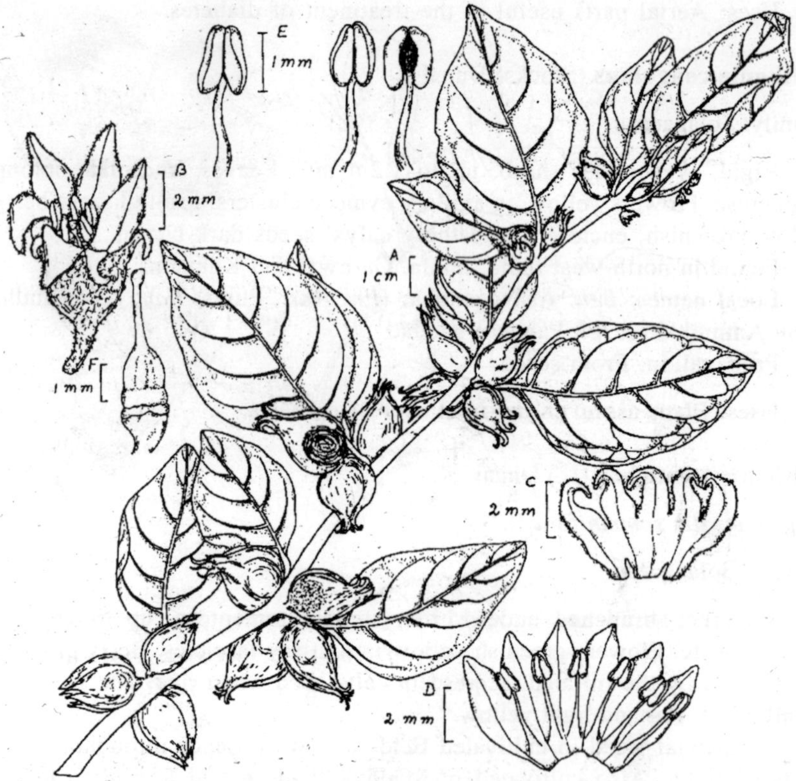


Fig. 91: *Withania somnifera* (L.) Dunal.
A. Twig; B. Flower; C. Calyx split open (Ventral view); D. Corolla split open with Stamens; E. Stamens; F. Pistil.

versely cut into smaller pieces for drying. The yield of roots is 500 kg per hectare when fresh and 150 kg per hectare when dried.

**Wrightia coccinea** Sims.

Family: Apocynaceae

Deciduous tree, up to 18m tall. Leaves elliptic or elliptic-lanceolate. Flowers deep red, in terminal cymes. Fruit follicles.

In hills of Sikkim, Eastern Himalayas, Assam, Arunachal Pradesh, Meghalaya and Nagaland.

Local names: *Ben*: Pallam.

Uses: Fruits are used to treat Diabetes mellitus

**Xanthium strumarium** L.

Family: Asteraceae (Compositae).

Annual erect subshrubs, up to 1.5m tall, stem hispid. Leaves broadly ovate, hispidulous. Flowers in terminal heads, heads monoecious, sessile, male heads many-flowered, female heads 2-flowered. Fruit oblong-ovoid achene enclosed in a 2-beaked utricle formed by the hardened involucral bracts and covered with hooked spines.

Common weed of road sides.

Fl. & Fr.: September–February.

Sanskrit: Arishta.

Local names: *Ben*: Banokra, Chotadhatura; *Guj*: Gadariun; *Hin*: Banokra, Gokhru, Chota-gokhru, Chota-dhatura, Adhasisi; *Kan*: Maruluummatti; *Mar*: Shankeshwara, Dutundi; *Tam*: Maruloomathum; *Tel*: Marlu Mathangi.

Trade name: Cocklebur, Bur weed.

Propagation: By seeds.

Uses: Roots, seeds and aerial parts useful in the treatment of diabetes.

**Zanthoxylum armatum** DC

Syn: *Zanthoxylum alatum* Roxb.

Family: Rutaceae.

Armed shrubs with dense foliage and pungent aromatic smell and taste. Leaves imparipinnate, petiole narrowly winged, leaves elliptic-lanceolate. Flowers in sparse panicles. Fruit pale red.

Occasional in forests in Visakhapatnam district.

Sanskrit: Tumburu, Gandhalu.

Local names: *Ben*: Gaira, Nepali thaniya, Tambul; *Ori*: Tundopoda; *Hin*: Darmar, Nepali dhaniya, Tejphal, Tumuru.

Propagation: By seeds, by cutting of half ripened shoots or root cutting.

Uses: Stem useful in the treatment of diabetes.

**Zanthoxylum ovalifolium** Wight

Family: Rutaceae.

Small, aromatic, armed or unarmed tree or shrub, up to 8m tall. Leaves trifoliolate, occasionally bi-or unifoliolate, leaflets ovate to elliptic. Flowers white in terminal and axillary paniculate cymes. Fruit follicle.

Eastern Himalayas in Sikkim, Khasi hills, Western Ghats and Andaman islands.

Local names: *Kan*: Armadalu.

Uses: Stem used in treatment of diabetes.

**Zea mays** L.

Family: Poaceae.

Robust, monoecious, annual grass, up to 5m tall. Leaves lanceolate. Male spikelets in long spike like terminal raceme, female spikelets in the axil of leaves, spikelets on thickened woody axis, enclosed by foliaceous bracts, styles long, silky. Fruit subglobose.

Cultivated all over India.

Local names: *Ben*: Janar, Bhutta, Jonal; *Hin*: Makai, Makka, Bhutta, Junri; *Guj*: Makkari, Makkai; *Kan*: Mekkejola, Musukojola; *Mal:* Cholam; *Mar*: Maka, Makai, Buta; *Ori*: Maka, Buta; *Tam*: Makka cholam; *Tel*: Mokka jonna.

Trade name: Maize, corn.

Uses: Styles useful in the treatment of diabetes.

**Zingiber officinale** Roscoe

Family: Zingiberaceae.

Rhizomatous perennial herb, aerial shoot leafy, up to 75 cm tall. Leaves sheathing, alternate, linear lanceolate. Flowers yellow with dark purplish spots in condensed spikes.

Fruit oblong capsule.

Cultivated for its rhizome.

Propagation: By rhizomes.

Sanskrit: Ardrakam.

Local names: *Hin*: Adrak, ada; *Kan*: Harisunti; *Mal*: Andrakam, Inchu; *Mar*: Ale; *Tam*: Allam, Inji; *Tel*: Allamu.

Trade name: Ginger.

Propagation: By rhizomes.

Uses: Aerial parts and rhizome useful in the treatment of diabetes.

**Zingiber zerumbet** Roscoe

Syn: *Amomum zerumbet* L.

Family: Zingiberaceae

Rhizomatous herb. Leaves oblong-lanceolate. Flowers yellow in terminal spike. Fruit ovoid, red.

Throughout India.

Sanskrit: Karpooraharidra.

Local names: *Ben & Hin*: Narkachur; *Tel*: Karrallamu; *Mal*: Kattinji.

Uses: Plant is useful in the treatment of diabetes.

**Ziziphus mauritiana** Lam.

Syn: *Ziziphus jujuba* (L.) Gaertn.

Family: Rhamnaceae.

Much branched, small, thorny trees, up to 8m tall, spines paired, one straight, another recurved. Leaves suborbicular, basally 3-nerved, glabrous above, rusty tomentose below. Flowers pale green in axillary pedicellate clusters. Fruit globose drupe, yellow or red when ripe, 1–2-celled.

Common in waste lands and scrub jungles.

Fl. & Fr.: October–January.

Sanskrit: Kola, Koli, Badari.

Local names: *Ben*: Kool, Ber; *Guj*: Bor, Bordi; *Hin*: Baer; *Kan*:Yalachi, Elanji; *Mal*: Elentha; *Mar*: Bor, Bera; *Ori*: Barkoli, Bodokjoli, Bodori; *Pun*: Amlai, Singli, Simli, Banari; *Tam*: Elandai, Yellande, Elladu; *Tel*: Regu.

Trade name: Indian Jujube, Chinese date.

Propagation: By seeds, air layering, bud grafting.

Uses: Leaves useful in the treatment of diabetes.

Active principle: A number of cyclopeptide alkaloids have been reported.

**Ziziphus rugosa** Lam.

Family: Rhamnaceae

Lianas, branches brown-pubescent. Leaves elliptic, ovate-oblong. Flowers pale-yellow or greenish–yellow in cymose panicles. Fruit globose drupe.

Fl. & Fr.: March–May.

Throughout India.

Uses: Stem bark useful in the treatment of diabetes.

## REFERENCES


Abdul Hamed Saheb, H. 1982. The complete Book of Home Remedies. Orient Paperbacks, Delhi.

Abdul Kareen, M. 1997. Plants in Ayurveda. FRLHT, Bangalore.

Agarwal, V.S. and Ghosh Barin. 1985. Drug Plants of India: Root Drugs. Kalyani Publishers, New Delhi.

Akhtar Hussain. 1993. Medicinal Plants and their cultivation. CIMAP, Lucknow.

Akhtar, M.S., M.A. Khan, M.T. Malik. 2002. Hypoglycaemic activity of *Alpinia galanga* rhizome and its extracts in rabbits. *Fitoterapia* 73: 623–628.

Aman. 1985. Medicinal Secrets of your food. Indo-American Hospital, Mysore.

Ambasta, S.P. 1986. The useful plants of India. Publication and Information Directorate, CSIR, New Delh.

Anonymous. 2000. PDR for Herbal Medicines. Medical & Economics company, Montvale, USA.

Atal, C.K. and B.M. Kapoor. 1982. Cultivation and utilization of Aromatic Plants. Regional Research Laboratory, Jammu.

Bakhru, H.K. 1992. Herbs that heal. Orient Paper backs, New Delhi.

Bakhru, H.K. 1995. Home Remedies. Orient Paper backs, New Delhi.

Batra, A., S. Mathur, S.Rajore, Gyan Singh, Shekhawat and Sandhya Goyal. 2002. Herbal Therapy for curing diabetes. In: Irfan A. Khan & A. Khanum (eds.) Role of Biotechnologym in Medicinal and Aromatic Plants. Vol. VI. 91–104.

Bhattacharjee, S.K 2001. Hand book of medicinal plants. Pointer Publishers, Jaipur.

Bonar, A.199. Herbs—A complete guide to their cultivation and use.Tiger books International, London.

Caius, J.F. 1986. The medicinal and poisonous plants of India. Scientific Publishers, Jodhpur.

Chadha, K.L. 2001. Handbook of Horticulture. ICAR, New Delhi.

Chandel, K.P.S. 1996. Biodiversity in medicinal and aromatic plants in India (Eds.) S.Ganesh & N. Sharma. ICAR, New Delhi.

Chopra, R.N., S.L. Nayar and I.C. Chopra. 1956. Glossary of Indian Medicinal Plants. CSIR, New Delhi.

Chopra, R.N., I.C. Chopra, K.L.Handa and L.D. Kapoor. 1982. Indigenous drugs of India. Academic Publishers, Calcutta.

Chopra, R.N., I.C.Chopra and B.S.Verma. 1968. Supplement to glossary of Indian Medicinal palnts, CSIR, New Delhi.

Dastur, J.F. 1952. Medicinal plants cf India and Pakistan. D.B. Tarapoorvala and Co. Ltd. Bombay.

Farooqi, A.A. and B.S. Sreeramu. 2001. Cultivation of medicinal and aromatic crops. Universities Press, Hyderabad.

Guha Bakshi, D.N. and P. Sensarma and D.C.Pal. 1999–2001. A lexicon of medicinal palnts in India. Vol. 1 & 2. Naya Prokash, Calcutta.

Handa, S.S. and M.K.Koul. 1982. Cultivation and Utilization of Medicinal Plants. CSIR, New Delhi.

Handa, S.S. and M.K. Koul. 1996. Supplement to cultivation and utilization of medicinal plants. Regional Research Laboratory, Jammu Tawi.

Hussain, A. O.P.Virmani, S.P.Poli 1992. Dictionary of Indian Medicinal Plants. CIMAP, Lucknow.

Jain, S.K.1968. Medicinal Plants. National Book Trust, New Delhi.

Jain, S.K. 1991. Dictionary of Indian Folk medicine and Ethnobotany. Deep publications, New Delhi.

Jain, S.K. and R.A. Defilips. 1991. Medicinal Plants of India. Reference Publ. Inc. Algonac, Michigan.

Jasrai, Y.T. and B.B. Wala. 2001. *Curculigo orchioides* Gaertn. (Kali Musli) an endangered medicinal herb. In: (Eds.) Irfan A.Khan & A.Khanum. 20001. Role of Biotechnology in Medicinal and Aromatic Plants. Ukaaz publications. Hyderabad.

Jayaweera, D.M.A. 1980. Medicinal plants used in Sri Lanka. The National Science Council of Sri Lanka.

Jordan,. J.M.Midgley, C.M.Thonoor and C.M.Williams.1987. *J. Pharm. Pharmacol.* **39**: 752.

Kamboj, V.P. 2000. *Curr. Sci.* **78**: 35–39.

Khanna Girija. 1986. Herbal Remedies. Tarang Paperbacks. New Delhi.

Kirtikar, K.R and B.D.Basu.1935. Indian Medicinal Plants 4.Vols.

Koul, M.K. 1997. Medicinal plants of Kashmir and Ladakh–Temperate and cold Arid Himalaya. Indus Publishing Co. New Delhi.

Kusu, F., X.D.Li and K.Takamura. 1992. *Chem. Pharm. Bull.* **40**: 3284.

Moulali, D.A., P.S.P. Babu and T. Pullaiah. 1997. Aphrodisiac root. *The Indian Express.*

Muddappa, A. 1992. Medicinal Plant source book. International Library Association. Dehra Dun.

Nadkarni, K.M. and A.K. Nadkarni. 1982. Indian Materia Medica. Popular Prakasan. Bombay.

Nair, C.K.N. and N. Mohanan. 1998. Medicinal plants of India. Nag publishers, Delhi.

Nayak, B.S., A.L. Udupa and S.L. Udupa. 1999. Effect of flowers on dead space wound healing in rats. *Fitoterapia* **70**: 233–236.

Parrotta, J.A. 2000. Healing Plants of Peninsular India. CABI Publishing, U.K.

Pullaiah, T. 1999. A multipurpose medicinal twine. *The Indian Express–Science Express.* 27th July 1999.

Pullaiah, T. and D. Muralidhara Rao. 2002. Little known medicinal herb. THE HINDU-Sunday Magazine, p. 7.

Rao, P.S., K. Venkaiah and R. Padmaja. 1999. Field guide on Medicinal Plants, Andhra Pradesh Forest Department.

Rasheeduz Zafar. 1994. Medicinal Plants of India. CBS Publishers & Distributors. New Delhi.

Satyavathi, G.V., K.G.Ashok and T. Neeraj. 1987. Medicinal Plants of India. Indian Council for Medical Research. New Delhi.

Shah, M.B. and G. Chauhan. 1996. Recent developments of some Natural products. In: S.S. Handa and M.K.Koul. (eds.). Supplement to cultivation and utilization of medicinal plants. Regional Research Laboratory. Jammu Tawi.

Shah, S. 1992. The selected Indian Medicinal Plants. Chemixil, Madras.

Srivastava, P.S., Deepsikha Pande, Aniruddha Datta and Sandip Das. 2002. Biotechnological approaches to potential anticancerous herbal drugs of the future. In: Irfan A. Khan and A. Khanum (eds.) Role of Biotechnology in Medicinal and Aromatic and Aromatic Plants. Vol. 5. pp 1–20.

Sivarajan, V.V. and Indira Balachandran. 1994. Ayurvedic drugs and their plant sources. Oxford & IBH Publ. Co., New Delhi.

Sunny Oommen, D.K. Ved and R. Krishnan. 2000. Tropical Indian Medicinal Plants. Propagation methods. FRLHT, Bangalore.

Ugochukwn, N.H. and N.E. Babady. 2002. Antioxidant effects of *Gongronema latifolium* in hepatocytes of rat models of non-insulin dependent diabetes mellitus. *Fitoterapia* 73: 612–618.

Warrier, P.K., V.P.K. Nambiar and C. Ramankutty.1994. In: P.S. Vaidyaratnam (ed.) Indian Medicinal plants. A compedium of 500 species. 5 vols. Orient Longman Ltd.

Watt, G. 1972. A Dictionary of economic Products of India. Periodical Experts, New Delhi.

Wijesekera, R.O.B. (ed.) 1991. The medicinal plant industry. CRC Press, Boca Raton.